Medical Genetics

in Pediatric Practice

AUTHOR

American Academy of Pediatrics
Committee on Genetics

EDITOR

Robert A. Saul, MD, FAAP, FACMG

American Academy of Pediatrics

DEDICATED TO THE HEALTH OF ALL CHILDREN™

American Academy of Pediatrics Department of Marketing and Publications Staff

Maureen DeRosa, MPA, Director, Department of Marketing and Publications

Mark Grimes, Director, Division of Product Development

Martha Cook, MS, Senior Product Development Editor

Carrie Peters, Editorial Assistant

Sandi King, MS, Director, Division of Publishing and Production Services

Theresa Wiener, Manager, Publications Production and Manufacturing

Kate Larson, Manager, Editorial Services

Linda Diamond, Manager, Art Direction and Production

Julia Lee, Director, Division of Marketing and Sales

Linda Smessaert, Manager, Clinical and Professional Publications Marketing

Library of Congress Control Number: 2010907077
ISBN: 978-1-58110-496-7
eISBN: 978-1-58110-497-4
MA0565

The recommendations in this publication do not indicate an exclusive course of treatment or serve as a standard of medical care. Variations, taking into account individual circumstances, may be appropriate.

Every effort has been made to ensure that the drug selection and dosage set forth in this text are in accordance with the current recommendations and practice at the time of publication. It is the responsibility of the health care provider to check the package insert of each drug for any change in indications and dosage and for added warnings and precautions.

The mention of product names in this publication is for informational purposes only and does not imply endorsement by the American Academy of Pediatrics.

The publishers have made every effort to trace the copyright holders for borrowed material. If they have inadvertently overlooked any, they will be pleased to make the necessary arrangement at the first opportunity.

Printed in the United States of America.
3-229/0313

1 2 3 4 5 6 7 8 9 10

American Academy of Pediatrics Committee on Genetics 2012–2013

Robert A. Saul, MD, FAAP, FACMG; Chairperson
Stephen R. Braddock, MD, FAAP, FACMG
Emily Chen, MD, PhD, FAAP, FACMG
Debra L. Freedenberg, MD, FAAP, FACMG
Marilyn C. Jones, MD, FAAP, FACMG
Beth A. Tarini, MD, MS, FAAP

Former Committee on Genetics Members

Marilyn J. Bull, MD, FAAP
Gregory M. Enns, MB, ChB, FAAP
Jeffrey R. Gruen, MD, FAAP
Nancy J. Mendelsohn, MD, FAAP, FACMG
James M. Perrin, MD, FAAP
Howard M. Saal, MD, FAAP, FACMG

Liaisons

Sara M. Copeland, MD
Health Resources and Services Administration
Katrina M. Dipple, MD, PhD, FAAP, FACMG
American College of Medical Genetics
Melissa A. Parisi, MD, PhD, FAAP, FACMG
National Institute of Child Health and Human Development
Nancy C. Rose, MD
American Congress of Obstetricians and Gynecologists
Stuart K. Shapira, MD, PhD, FACMG
Centers for Disease Control and Prevention

AAP Staff

Paul Spire

American Academy of Pediatrics Reviewers

Marilyn Bull, MD, FAAP, Board of Directors

Committee on Bioethics

Committee on Drugs

Committee on Health Information Technology Initiatives

Committee on Medical Liability & Risk Management

Committee on Pediatric Dentistry

Committee on State Government Affairs

Committee on Substance Abuse

Council on Community Pediatrics

Section on Administration & Practice Management

Section on Bioethics

Section on Clinical Pharmacology & Therapeutics

Section on Hospice & Palliative Medicine

Section on Nephrology

Section on Neurological Surgery

Section on Ophthalmology

Section on Orthopaedics

Section on Plastic Surgery

Section on Urology

Contributors

Lynne M. Bird, MD, FAAP, FACMG
Professor of Pediatrics
University of California, San Diego
Clinical Geneticist, Rady Children's Hospital
San Diego, CA

Leah Weyerts Burke, MD, FAAP, FACMG
Professor
University of Vermont College of Medicine
Director, Vermont Regional Genetics Center
Burlington, VT

Emily Chen, MD, PhD, FAAP, FACMG
Chief, Department of Genetics
Kaiser Permanente San Francisco Medical Center
Codirector, Regional Molecular Genetics Laboratory
Kaiser Permanente, San Jose
Clinical Professor, UCSF Medical Center, Department of Pediatrics and Genetics
San Francisco, CA

Ellen Wright Clayton, MD, JD, FAAP, FACMG
Craig-Weaver Chair and Professor of Pediatrics
Professor of Law
Cofounder, Center for Biomedical Ethics and Society
Vanderbilt University
Nashville, TN

Sarah L. Dugan, MD, FACMG
Clinical Geneticist
Children's Hospitals and Clinics of Minnesota
University of Minnesota
Department of Pediatrics
Minneapolis, MN

James Flory, MD, MSCE
Fellow in Endocrinology
New York Presbyterian Hospital-Weill Cornell Medical Center
Division of Endocrinology, Diabetes and Metabolism
New York, NY

Carol L. Greene, MD, FAAP, FACMG
Professor of Pediatrics and of OB/Gyn and Reproductive Medicine
University of Maryland School of Medicine
College Park, MD

Hakon Hakonarson, MD, PhD
Associate Professor of Pediatrics
Division of Human Genetics
Director, Center for Applied Genomics
The Children's Hospital of Philadelphia
University of Pennsylvania, School of Medicine
Philadelphia, PA

R. Rodney Howell, MD, FAAP, FACMG
Professor of Pediatrics
Chairman Emeritus
Department of Pediatrics
Miller School of Medicine
University of Miami
Miami, FL

H. Eugene Hoyme, MD, FAAP, FACMG
Chief Academic Officer
Sanford Health
President and Senior Scientist
Sanford Research
Sioux Falls, SD

Tamison Jewett, MD, FAAP, FACMG
Professor
Section on Medical Genetics
Department of Pediatrics
Wake Forest School of Medicine
Director of Clinical Genetics Services
Winston-Salem, NC

Alex R. Kemper, MD, MPH, MS, FAAP
Associate Professor
Department of Pediatrics
Duke University
Durham, NC

Kim M. Keppler-Noreuil, MD, FACMG
Clinical Professor of Pediatrics
Division of Medical Genetics
Program Director for the Medical Genetics Residency Program & Clinical Director of Birth Defects
Iowa Registry for Congenital & Inherited Disorders
University of Iowa Hospitals & Clinics
Iowa City, IA

Michelle Huckaby Lewis, MD, JD
Research Scholar
Berman Institute of Bioethics
Johns Hopkins University
Baltimore, MD

Michele A. Lloyd-Puryear, MD, PhD, FAAP
Senior Medical and Science Advisor
Eunice Kennedy Shriver National Institute of Child Health and Human Development
National Institutes of Health
Bethesda, MD

Michael J. Lyons, MD, FAAP, FACMG
Clinical Geneticist
Greenwood Genetic Center
North Charleston, SC

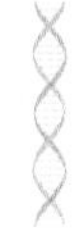

Gustavo H. B. Maegawa MD, PhD, FACMG
Assistant Professor
McKusick-Nathans Institute of Genetic Medicine
Department of Pediatrics
Johns Hopkins University School of Medicine
Baltimore, MD

Nancy J. Mendelsohn, MD, FAAP, FACMG
Director, Medical Genetics
Children's Hospital and Clinics of Minnesota
Assistant Professor, University of Minnesota
Minneapolis, MN

John B. Moeschler, MD, MS, FAAP, FACMG
Professor of Pediatrics (Medical Genetics)
Geisel School of Medicine at Dartmouth
Dartmouth Hitchcock Medical Center
Lebanon, NH

Melissa A. Parisi, MD, PhD, FAAP, FACMG
Chief, Intellectual and Developmental Disabilities Branch
Eunice Kennedy Shriver National Institute of Child Health and Human Development
National Institutes of Health
Bethesda, MD

Dinel Pond, MS, CGC
Genetic Counselor
Children's Hospitals and Clinics of Minnesota
Minneapolis, MN

Francis Edwards Rushton Jr, MD, FAAP
Beaufort Pediatrics PA
Beaufort, SC

Howard M. Saal, MD, FAAP, FACMG
Director, Clinical Genetics
Cincinnati Children's Hospital Medical Center
Professor of Pediatrics
University of Cincinnati College of Medicine
Cincinnati, OH

Robert A. Saul, MD, FAAP, FACMG
Senior Clinical Geneticist
Training Program Director
Greenwood Genetic Center
Greenwood, SC

Robert D. Steiner, MD, FAAP, FACMG
Credit Unions for Kids Professor of Pediatrics and Vice Chair for Research in Pediatrics
Faculty, Program in Molecular and Cellular Biosciences, Pediatrics, and Molecular and Medical Genetics
Doernbecher Children's Hospital and Institute on Development and Disability
Oregon Health & Science University
Portland, OR

Lori Terry, MS, CGC
Certified Genetic Counselor
Wake Forest University Health Sciences
Department of Pediatrics
Section on Medical Genetics
Winston-Salem, NC

Brad T. Tinkle, MD, PhD, FACMG
Clinical Geneticist
Division of Human Genetics
Cincinnati Children's Hospital Medical Center
Associate Professor of Pediatrics
University of Cincinnati
Cincinnati, OH

Tracy L. Trotter, MD, FAAP
Senior Partner
San Ramon Valley Primary Care
Associate Professor, UCSF School of Medicine
San Ramon, CA

Tiina K. Urv, PhD
Program Director
Eunice Kennedy Shriver National Institute of Child Health and Human Development
National Institutes of Health
Bethesda, MD

Marc S. Williams, MD, FAAP, FACMG
Director, Genomic Medicine Institute
Geisinger Health System
Danville, PA

Table of Contents

Introduction

One of the joys of the practice of medicine is the application of new and exciting advances to primary care of pediatric patients and their families. One of the difficulties in the practice of medicine is the need to continually update one's knowledge base and skill set in primary care of pediatric patients and their families. This dichotomy is a constant challenge for primary care physicians (PCPs), yet it signals the ever-present reminder of the importance of research and its application to clinical care.

The practice of primary care pediatrics has always combined acute illness with prevention and anticipatory guidance. With advances in our understanding of the genetic basis for disease come public awareness and interest in what these advances have to offer. Public awareness of genetic and genomic information requires PCPs to effectively and responsively integrate genetics into their daily practice.

This American Academy of Pediatrics (AAP) manual, *Medical Genetics in Pediatric Practice*, attempts to bridge the gap between the perceived rarity of genetic issues in pediatric practice and the practical application of omnipresent genetic issues to primary care, whether via treatment of acute illness or prevention and anticipatory guidance. Conceived by the AAP Committee on Genetics, this manual presents a broad range of topics (overview of genetics; implementation of genetics in pediatric practice; genetic testing; counseling, community, and ethical issues; trends in genetics; and resources in genetics) to assist in the integration of this information. The emerging understanding of the genetics of common diseases coupled with increased availability of DNA-based tests has led to a demand by patients and families for genetic information and advice from their PCP. This combination of rapidly expanding genetic science and its translation to clinical medicine requires PCPs to increasingly integrate genetics into their daily practice.

Francis Collins, MD, PhD, current director of the National Institutes of Health and previous director of the Human Genome Project, believes that the next revolution in medicine will fall on the shoulders of physicians who provide primary care. His successor, Alan Guttmacher, MD, expanded on this by stating that "for decades, knowledge of genetics has had a large role in the health care of a few patients and a small role in the health of many. We have recently entered a transition period in which specific genetic knowledge is becoming critical to the delivery of effective health care for everyone."[1] According to Centers for Disease Control and Prevention data from 2004, approximately 48% of the 1.1 billion ambulatory care visits that occurred in the United States were in a primary care setting. This contrasts with about 18% occurring in medical specialty settings, of which visits to medical geneticists likely represent a very small percentage.[2] The US public expects its PCPs to know something about genetics, with 72% of 1,000 individuals in the United States surveyed in 1998 saying that they would turn first to their PCP with a question about a genetic disorder.[3]

Primary care physicians recognize the multifactorial origins of disease and focus on prevention, early identification, and family-centered care. Overwhelming evidence suggests that gene-environment interactions very early in development have profound effects on the emergence of adult disease such as cardiovascular disease, cancer, and psychiatric illness.[4] It is likely that the individual genetic code that predisposes to these common diseases and the epigenetic mechanisms that control gene expression will likely be available prenatally or in the first months or years of life. Pediatricians will have the first opportunity to actively intercede in the progression of these disorders, thus translating genetics into practice, policy, and communities.[5]

Rapid expansion of the number of congenital conditions included in state newborn screening programs and the robust public health support for these programs have provided a model for early diagnosis and treatment of genetic diseases.[6] These exciting developments will continue to blossom with predictably more conditions diagnosed and more therapeutic interventions possible. Primary care physicians will need to be an integral part of these processes to the benefit of their patients and families.

As clinicians, we live and practice in the molecular age of medicine. To use the exciting products of the Human Genome Project, PCPs must be able to identify those patients or families for whom testing or intervention would be beneficial. An accurate family history represents the gateway to the molecular age of medicine for PCPs.[7] The ability to collect and use family history information will become increasingly important in primary care.

Rapid advances in genetic research are leading to an expanding array of genetic tests. Primary care physicians will increasingly be challenged to identify patients whose symptoms, physical findings, or family history

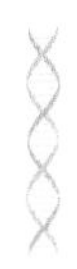

indicate the need for genetic testing and to determine how to use genetic information most effectively to improve disease prevention.[8]

Primary care physicians need to change their paradigm of care in the age of genetics. This change moved pediatrics beyond treating diseases to treating individuals with inherited and acquired risks for disease. An understanding of genetic information and access to genetic resources aid pediatricians as they seek to bring the best care possible to their patients and families.

The 5 sections of this manual (Overview of Genetics; Implementing Genetics in Pediatric Practice; Genetic Testing; Counseling, Community, and Ethics; and Trends in Genetics) are intended to address these issues and provide an initial resource for the PCP.

It is the sincere wish of the AAP Committee on Genetics that this manual become a valuable tool for pediatricians and related health care professionals in primary care pediatrics. Any comments or concerns should be directed to the committee as future editions are prepared.

I am grateful to the Greenwood Genetic Center for providing the time necessary to shepherd this manual through the writing, editing, and publishing process. I have accepted a new position at Children's Hospital, Greenville Health System (Greenville, SC), where I hope to further my efforts in child advocacy.

Robert A. Saul, MD, FAAP, FACMG, Editor

References

1. Guttmacher AE, Collins FS, Carmona RH. The family history—more important than ever. *N Engl J Med*. 2004;351(22):2333–2336
2. Burt CW, McCaig LF, Rechtsteiner EA. NCHS Health E-Stat. Ambulatory medical care utilization estimates for 2004. http://www.cdc.gov/nchs/data/hestat/estimates2004/estimates2004.htm. Updated April 6, 2010. Accessed March 21, 2013
3. Mitka M. Genetics research already touching your practice. *Am Med News*. April 6, 1998; News section:3
4. Eriksson JG. Gene polymorphisms, size at birth, and the development of hypertension and type 2 diabetes. *J Nutr*. 2007;137(4):1063–1065
5. Cheng TL, Cohn RD, Dover GJ. The genetics revolution and primary care pediatrics. *JAMA*. 2008;299(4):451–453
6. Newborn Screening Authoring Committee. Newborn screening expands: recommendations for pediatricians and medical homes—implications for the system. *Pediatrics*. 2008;121(1):192–217
7. Trotter TL, Martin HM. Family history in pediatric primary care. *Pediatrics*. 2007;120(Suppl 2):S60–S65
8. Burke W. Genetic testing in primary care. *Annu Rev Genomics Hum Genet*. 2004;5:1–14

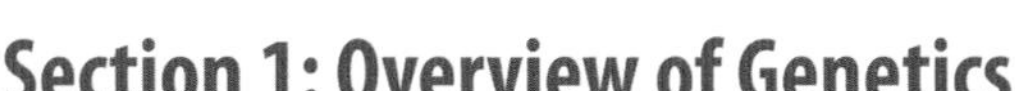

Section 1: Overview of Genetics

Chapter 1

Fundamentals of Genetics and Genomics

Lynne M. Bird, MD

Definitions

Genetics is the science of heredity and phenotypic and genotypic variation in organisms, including the investigation of the roles and function of individual genes. Classical genetics arose from Gregor Mendel's experiments with pea plants, through which he described the inheritance pattern of specific traits (known as Mendelian genetics). The term *genetics* was coined and popularized by William Bateson, who rediscovered Mendel's work in the early 1900s. The structure of DNA was determined in 1953, giving birth to the field of molecular genetics. Shortly thereafter it was determined that DNA acts as a template to create messenger RNA (mRNA), which acts as a template to create a protein made up of a specific sequence of amino acids. The genetic code is the set of rules by which DNA is translated to an amino acid sequence.

Genomics is the study of the genome, the totality of the DNA in an organism, including genes, regulatory sequences, and noncoding sequences. Most DNA is located in the nucleus, and a small amount is contained in the mitochondria. The field of genomics encompasses structural genomics (determining the primary structure of DNA by sequencing) and functional genomics (determining the pattern of gene expression during development or under specific conditions).

Somatic cells in the body reproduce by the process of *mitosis* with the normal result being 2 identical daughter cells. The 5 stages of mitosis follow interphase during which the genome is replicated (Figure 1-1). As the mitotic phase is completed, the cell's membrane pinches inward and separates the

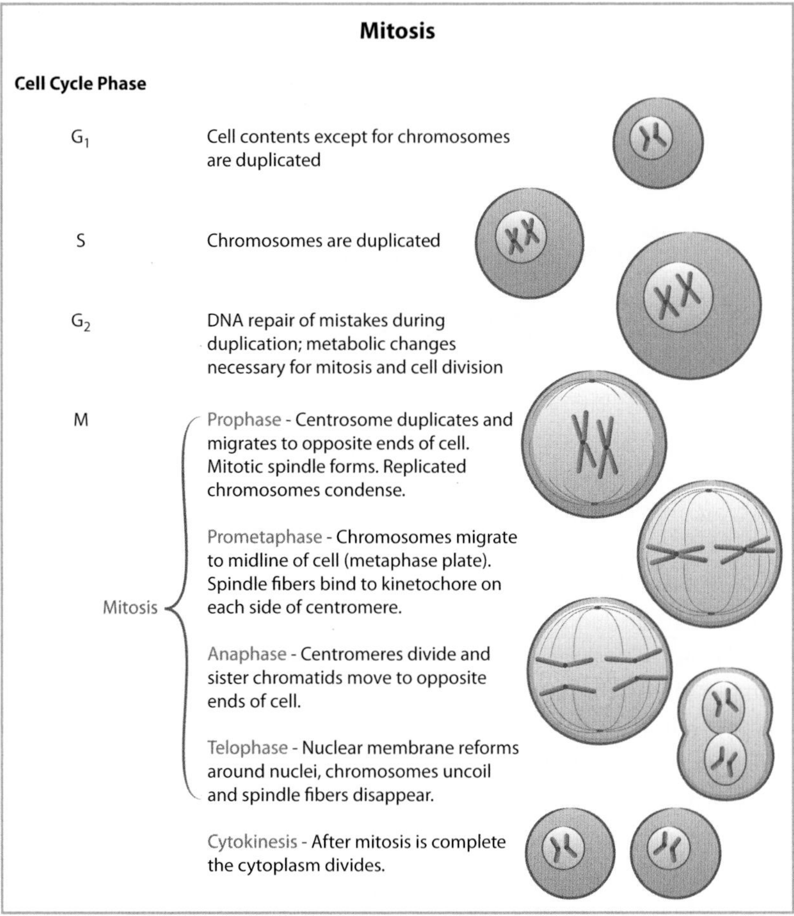

Figure 1-1. Mitosis is essential for growth and development, cell replacement, wound healing, and tumor formation.

developing nuclei and cellular contents into 2 cells. This process is known as cytokinesis.

Meiosis is the process of the creation of haploid cells (spermatocytes and ova) for sexual reproduction, and ultimately the fertilized diploid egg cell. Meiosis allows for a high degree of genetic variation that results from recombination of chromosomal material from parental chromosomes. Meiosis is divided into 2 phases known as MI and MII (Figure 1-2 and 1-3). In females, meiosis begins during gestation and results in the production of primary oocytes, which are suspended in MI. At the time of ovulation, typically one oocyte completes the MI stage. If a sperm cell penetrates the

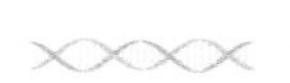

Interphase - 46 chromosomes replicate.

Spermatogonium

Oogonium

Growth/Maturation

MI - Duplicated sister chromatids pair with homologous chromosomes and crossover occurs (see Fig 1-3). Homologous chromosomes separate and haploid cells are formed. Primary oocyte is arrested in MI until ovulation.

Primary spermatocyte

Primary oocyte

Meiosis I

Secondary spermatocyte

First polar body

Meiosis II

MII - Similar to mitosis except the cells are haploid. Sister chromatids separate.

Spermatids

Ootid

Second polar bodies

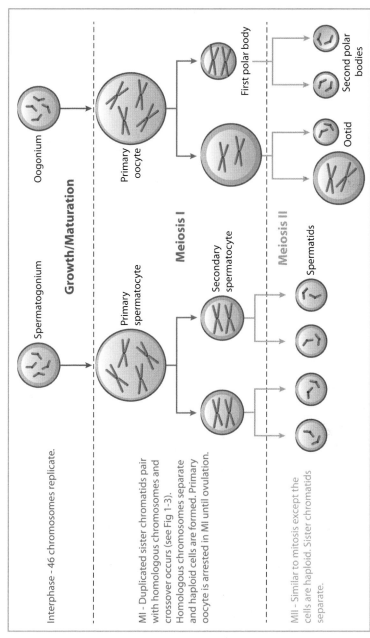

Figure 1-2. Meiosis occurs in 2 stages, MI and MII. MI is a reduction to the haploid state, though copies of sister chromatids remain together until MII.

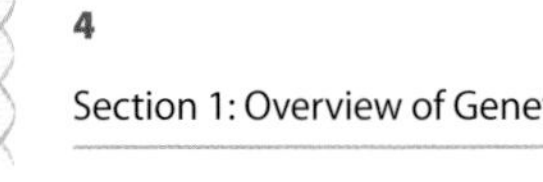

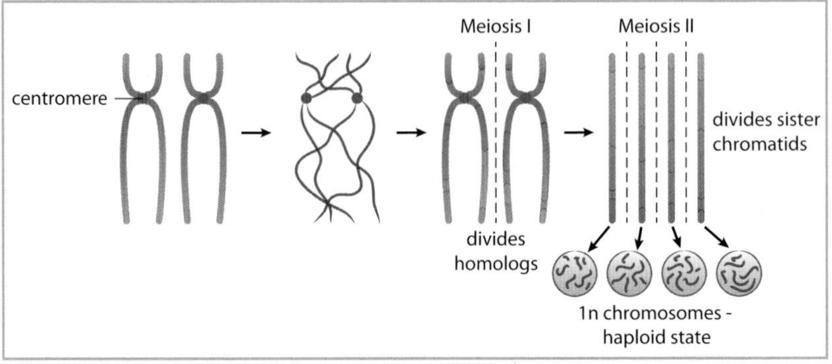

Figure 1-3. Crossover between duplicated homologous pairs occurs during the first meiotic stage. Random assortment of sister chromatids adds to diversity of the resulting haploid gametes.

egg, MII takes place generating a zygote. In males, spermatogonial stem cells divide by mitosis to form diploid primary spermatocytes. Meiosis of spermatocytes then results in secondary spermatocytes and, after MII, haploid spermatids.

An *allele* is 1 of 2 or more forms of a gene. Alleles determine the genotype (genetic makeup) and the phenotype (observable characteristic). A person *homozygous* at a particular allele or gene means they have 2 identical copies of an allele, and a person *heterozygous* for a particular allele means that their 2 genes are different. For example, at the gene locus determining the ABO blood group, there are 3 alleles (A, B, and O) that result in 6 possible genotypes (AA, AO, BB, BO, AB, and OO). This yields 4 possible phenotypes: type A, determined by genotype AA or AO; type B, determined by genotype BB or BO; type AB, determined by genotype AB; and type O, determined by genotype OO. The term *hemizygous* is reserved for males who carry a single copy of an X-linked allele. Females can be homozygous or heterozygous for X-linked genes.

Genetic abnormalities can be constitutional (present in every cell in the organism) or mosaic (present only in some cells). *Mosaicism* is the result of a post-zygotic event (ie, one that occurs after the union of the egg and sperm), and typically any 2 parents have a low risk for repeat recurrence of the same genetic abnormality in subsequent offspring. Individuals with mosaicism often exhibit an atypical pattern of involvement for a genetic condition. Individuals with mosaic genetic abnormalities who carry the abnormality in their germ cells (ie, gametes, oocytes, or spermatocytes) have an increased likelihood of passing on the genetic abnormality, which would then be present in every cell in the offspring. This type of mosaicism is called germline mosaicism.

The Organization of the Genome

Chromatin is a general term for DNA and its associated proteins (histones and others). Chromatin is loosely packaged until mitosis or meiosis, when it becomes condensed into a chromosome (Figure 1-4). The chromosome is made up of a single linear unduplicated strand until the DNA is replicated, after which it consists of 2 identical sister chromatids joined at the centromere until cell division occurs. The tight packaging of DNA into chromosomes allows for precise division of the genetic material during the cell cycle and permits examination of chromosomal structure with light microscopy. There are 23 chromosomes in the haploid human gamete (22 autosomes and a sex chromosome [X or Y]). Haploid gametes from the mother and father combine to form a diploid zygote with 46 chromosomes. A karyotype is the complete set of diploid chromosomes in a species, displayed pictorially as a karyogram. The convention for reporting normal karyotypes consists of stating the total number of chromosomes and the sex chromosome complement (46,XX or 46,XY) (Figure 1-5A and 1-5B). Abnormal karyotypes are reported according to standards known as the International System for Human Cytogenetic Nomenclature.[1]

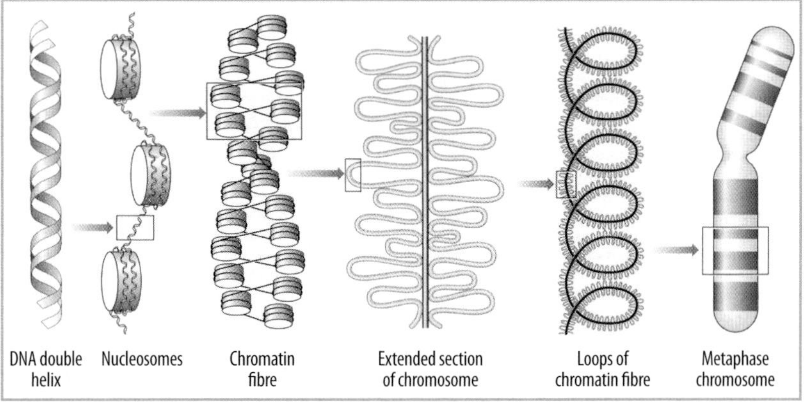

Figure 1-4. Solenoid model of DNA coiling that leads to visible structure of the chromosome. Turnpenny P, Ellard S. *Emery's Elements of Medical Genetics*. 13th ed. London: Churchill Livingstone; 2007:15

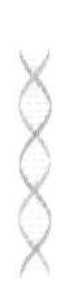

A

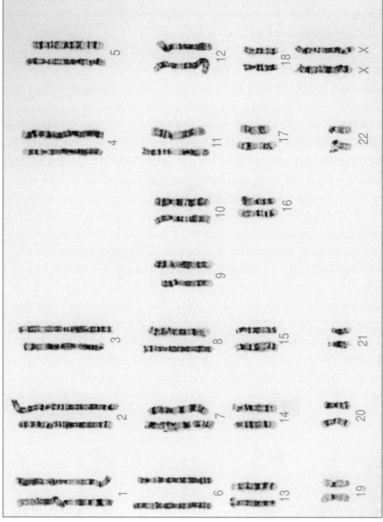

Figure 1-5. Normal karyograms (**A,** female and **B,** male). From *Genetic Counseling Aids,* 5th ed. Greenwood Genetic Center, Greenwood SC, p 4-5

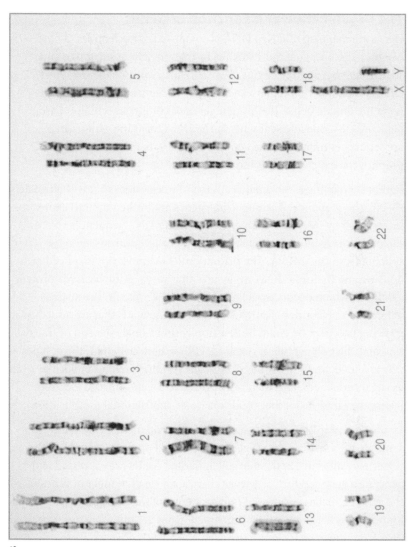

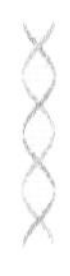

B

The Organization and Function of Genes

Genes are made up of DNA. DNA is composed of nucleotides (a base of either adenine, guanine, cytosine, or thymine plus a sugar phosphate) strung together in long chains. Two polynucleotide chains wrapped around each other (and paired adenine to thymine, cytosine to guanine) form the double helix. The human genome comprises 3 billion base pairs of DNA. Specific segments of the DNA form the genes. There are sequences outside of the gene boundaries that are necessary for proper gene expression (promoters, enhancers).

Rather than being a continuous stretch of nucleotides that will ultimately specify the sequence of amino acids, genes are broken up into exons interrupted by introns, which are intervening DNA sequences that do not code for amino acids in the resultant protein. Introns are removed by splicing from the mRNA. The primary mRNA transcript is spliced into one or more mature mRNA molecules that serve as the basis for protein synthesis, which occurs in the cytoplasm rather than in the nucleus. Triplets of nucleotides of mRNA specify amino acids that are added to a growing polypeptide chain until a stop codon signals the end of translation and the polypeptide is released. Following translation, the polypeptide is folded, and sometimes chemically modified (small molecules such as sugars attached), and then transported to an appropriate location, where they may be further modified (post-translational modification).

In addition to mRNA that is translated into protein, there are many non-translated RNAs that control gene expression. For most genes, both the maternally inherited and paternally inherited copies are expressed and generate a gene product. However, there are a small number of genes in the genome that are expressed only from one of the copies, a phenomenon known as genetic imprinting. Imprinted genes are ones that are expressed only from the gene (or more precisely the allele) inherited from the mother or only from the father's allele.

Disorders Caused by Chromosomal Abnormalities

Disorders caused by chromosomal abnormalities have a birth incidence of 6 per 1,000, and a population prevalence of 3.8 per 100. Chromosomal abnormalities involve gain or loss of one or more chromosomes (aneuploidy), gain of a complete set of chromosomes (polyploidy), or structural aberrations resulting from chromosome breakage and

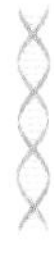

reunion. Aneuploidy is usually the result of nondisjunction, the failure of equal segregation of chromosomes to daughter cells at meiosis. The risk of nondisjunction rises with advancing maternal age. At age 20, 10% of human oocytes have nondisjunction events, rising to 40% at age 40 (most of these events result in nonviable conceptuses).[2] Nondisjunction may result in trisomy, 3 copies of an individual chromosome, or monosomy, a single copy of an individual chromosome. Autosomal monosomy is generally lethal. Examples of chromosomal disorders arising from nondisjunction are Down syndrome caused by having 3 copies of the 21st chromosome and Turner syndrome caused by having a single X chromosome. The most common example of polyploidy in humans is triploidy (3 copies of all chromosomes), which is found in 20% of spontaneous pregnancy losses.[3]

Most structural abnormalities (translocations, deletions, duplications, inversions, ring chromosomes, isochromosomes) are the result of chromosome breaks, which occur nonrandomly through the genome. Structural abnormalities can be balanced (genetic material is neither added nor missing) or unbalanced (genetic material is missing or extra resulting in pathology). A balanced chromosome abnormality most often does not affect the person who carries it, unless the chromosome break renders a gene dysfunctional. An example is a balanced translocation between chromosomes 11 and 22; those who carry this balanced rearrangement have no health effects, but are at risk to have children with unbalanced chromosomal disorders.

Patterns of Single-Gene Inheritance

In classical genetics, inheritance was thought to be limited to autosomal (dominant, co-dominant, or recessive) and X-linked (dominant or recessive). Although other forms of inheritance exist (see pages 14–17), single gene inheritance patterns outlined by Gregor Mendel remain true. In an individual who has 2 different alleles of a certain gene (heterozygous), when one allele expresses itself as the phenotype, and the other allele does not produce a phenotype, the expressed allele is dominant and the non-expressed allele is recessive. Sometimes both alleles are expressed, a situation called co-dominance. Taken together, disorders attributed to single-gene mutations have an incidence of 1% at birth and a population prevalence of 2% (Table 1-1.)

Table 1-1. Modes of Inheritance

Mode of Inheritance	Expression of Phenotype	Examples	Recurrence Risk
Autosomal dominant	Phenotype expressed in heterozygotes (Aa)	Neurofibromatosis, achondroplasia, Marfan syndrome	50% for offspring of affected individual
Autosomal recessive	Phenotype expressed only in homozygotes (aa)	Cystic fibrosis, sickle cell disease	25% for siblings of affected individual; very low to offspring of affected individual
X-linked dominant	Phenotype expressed in both heterozygous females (XaX) and hemizygous males (XaY)	Incontinentia pigmenti, Rett syndrome	33% for offspring of affected females (due to lethality of affected males)
X-linked recessive	Phenotype expressed only in male hemizygotes (XaY)	Hemophilia, Duchenne muscular dystrophy, fragile X syndrome	25% (50% males, 0% females) for offspring of carrier female; 0% to male offspring of affected male; 100% of females born to affected male are carriers
Mitochondrial	Phenotype depends on load of genetically abnormal mitochondria	Leber hereditary optic neuropathy	Risk transmitted only through affected females; severity varies depending on load of abnormal mitochondria transmitted
Imprinting	Phenotype expressed depending on parent of origin of mutation	Angelman syndrome, Prader-Willi syndrome, Beckwith-Wiedemann syndrome	Risk for siblings and offspring varies with sex of individual transmitting mutation

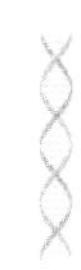

Autosomal Dominant Inheritance

In dominantly inherited disorders, a single abnormal allele (ie, heterozygous state) results in expression of the phenotype. Hallmarks of dominantly inherited disorders are vertical transmission (trait passing through multiple generations in a family), and male and female offspring are equally likely to be affected. Father-to-son transmission is another feature (since a trait transmitted from father to son cannot be located on the X chromosome) (Figure 1-6).

Some dominantly inherited disorders have a high proportion of new gene mutations, therefore the parents of the affected child might not carry the gene and vertical transmission may not be observed. In general, conditions that impair reproductive fitness of the affected individual are associated with a high frequency of new mutations, and those that do not affect fitness are rarely the result of new mutations. The risk of new mutations rises with advancing paternal age for many, but not all, dominantly inherited disorders.[4]

Another common feature of dominantly inherited disorders is *variable expressivity,* which is the observation that even within the same family, clinical features of the disorder can vary widely. If a gene mutation can be carried without producing any recognizable clinical manifestations whatsoever, the gene is said to show *incomplete penetrance.* This leads to the often misunderstood observation that a condition may "skip a generation."

Co-dominance is the expression of both alleles in the heterozygous state. The A and B blood group alleles exhibit co-dominance, because individuals who are AB exhibit both types of antigens on the surface of their red blood cells.

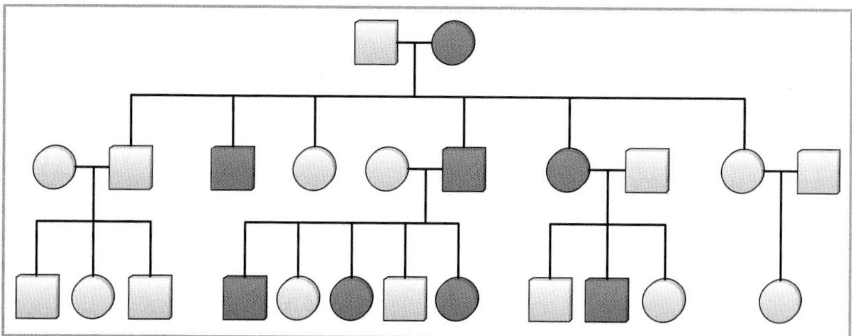

Figure 1-6. Autosomal dominant inheritance pedigree.

On rare occasion, an unaffected couple may have more than one child affected with a dominantly inherited disorder. Rather than this being the result of 2 separate spontaneous mutation events, most often these instances are the result of mosaicism in one parent. When the mutation is present in some proportion of the parental germ cells, but not in enough somatic cells to produce a phenotype, this is called germ-line mosaicism (sometimes called gonadal mosaicism). An example of germline mosaicism can be found in parents who are unaffected by achondroplasia but have more than one child with the disorder.

Some autosomal dominant disorders, such as Huntington disease and myotonic dystrophy, exhibit *anticipation,* or increasing severity and decreasing age of disease onset in subsequent generations. Anticipation is explained by an unstable area of DNA repeats causing a dynamic gene mutation that can be altered during meiosis. A triplet repeat sequence (CTG in the case of myotonic dystrophy) of a certain size is unstable and prone to expansion, such that offspring have higher repeat numbers than parents. For some disorders due to triple repeat expansion, expansion is limited to female meiosis (as in myotonic dystrophy) or male meiosis (as in Huntington disease) so only one sex is capable of transmitting a more severe neonatal or juvenile form of the condition.

Autosomal Recessive Inheritance

Recessive traits are those that manifest when a mutant allele is present in 2 copies. For most recessively inherited conditions, individuals who are heterozygous with one copy of a mutant allele and one normal copy are generally asymptomatic and referred to as carriers. Hallmarks of recessively transmitted disorders are horizontal transmission (a misnomer that refers to all affected individuals being seen in a single generation) and parental consanguinity (because of inheritance of the same mutation from a common ancestor). Although the prevalence of autosomal recessive disorders is higher in consanguineous populations, autosomal recessive disorders occur most frequently in nonconsanguineous couples. When 2 carriers of the same mutant allele reproduce, the likelihood of producing an affected child is 1 in 4 (25%), an unaffected carrier is 2 in 4 (50%), or an unaffected noncarrier is 1 in 4 (25%).

In some cases, a recessive trait may carry clinical significance even in the heterozygous state where one normal allele is present. Examples of this are sickle cell trait and rhabdomyolysis. Some argue that these are not truly recessive conditions.

A homozygous individual with a recessive condition carries the same mutation on both alleles (eg, delta-F508 homozygote, which accounts for 50% of those with cystic fibrosis). *Compound heterozygotes* are those that carry 2 different mutant alleles (eg, delta-F508 mutation on one allele and a different mutation on the other allele). See Figure 1-7 for a pedigree demonstrating autosomal recessive inheritance.

X-linked Recessive Inheritance

An X-linked recessive trait is one that is determined by a gene that resides on the X chromosome and produces symptoms usually in males. Of course, females can also express X-linked recessive conditions by being homozygous for the X-linked recessive trait, but this is statistically rare because the homozygous state requires a carrier mother and an affected father. Red-green colorblindness can occur in females for this reason.

Figure 1-8 demonstrates the pedigree of an X-linked recessive condition. Hemizygous, affected males are linked in the pedigree by healthy heterozygous female carriers. An affected male who reproduces will have no affected sons, but all of his daughters will be obligate carriers. Some X-linked conditions such as Duchenne muscular dystrophy impair reproductive fitness, so are transmitted nearly exclusively by female carriers.

On occasion, female carriers of an X-linked disorder may express a mixture of phenotypes, or a mixture of features of the normal allele and abnormal allele. An example of this is a female carrier of X-linked hypohidrotic ectodermal dysplasia exhibiting hairless patches of skin. This is due to the

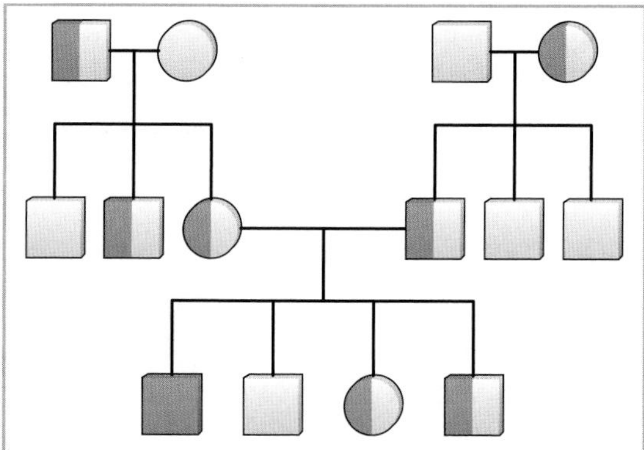

Figure 1-7. Autosomal recessive inheritance pedigree.

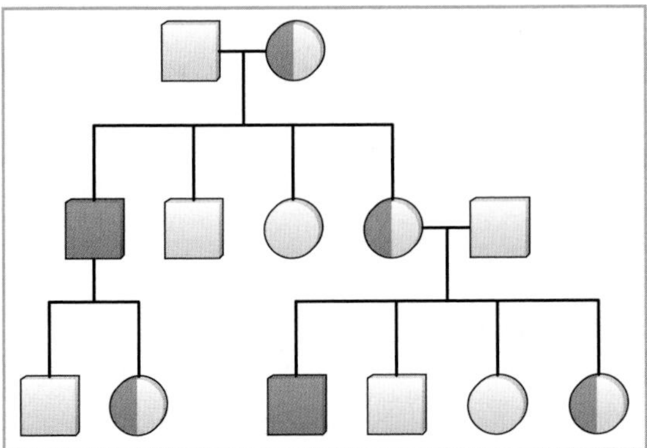

Figure 1-8. X-linked recessive inheritance pedigree.

usually random process of X inactivation (also known as lyonization), whereby most of the genes of one X chromosome are inactivated (silenced) early in development. Females can express X-linked recessive disorders even when they carry a normal allele if their X chromosome inactivation pattern is highly skewed in favor of inactivating the X chromosome with the normal allele.

X-Linked Dominant Inheritance

X-linked dominant traits are uncommon and result in both XX and XY individuals expressing a phenotype. The presence of more affected females than males and the absence of male-to-male transmission allow X-linked dominant pedigrees to be distinguished from those of autosomal dominant conditions. In X-linked dominant disorders where affected males die in utero, more miscarriages and females in the pedigree (half of whom are affected) are seen. One example of this is incontinentia pigmenti, in which the altered X chromosome inactivation pattern can be seen readily in the skin pigmentation of affected females.

Nontraditional Inheritance Patterns

Mitochondrial Inheritance

The mitochondrial DNA is inherited almost exclusively from the mother through the oocyte during the replication and division of cellular contents in cytokinesis. *Matrilineal inheritance* (Figure 1-9) occurs for disorders

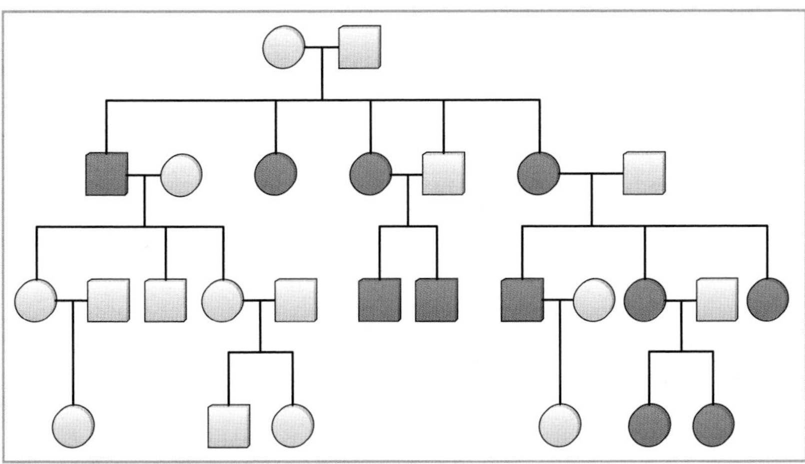

Figure 1-9. Matrilineal (mitochondrial) inheritance.

that are caused by mutations in mitochondrial genes. Both sexes can be affected, but only females transmit the condition. Having a combination of normal mitochondria and mitochondria with a DNA mutation is referred to as heteroplasmy. The relative proportion of normal and abnormal mitochondria is a possible explanation for the range of phenotypic severity in persons with mitochondrially inherited disorders. Most genes that contribute to mitochondrial function are in the nuclear DNA. Because of this, there are many disorders of mitochondrial function that have inheritance patterns similar to Mendelian patterns, autosomal or X-linked, rather than matrilineal inheritance.

Genomic Imprinting and Uniparental Disomy

Genomic imprinting refers to a process of DNA methylation and histone modification that occurs in the germline cells and regulates expression of genes while leaving the DNA sequence intact. This process is independent of Mendelian genetics and is explained in further detail in Chapter 2. Briefly, it is the mechanism whereby a gene may be active when inherited from one parent but inactive when inherited from the parent of the opposite sex. While a common phenomenon in general, genomic imprinting is observed for a minority of genes recognized to cause human disease. This is because an abnormal phenotype is expressed only when a mutated gene is inherited from the parent responsible for contributing the active gene. Examples of this include Angelman syndrome (the paternal allele of *UBE3A* is inactive, so absence or aberrations of the maternal allele result in Angelman syndrome), Prader-Willi syndrome (the maternal gene cluster at chromosome 15q11-13 is not expressed, so a defect in genes in this region from the paternal allele causes Prader-Willi syndrome), Beckwith-Wiedemann syndrome (some genes within 11p15 are expressed only from the paternally inherited allele, and others are only maternally expressed), and Russell-Silver syndrome (some cases of which are due to aberrant expression of the same gene cluster at 11p15).

Uniparental disomy refers to the situation in which an individual inherits both members of a chromosome pair from one parent. This can occur due to an error in MII, in which case the individual receives 2 identical copies of the chromosome (uniparental isodisomy), or due to an error in MI, in which case the individual receives 2 different homologues from the same parent (uniparental heterodisomy) (Figure 1-10). The 2 mechanisms thought to result in the phenomenon of uniparental disomy

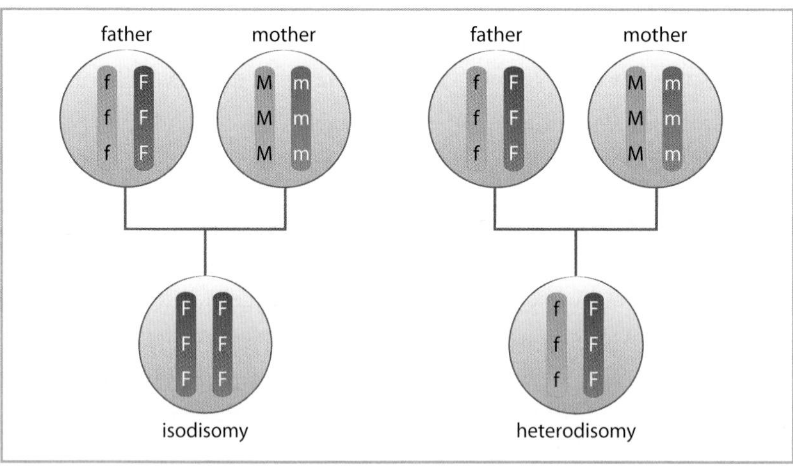

Figure 1-10. Uniparental disomy.

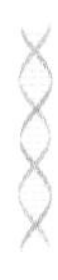

are (1) trisomic conceptus (an embryo/fetus with trisomy instead of disomy for one of the chromosomes) with early loss of the single chromosome contributed by one parent and (2) nullisomic gamete (lacking a certain chromosome) being fertilized by a gamete that is disomic for the same chromosome. Uniparental disomy only produces a phenotype if there are imprinted genes on the involved chromosome.

Multifactorial Gene Inheritance

Multifactorial conditions or traits are those that are determined by the interaction of many genes, each individually having a small effect, with environmental influences. Stature, skin color, and intelligence are multifactorial, or polygenic, traits, where many genes at different loci exert a small additive effect. Multifactorial conditions cluster in families but do not conform to any of the recognized patterns of inheritance listed above, and typically have a 2% to 4% incidence in close relatives of an affected individual. Many congenital malformations, such as cleft lip, congenital heart disease, neural tube defects, and club foot, show multifactorial (or complex) inheritance.

Such recognizable disorders at birth can be attributed to multifactorial inheritance approximately 3% of the time. Most common adult-onset disorders (hypertension, diabetes, Alzheimer disease, mental illness) are likely due to a multifactorial mechanism, whereby several different genes interact to generate a susceptibility or predisposition to a condition, which may be manifest in the setting of appropriate environmental triggers. In adulthood, disorders with multifactorial basis that begin in adolescence or adulthood account for a population prevalence of greater than 60%. Multifactorial inheritance is therefore responsible for most genetic disease in the population.[5]

In some multifactorial disorders, genes that contribute risk have been identified, but in most, the underlying genetic mechanisms are unknown. Some multifactorial disorders have high heritability (ie, most of the etiology can be ascribed to genetic rather than environmental factors). Heritability estimates are derived from the degree of resemblance between relatives and from rates of concordance of monozygotic and dizygotic twins (Table 1-2).

Table 1-2. Examples of Conditions Exhibiting Complex Inheritance Pattern

Disorder	% Heritability	Relative Risk for Sibling Compared to Population
Cleft lip/palate	76	40
Club foot	68	10–30
Congenital hip dysplasia	60	2–22 (higher for females)
Congenital heart defects	35	25–60
Hirschsprung disease	High (depends on length of involved segment)	200 (higher for males)
Neural tube defects	60	4–20
Pyloric stenosis	75	8–38 (depending on sex of proband and sibling)
Alzheimer disease	80	4–5
Asthma	80	Unknown
Autism	90	150
Bipolar disorder	85	31
Coronary artery disease	65	2.5–11.4 (depending on age and sex of proband)
Diabetes mellitus, type I	88	15–35
Hypertension, essential	62	3
Multiple sclerosis	25–76	24
Schizophrenia	85	11

Key Points

- Genomics is the study of the genome, which includes genes, regulatory sequences, and noncoding sequences.
- Chromosomal errors can be numeric or structural. Numeric errors result from segregation errors during meiosis. Structural errors occur during chromosome breakage and reunion (Figure 1-2 and 1-3).
- Dominant inheritance is characterized by vertical transmission through generations, equal sex predilection, father-to-son transmission, and often variable expressivity. Anticipation (increasing severity in subsequent generations) is seen in some dominantly inherited disorders.
- Recessive inheritance usually affects individuals in the same generation and occurs more frequently with parental consanguinity.

- X-linked recessive inheritance produces symptoms in the hemizygous male, and heterozygous female carriers are often healthy, unless X inactivation is very skewed.
- X-linked dominant inheritance expresses in both males and females, unless the trait is lethal in males, in which case an excess of females are affected and generally numerous miscarriages, male offspring often, are seen in the pedigree.
- Mitochondrial disorders are seen with all patterns of inheritance. Those due to defects in mitochondrial genes are characterized by expression in both males and females, but are passed to offspring only through females.
- Genomic imprinting refers to differential gene expression depending on parent of origin.
- Uniparental disomy results when both copies of a chromosome are inherited from the same parent.
- Multifactorial inheritance results from the interaction of genes and environmental factors, and is the most common form of inheritance for recognized disorders. For a given multifactorial trait or disorder, there are many genes that contribute a small additive effect to the overall expression.

Resources

Harper PS. *Practical Genetic Counseling.* 6th ed. London: Hodder Arnold; 2004

Nussbaum RL, McInnes RR, Willard HF. *Thompson & Thompson Genetics in Medicine.* 7th ed. Philadelphia, PA: Saunders Elsevier Limited; 2007

Read A, Donnai D, eds. *New Clinical Genetics.* Oxfordshire: Scion Publishing Limited; 2007

Schlessinger D. Genome sequencing projects. *Nat Med.* 1995;1(9): 866–868

Turnpenny P, Ellard S, eds. *Emery's Elements of Medical Genetics.* Philadelphia, PA: Churchill Livingstone Elsevier Limited; 2007

References

1. Shaffer LG, Slovak ML, Campbell LJ, eds. *ISCN 2009: An International System for Human Cytogenetic Nomenclature (2009): Recommendations of the International Standing Committee on Human Cytogenetic Nomenclature.* Basel, Switzerland: S. Karger AG; 2009

2. Pellestor F, Andréo B, Anahory T, Hamamah S. The occurrence of aneuploidy in human: lessons from the cytogenetic studies of human oocytes. *Eur J Med Genet.* 2006;49(2):103–116
3. Warren JE, Silver RM. Genetics of pregnancy loss. *Clin Obstet Gynecol.* 2008;51(1): 84–95
4. Toriello HV, Meck JM. Statement on guidance for genetic counseling in advanced paternal age. *Genet Med.* 2008;10(6):457–460
5. Nussbaum RL, McInnes RR, Willard HF. *Thompson & Thompson Genetics in Medicine.* 7th ed. Philadelphia, PA: Saunders Elsevier Limited; 2007:151

Chapter 2

Genetics Over the Life Cycle

Melissa A. Parisi, MD, PhD

Introduction

The observation that monozygotic twins are not truly identical in appearance, personality, and disease susceptibility suggests that human development and disease are not dictated solely by the sequence of bases in DNA. Epigenetic changes and genetic and environmental factors affect the growing child. In fact, there is increasing evidence that prenatal factors influence the susceptibility to diseases such as heart disease and diabetes in adulthood. Here we elucidate how genetics, epigenetics, and environment affect human development over the life cycle.

Epigenetics

Epigenetics is the study of changes in chromosome or gene function that are stable and potentially heritable, but do not change the DNA sequence.[1] Epigenetic changes can have a major effect on how genes are expressed, and can be passed on to future generations without an identifiable difference in the nucleic acid sequence. In combination with genetics, environmental factors, and random or stochastic events, epigenetic factors can profoundly influence the development of a child (Figure 2-1).

Mechanisms of Epigenetic Processes

There are a number of fundamental epigenetic processes that affect chromatin structure, thereby regulating gene expression. The 2 most common are methylation of cytosine residues in DNA and histone modification (Figure 2-2). The addition of a methyl ($-CH_3$) group to a cytosine base, most typically at CpG dinucleotides in DNA, is accomplished by methyltransferases. These cellular enzymes specifically methylate genes in a cell- and tissue-specific manner in regulatory regions that reduce their

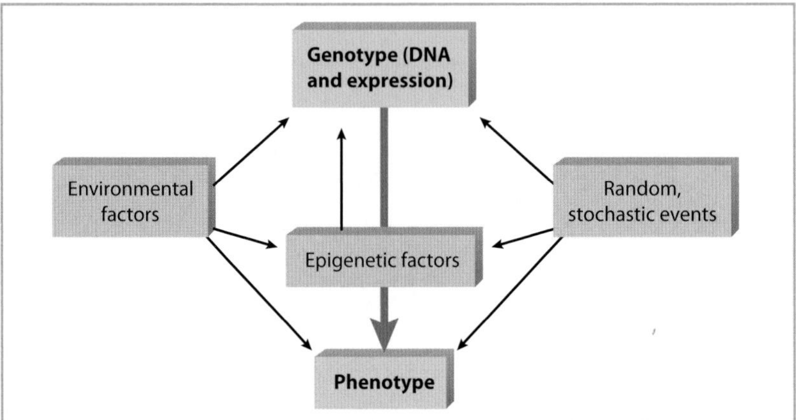

Figure 2-1. The complex interplay between genetics, random events, epigenetics, and environmental factors on health and disease. Modified from Beaudet AL. Is medical genetics neglecting epigenetics? *Genet Med.* 2002;4:399–402. Reprinted with permission from Macmillan Publishers Ltd.

transcription and essentially turn them "off." CpG islands are GC-rich regions more than 500 nucleotides in length that are found near approximately 70% of promoter regions of human genes. Unmethylated CpG islands are associated with actively expressed genes in a cell. The presence of methyl groups interferes with the binding of transcription factors to the DNA and prevents the polymerase machinery from accessing the gene promoter. The methylation pattern is stably maintained via DNA methyltransferases that are sequence-independent and prefer hemimethylated templates, thus preserving gene expression patterns during DNA replication and allowing stable propagation of the methylation status during cell division.[1,2]

Another mechanism of epigenetic gene control occurs via modification of histone proteins, which wrap DNA into units known as nucleosomes that modulate access to DNA by the transcriptional apparatus and thereby affect gene expression. The most common form of histone modification is acetylation (typically of lysine residues at the cytoplasmic tails of histone proteins), but methylation, phosphorylation, ubiquitination, and other alterations have also been described.[1] Mechanisms of propagation of histone modifications during cell division are not known. In general, methylation patterns are believed to represent a more long-term and stable mechanism of regulating gene expression than the short-term and more flexible histone modifications.[3]

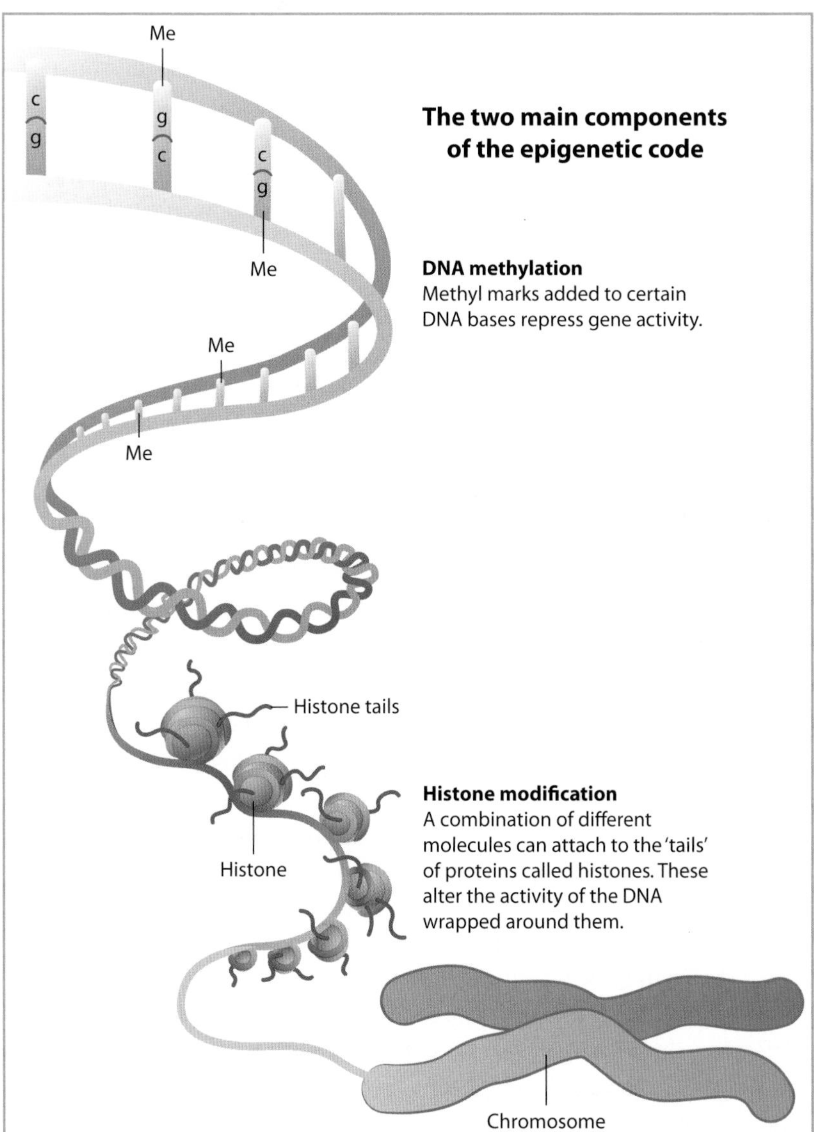

Me
c
g
g
c
c
g
Me
The two main components of the epigenetic code
DNA methylation
Methyl marks added to certain DNA bases repress gene activity.
Me
Me
Histone tails
Histone modification
A combination of different molecules can attach to the 'tails' of proteins called histones. These alter the activity of the DNA wrapped around them.
Histone
Chromosome

Figure 2-2. Epigenetic processes include methylation of DNA and histone modifications. From Qiu J. Epigenetics: unfinished symphony. *Nature.* 2006;441:143–145. Reprinted with permission from Macmillan Publishers Ltd.

Imprinting

Genomic imprinting is an epigenetic form of gene regulation in which a gene is selectively expressed from either the copy inherited from the mother or the copy inherited from the father, but not both parental copies.[2] More than 200 genes are estimated to be imprinted, with many of these genes playing a role in growth, metabolism, or development, and some associated with tumor suppression.[4] Approximately 80% of imprinted genes cluster together in specific regions of the genome and are often bound by small noncoding RNA (ncRNA) molecules encoded within the same region that likely play a regulatory role.[5] For imprinted genes, the degree of methylation (and to a lesser extent, histone modification) at a nearby imprinting control element (ICE) distinguishes the parental copies of the gene with the more heavily methylated copy associated with transcription repression. The status of an imprinted gene is maintained throughout development, and the parental imprint is specific for a particular gene. This imprinting pattern is erased only in the primordial germ cells during gametogenesis and is reset before the maturation of egg or sperm, as illustrated in Figure 2-3.

Because imprinted genes are only expressed from one chromosome, they are functionally haploid and are at high risk of contributing to disease because a single mutation or epigenetic change can alter their function. In addition, the close proximity of several imprinted genes on a chromosome makes them vulnerable to a single genetic change in the region, such as at the ICE. Examples of disorders that can be caused by errors in epigenetic regulation at imprinted genes include Beckwith-Wiedemann, Prader-Willi, Angelman, and Russell-Silver syndromes, all of which are associated with growth abnormalities (Table 2-1).[6] The mechanisms of disease causality for the disorders associated with reciprocal imprinting defects on chromosome 15, Prader-Willi and Angelman syndromes, are illustrated in Figure 2-4.[7] The mechanisms that underlie these conditions are very complicated and still being elucidated.

X-Chromosome Inactivation

Another example of a developmental form of epigenetic regulation is X chromosome inactivation in females. X inactivation is necessary to maintain equal dosage of X-linked genes between males (with a single copy of the X chromosome and XY sex chromosomes) and females (with 2 copies of the X chromosome, XX). The inactivation of 1 of the 2 X chromosomes occurs in the inner cell mass of the blastocyst

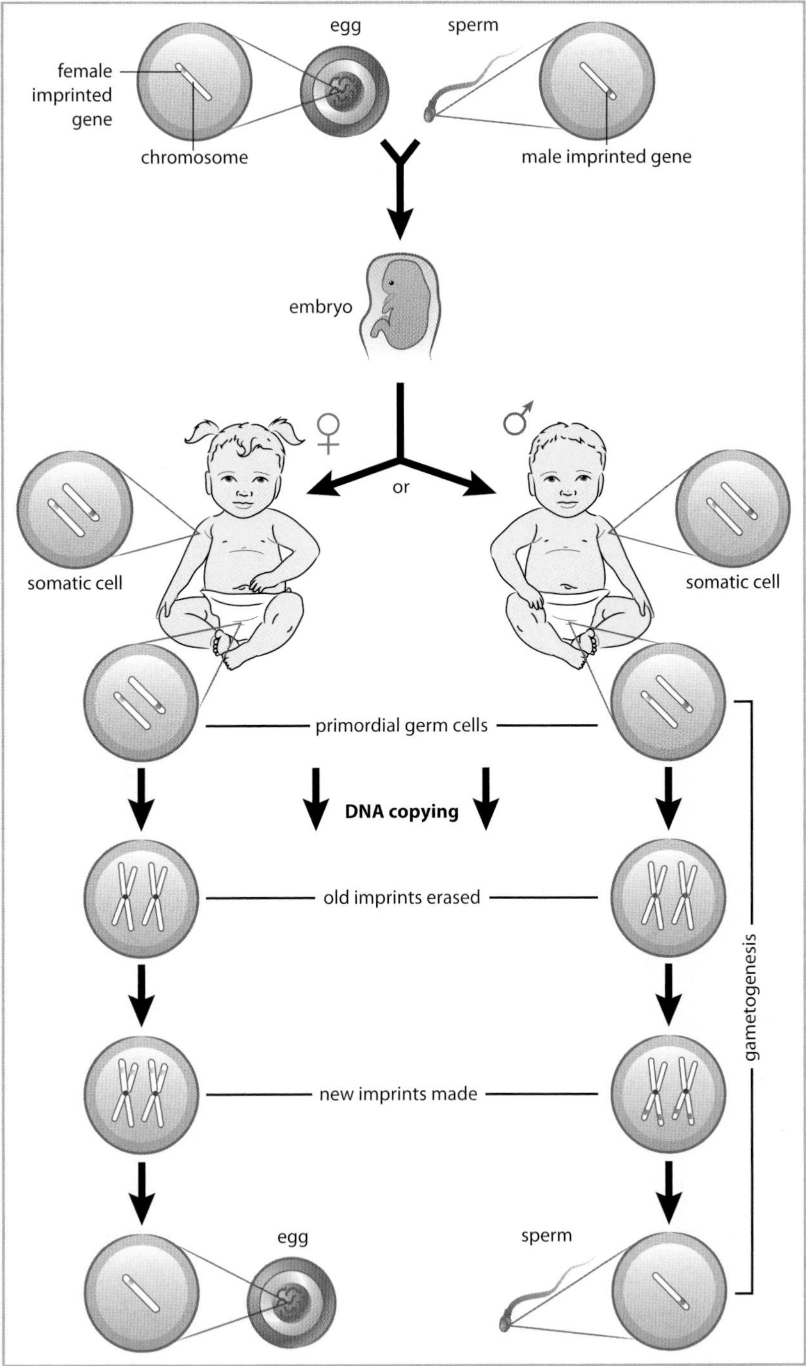

Figure 2-3. Imprints must be reset in each new generation to ensure appropriate gene activity. The sex-specific imprints on DNA from the sperm and the egg persist in somatic cells throughout the body—every cell except those destined to become gametes. In primordial germ cells, DNA copying is followed by the erasing of old imprints and the reestablishment of new uniform imprints that reflect the offspring's own sex. From Jirtle RL, Weidman JR. Imprinted and more equal. *Am Sci.* 2007;95:143–149. Reprinted with permission.

Table 2-1. Disorders Caused by Errors in Epigenetic Regulation at Imprinted Genes

Syndromes Involving Imprinted Genes	Clinical Features	Chromo-somal Location	Birth Prevalence	Parental Origin of Normal Expressed Allele (Imprinted Gene)
Albright hereditary osteodystrophy	SS, obesity, LD, brachydactyly of 4th/5th digits, facial features, cutaneous ossification, hypocalcemia, hypothyroid	20q13	Rare	Maternal and paternal transcripts distinct (*GNAS*)
Angelman syndrome	ID, ataxic gait, absent speech, hand flapping, acquired microcephaly, seizures	15q11-q12	1:12,000	Maternal (*UBE3A*)
Beckwith-Wiedemann syndrome	Overgrowth, hemihyperplasia, omphalocele, macroglossia, facial features, embryonal tumors	11p15	1:13,700	15% inherited; maternal (*CDKN1C*, others)
Hereditary paraganglioma-pheochromocytoma syndrome	Paragangliomas (neuroendocrine tumors of the spine), pheochromocytomas (adrenal medulla), malignant tumors	11q23	Rare	Paternal (*SDHD*)
Prader-Willi syndrome	FTT in infancy, SS, ID, hyperphagia, obesity (childhood), hypogonadism, small hands/feet	15q11-q12	1:10,000	Paternal (*SNURF-SNRPN* locus)
Russell-Silver syndrome	GR (prenatal and postnatal), SS, limb hemihypotrophy, inverted triangular facies, 5th digit clinodactyly, LD/ID	11p15.5, chromosome 7	1:100,000	Paternal (*H19-IGF2;* unknown genes)
Transient neonatal diabetes mellitus	GR, diabetes in first week of life, remission by 3 mo	6q24	Rare	Paternal (*ZAC/PLAGL1*)
UPD14 syndromes	Overgrowth or GR depending on the parent of origin	14	Rare	Both maternal and paternal genes

Abbreviations: FTT, failure to thrive; GR, growth restriction; ID, intellectual disability; LD, learning disability; SS, short stature.

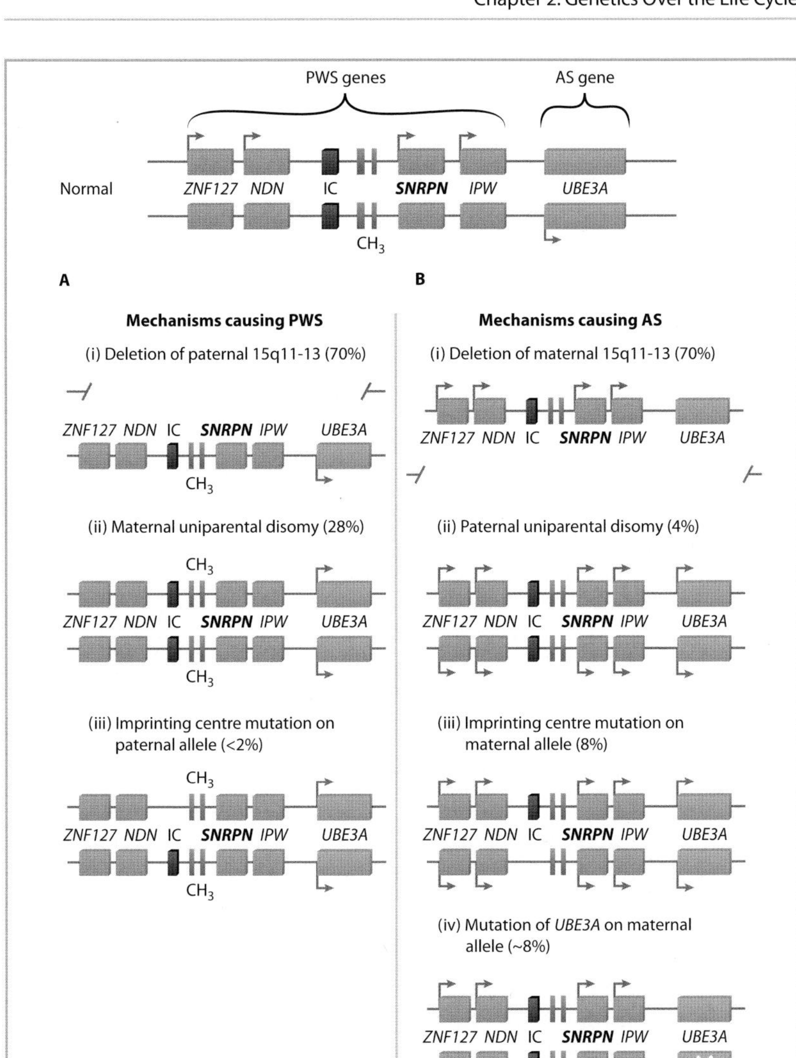

Figure 2-4. Diagrammatic representation of the mechanisms causing Prader-Willi syndrome (PWS) and Angelman syndrome (AS). **A.** The paternal (blue line) and maternal (red line) homologues of the human 15q11-13 region are shown. Paternally expressed genes involved in PWS are represented by blue boxes, and the UBE3A gene, which is maternally expressed in the brain, is represented by a red box. Arrows denote functional activity. The imprinting center (IC) is shown as a black box. The parental epigenotype is represented by vertical black lines; methylated loci are labeled CH3. **B.** The mechanisms causing PWS and AS are similar, involving the same region, but occur on opposite alleles. Either disorder is caused by absence of imprinted genes on the respective alleles. AS is also caused by mutations of *UBE3A*. PWS is a multigene disorder. The frequency (%) of each mechanism among patients is given. From Hitchins MP, Moore GE. Genomic imprinting in fetal growth and development. *Expert Rev Mol Med.* 2002;4(11):1–19. Reprinted with permission from Cambridge University Press.

in a random pattern established early during female embryogenesis in a complex process that persists for all the progeny of a given cell.[8] Inactivation is initiated at the X inactivation center, which encodes 2 genes for non–protein-coding RNA molecules, *XIST* and *TSIX*. The X chromosome that is inactivated expresses the approximately 17kb *XIST* (X inactivation–specific transcript) RNA, which coats and silences its adjacent chromosome, recruiting histones and other proteins that cause DNA condensation and creating the Barr body visible at the periphery of the nucleus in buccal smears.[9] In contrast, *TSIX (XIST* antisense RNA) transcription from the active X chromosome prevents its inactivation.[10] The process is decidedly more complex than presented here, because approximately 15% of genes escape X inactivation (and are thus expressed from both X chromosomes in females), but these are distributed throughout the X chromosome and may vary between tissues and between individuals.[11] In addition, the randomly chosen inactivated X chromosome must be reactivated in migrating germ cells in the female embryo postimplantation.[8]

Although X chromosome inactivation is generally a random process with equal inactivation of the maternally or paternally inherited X chromosome, for some individuals there is preferential inactivation of one X chromosome in at least 75% of cells, known as skewed X inactivation.[11] About 5% of women have extreme skewing in at least 90% of their cells, a finding that seems to be more common in blood-derived cells and as women age. For some X-linked disorders, there is preferential inactivation of the X chromosome containing the mutated gene, perhaps reflecting a selective advantage of cells in which the normal X is active, with the consequence that female carriers will have a less severe or normal phenotype.[11] Other X-linked disorders, such as hemophilia or Duchenne muscular dystrophy (DMD), are usually not associated with skewing, resulting in variable manifestations in carrier females depending on the degree of inactivation of the mutant allele. For example, female DMD carriers with preferential inactivation of the normal allele of the *DMD* gene in cardiac or skeletal muscle precursor cells often have elevated levels of serum creatine kinase, muscle weakness, and cardiomyopathy. Female carriers of some X-linked intellectual disability genes also exhibit skewed X chromosome inactivation, so this finding in the mother of a boy with an unknown form of intellectual disability may provide clues regarding the underlying etiology.[11]

Noncoding RNA

Of the 3 billion nucleotides that comprise the human genome, only 1% to 2% of this DNA encodes proteins, corresponding to an estimated 20,000 to 30,000 total protein-coding genes.[12] Although the remainder of the genome has been previously dismissed as "junk DNA," it seems that most of the RNA species transcribed from it comprise ncRNAs that may play a role in gene regulation. The regulatory roles for ncRNA include dosage compensation, genomic imprinting, developmental patterning, and cellular differentiation.[13] There are many classes of ncRNAs depending on their size, function, and polarity (sense or antisense). Although a comprehensive review of ncRNA is outside the scope of this chapter, some examples from known biological processes have helped elucidate disease mechanisms and provide tantalizing prospects for therapeutic targets. The class of long ncRNAs (>200 nucleotides in length) includes the *XIST* gene on the X chromosome that coats the inactive X chromosome in female cells and recruits histone-modifying enzymes that promote chromatin condensation (Figure 2-2). Other long ncRNAs are found concentrated within the HOX (homeobox) cluster of 39 genes in humans and other mammals that are essential for many developmental processes.[14] Small ncRNAs, known as RNAi (interfering RNA), play an essential role in gene silencing. In fact, some investigators are developing RNAi-based molecules to treat human diseases (eg, age-related macular degeneration[15] and Duchenne muscular dystrophy[16]).

Critical Periods During the Life Span

Conditions in the fetal environment, such as nutrition and stress, can lead to permanent changes in the epigenome that increase the risk of developing chronic metabolic and cardiovascular diseases in adulthood. Barker et al[17] first identified the correlation between infants with low birth weight who demonstrated rapid weight gain in childhood when nutrients were plentiful and later developed adult-onset coronary heart disease, hypertension, and type 2 diabetes mellitus (the Barker hypothesis). Apparently, these changes in gene expression are mediated by epigenetic processes and become stably established. For example, pregnant rats fed a low-protein diet give birth to offspring who develop hypertension and have associated hypomethylation and overexpression of metabolic and endothelial genes, such as the angiotensin and glucocorticoid receptors.[1] Conversely, maternal obesity and a hyperglycemic uterine environment contribute to an increased risk of metabolic disorders, particularly type 2 diabetes, in their offspring.[1] The study of the developmental origins of health and disease via fetal programming is an emerging area of investigation. Specific genetic, epigenetic, and environmental influences occur over the life cycle; some have particular pediatric relevance, including modifications that occur during gametogenesis, periconceptional and prenatal period, childhood, and adulthood and aging (Figure 2-5).[1]

Gametogenesis

Nondisjunction

The process of gametogenesis lends itself to potential errors that result in many genetic disorders (Table 2-2). Nondisjunction errors during meiosis result in miscarriage in most cases, because the addition or loss of a complete chromosome is incompatible with normal development and survival of the embryo to term; the exceptions are the chromosomal aneuploidy conditions such as trisomy 21, Turner syndrome, and Klinefelter syndrome. The most common disorder arising from nondisjunction of an autosome (non-sex chromosome), Down syndrome or trisomy 21 (see Chapter 9), occurs in 1:691 live births. The risk of nondisjunction increases with advanced maternal age, presumably because the paired homologous chromosomes fail to separate after a long period of gamete arrest in prophase I of meiosis (which is when meiosis arrested when the pregnant woman was an embryo).

Spontaneous Mutation

In contrast to chromosomal aneuploidy disorders that arise from maternal nondisjunction during meiosis, new autosomal dominant genetic syndromes are likely to result from spontaneous mutations during gametogenesis. The estimated neutral mutation rate in the human genome is 2.3×10^{-8} mutations per nucleotide site per generation,[18] with evidence that the mutation rate is about twice as high in male as in female meiosis. Thus most new mutations occur in the male germline.[12] It is hypothesized that these mutations (generally nucleotide base substitutions comprising DNA point mutations) arise in the self-renewing spermatogonia that divide continuously throughout a man's life, whereas a woman's oogonia stop replicating during fetal life after about 30 cell generations. As a consequence, the increased cell generations during male meiosis are more likely to accumulate point mutations associated with advanced paternal age that result in disease in their progeny.[18] For some conditions, such as achondroplasia and Apert syndrome, there seem to be specific mutations that occur

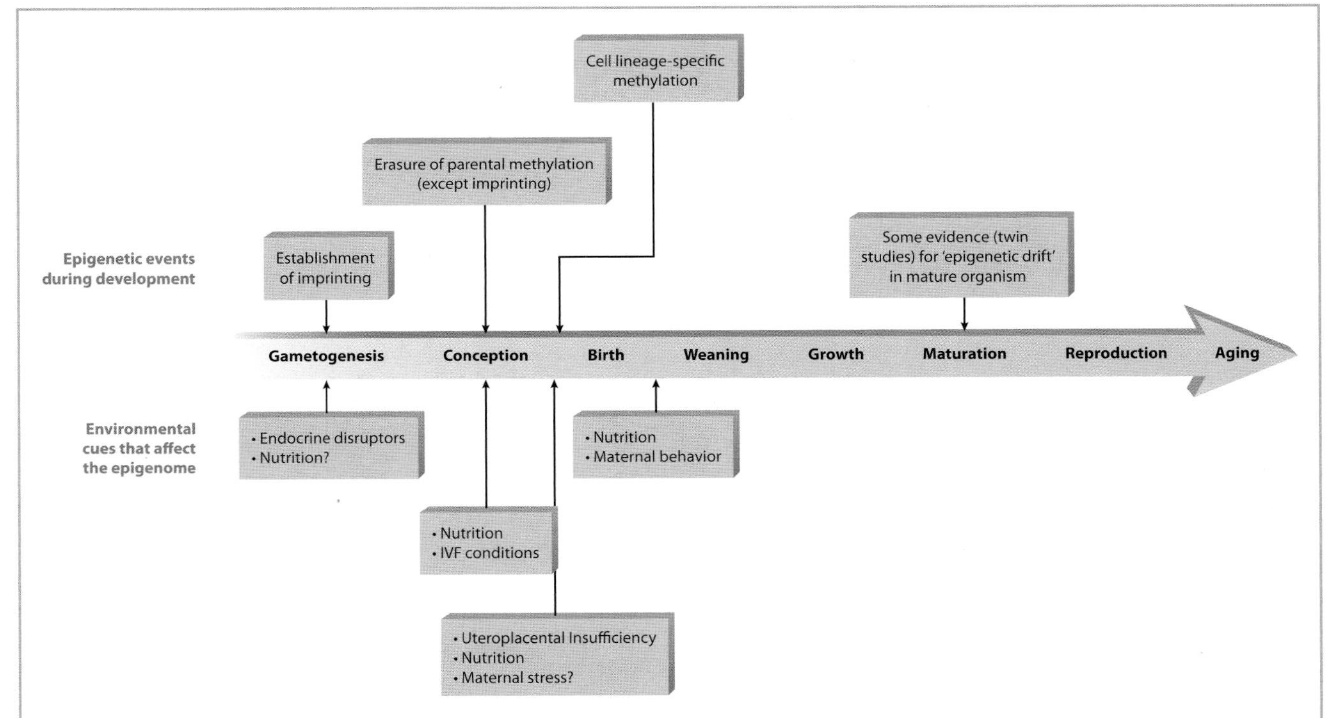

Figure 2-5. Timeline with susceptible periods for epigenetic changes throughout the life span. IVF, in vitro fertilization. From Gluckman PD, Hanson MA, Buklijas T, et al. Epigenetic mechanisms that underpin metabolic and cardiovascular diseases. *Nat Rev Endocrinol.* 2009;5(7):401–408. Reprinted with permission from Macmillan Publishers Ltd.

Table 2-2. Select Disorders Caused by Nondisjunction During Gametogenesis

Genetic Disorder	Clinical Features	Birth Prevalence	Comments
Autosome Disorders			
Trisomy 16	Most common aneuploidy that results in miscarriage	0	Not viable
Trisomy 21 (Down syndrome)	ID, SS, CHD, hypotonia, GI malformations, hypothyroid, facial features, STPC, leukemia, early dementia	1:691 live births	Maternal nondisjunction, associated with AMA
Trisomy 18 (Edwards syndrome)	Profound ID, GR, CHD, facial features, clenched fist, rocker bottom feet, prominent occiput, mean life expectancy 4 days, only 5% survive to 1 y	1: 8,000 live births	Maternal nondisjunction, associated with AMA
Trisomy 13 (Patau syndrome)	Profound ID, GR, cutis aplasia, holoprosencephaly, CHD, polydactyly, facial features, mean life expectancy 7–10 days, only 5%–10% survive to 1 y	1:10,000 live births	Maternal nondisjunction, associated with AMA
Sex Chromosome Disorders			
Klinefelter syndrome (47,XXY)	Tall stature, hypogonadism, infertility, gynecomastia, mild LD, normal life span	1:600–1:800 male births	Associated with AMA
Turner syndrome (45,X; other variants)	SS, facial features, gonadal dysgenesis/primary ovarian failure, CHD, renal anomalies, hypothyroid, mild LD, HL, fetal edema, facial features	1:2,500 female births	Most due to paternal meiotic errors
Triple X syndrome (47,XXX)	Tall stature, mild LD, normal fertility	1:1,000–1:1,200 female births	Often undiagnosed
47,XYY	Tall stature, mild LD, behavioral problems, normal fertility	1:1,000 male births	Often undiagnosed, no APA effect

Abbreviations: AMA, advanced maternal age; APA, advanced paternal age; CHD, congenital heart defects; GI, gastrointestinal; GR, growth restriction; HL, hearing loss; ID, intellectual disability; LD, learning disability; SS, short stature; STPC, single transverse palmar crease.

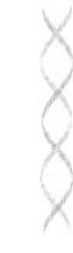

with high frequency in the DNA of sperm cells, potentially because these mutations confer a selective advantage for the spermatogonia that harbor them.[18] Table 2-3 includes a list of conditions with high mutation frequency that might reflect positive germline selection; many of these are dominant disorders and some have poor reproductive fitness.

Although the recurrence risk for a couple with a child with a dominant disorder arising from a spontaneous mutation is generally low in a subsequent pregnancy, the couple should be made aware that the disorder may have arisen from germline mosaicism. Germline mosaicism is the presence of a mixture of normal and abnormal gametes in the gonads of one of the parents. This phenomenon has been documented in several conditions. In one family with a lethal dominant brittle bone disease, osteogenesis imperfecta (OI), a man fathered 2 children with lethal OI with 2 different partners and was later found to have a collagen gene *(COL1A2)* point mutation detected in a proportion of his sperm cells.[19] Thus the possibility of germline mosaicism in an otherwise unaffected parent should be considered when counseling couples with a child with what appears to be a new, non-inherited dominant disorder.

Epigenetics and Assistive Reproductive Technologies

During gametogenesis, epigenetic marks are reestablished for each generation after global demethylation wipes the methylation pattern clean in the primordial germ cells (Figure 2-3). There seem to be differences between male and female germ cells with regard to the timing and extent of reestablishment of methylation. In the germline of developing male embryos, the male pattern of methylation is restored during a subsequent stage of embryogenesis and allows mitosis and later meiosis to occur. In contrast, remethylation of the female germline occurs after birth during the growth of oocytes, which remain in meiotic arrest.[2] These differences may predispose to differences in vulnerability to epigenetic changes. Reprogramming in the germ cells is necessary to reset the imprints for genes subject to parent-specific expression, and it probably also serves to remove acquired epigenetic modifications due to environmental or genetic factors.[2] However, some epigenetic changes in eggs and sperm may persist and be passed on to subsequent generations, although whether this represents true transgenerational transmission or the influence of a similar environmental milieu across generations remains an open question.[1]

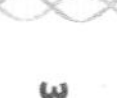

Table 2-3. Disorders Caused by New Point Mutations During Gametogenesis[a]

Genetic Disorder	Clinical Features	Mode of Transmission (Gene)[b]	Almost Always of Paternal Origin	Birth Prevalence
Achondroplasia	Disproportionate SS, short limbs, other skeletal anomalies, facial features, risk of cervical cord compression	AD (*FGFR3*)[c]; associated with APA	Yes	1:27,000
Apert syndrome	Coronal craniosynostosis, severe digital syndactyly ("mitten hand"), ID	AD (*FGFR2*)[c]; associated with APA	Yes	1:100,000
CHARGE syndrome	Coloboma, CHD, choanal atresia, GR, genital anomalies, ear anomalies, HL, ID	AD (*CHD7*)		1:12,000
Congenital central hypoventilation syndrome	Poor respiratory effort especially while asleep, autonomic disturbance, Hirschsprung disease, neuroblastoma	AD (*PHOX2B*) polyalanine expansion		Unknown
Marfan syndrome	Tall stature, aortic root dilation, MVP, lens dislocation, facial features, arachnodactyly, skeletal anomalies, hypermobility	AD (*FBN-1*)		1:3,000–5,000
Multiple endocrine neoplasia type 2B	Medullary thyroid cancer, pheochromocytoma, mucosal neuromas, facial features, GI ganglioneuromatosis, thin body habitus	AD (*RET*)[c]; associated with APA	Yes	1:30,000 for all MEN2; much lower for MEN2B
Neurofibromatosis I	Café au lait spots, axillary freckles, dermal and plexiform neurofibromas, Lisch nodules of the eye, optic gliomas, LD	AD (*NF1*)	Yes	1:4,000
Osteogenesis imperfecta (OI) (severe forms)	Brittle bones with multiple fractures, Wormian bones, blue sclera, dentinogenesis imperfecta, HL	AD (*COL1A1* and *COL1A2* genes)		1:20,000 for all OI; much lower for severe forms

Table 2-3. Disorders Caused by New Point Mutations During Gametogenesis[a] *(continued)*

Genetic Disorder	Clinical Features	Mode of Transmission (Gene)[b]	Almost Always of Paternal Origin	Birth Prevalence
Rett syndrome	Normal development with regression at 6–18 mo, ID, stereotypic hand movements, acquired microcephaly, seizures, autistic-like features	XL-females only affected *(MECP2)*	Yes	1:10,000 females
Tuberous sclerosis complex	Hamartomas of brain, skin, retina; infantile spasms; epilepsy; LD/ID; subependymal nodules; renal angiomyolipomas; facial angiofibromas; hypomelanotic macules; ungual fibromas; cardiac rhabdomyomas	AD (*TSC1* or *TSC2*)		1:10,000
von Hippel-Lindau disease	Hemangioblastomas of cerebellum/spinal cord, retinal angiomas, renal cell carcinoma, pheochromocytomas, renal and pancreatic cysts	AD (*VHL*)		1:36,000

Abbreviations: AD, autosomal dominant; APA, advanced paternal age; CHD, congenital heart defects; GI, gastrointestinal; GR, growth restriction; HL, hearing loss; ID, intellectual disability; LD, learning disability; MVP, mitral valve prolapse; SS, short stature; XL, X-linked.

[a] This list is not exhaustive, and other disorders result from new point mutations: Holt-Oram, renal-coloboma, campomelic dysplasia, and Crouzon syndromes, among others.

[b] Inheritance from an affected parent has been reported for all of these but congenital central hypoventilation syndrome, CHARGE syndrome, severe osteogenesis imperfecta, and Rett syndrome.

[c] An unexpectedly high mutation frequency of a specific nucleotide substitution(s) has been observed.

In developed countries, 1% to 3% of births are the result of assisted reproductive technologies (ART).[20] Although most children conceived by ART are healthy, more than 30% of ART pregnancies constitute multifetal gestations (twins or higher), with associated complications, such as preterm birth and low birth weight, that themselves represent epigenetic programming risks.[21] Assisted reproductive technologies may be associated with an increased risk of epigenetic disorders such as Beckwith-Wiedemann syndrome (BWS), a disorder with features of overgrowth, omphalocele, large tongue, and hypoglycemia associated with an imprinted region on chromosome 11. (See Table 2-1.) This association suggests that manipulations of egg, sperm, or the fertilization process may affect normal developmental processes. The studies are limited by small sample size given the low frequency of epigenetic disorders in general (<1:12,000 births), but compiled data suggest that more than 90% of children with BWS conceived using ART had imprinting defects rather than other causative mechanisms; whereas only 40% to 50% of children with BWS who were conceived *without* the use of ART had imprinting defects. Similar data suggest imprinting defects as the mechanism in most children with Angelman syndrome born after ART.[20]

Periconceptional and Prenatal Period

Effect of Inadequate Nutrition

The periconceptional period and prenatal period play important roles in subsequent metabolic dysfunction, as underscored by retrospective studies of adults exposed prenatally to famine during the Dutch Hunger Winter (a limited famine in 1944–1945 at the end of World War II). Based on studies of 300,000 males at the age of military conscription (19 years), those exposed to famine during the first half of gestation had a much higher rate of obesity than those who were not.[22] The effects of caloric restriction were not limited to infants born small-for-gestational age, because those exposed to famine in the periconceptional period and the first trimester of pregnancy did not exhibit low birth weights, but as adults they experienced obesity and coronary artery disease.[1] Remarkably, decreased levels of methylation of specific imprinted genes associated with growth (such as *IGF2)* were measured in these men when they reached their 60s, suggesting the persistence of epigenetic modifications arising in the periconceptional period.[23] Conversely, those men exposed to limited nutrients in the last trimester of pregnancy and the first few months of life had low birth weights and significantly lower obesity rates in adulthood, but increased risk of insulin resistance and hypertension.[1,22]

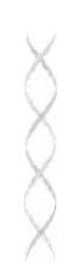

Some studies show a correlation between prenatal exposure to famine and the development of congenital anomalies of the central nervous system, as well as schizophrenia and related personality disorders. In fact, the risk of developing schizophrenia in adulthood was 2-fold higher in those children conceived during the height of the Dutch Hunger Winter.[24] These studies were replicated by studies in a Chinese province that experienced a limited but extreme famine in 1959–1961, with a comparable increased risk of developing schizophrenia for individuals conceived during this period.[25] Conceptually, these data are not too surprising if one considers schizophrenia a neurodevelopmental disorder subject to environmental influences during early brain development that may modify an underlying genetic predisposition.

These studies suggest that environmental factors in utero (eg, nutritional status) that affect birth weight play a role in susceptibility to the adult disorders of hypertension, cardiovascular disease, insulin resistance, diabetes, and obesity. Perhaps fetal metabolic adjustments under dire nutritional circumstances that conserve nutrients to protect brain development have unfortunate deleterious effects in adulthood and cause chronic disease. Similarly, there is evidence that fetuses exposed to a hyperglycemic environment or whose mothers are obese during pregnancy are at increased risk to later develop metabolic disorders such as type 2 diabetes mellitus.[1] Moreover, these effects may be transmitted to subsequent generations, so the child in the pediatrician's office may reflect environmental effects of the prior 1 or 2 generations.

Effect of Inadequate Nutritional Cofactors

Other nutritional factors during a woman's pregnancy play a role in the physiology, metabolism, and health of her children. A prime example of a public health effort to improve prenatal nutritional status and reduce birth defects is the recommendation that women of reproductive age take folic acid supplements in the preconceptional period to prevent neural tube defects (NTDs).[26] Low circulating folate levels during pregnancy were also known to be associated with an increased risk for preterm delivery, fetal growth restriction, and low birth weight.[27] In 1998 the US Food and Drug Administration began requiring the fortification of enriched cereal grain products with folic acid at a level that would increase the folate consumption of the general population.[26] Based on decades of research, including randomized, controlled trials that showed a reduction in NTDs in pregnancies supplemented with folic acid, the hypothesis for the effect is that folate serves as a cofactor for methyl group metabolism and production of the primary methyl donor used in purine and pyrimidine synthesis and DNA methylation, likely critical during neural tube closure in the early embryo. Since mandatory food fortification, the prevalence of NTDs in the United States has decreased by 19%.[26] However, critics have warned that there may be unintended consequences of population-wide folate supplementation because of its potential unknown effects on methylation, imprinting, and other epigenetic processes during human development.[27]

These studies underscore a developmental plasticity in which changes in metabolism and function can occur irreversibly during a critical period in response to fetal nutrition and environmental cues.[27] In fact, an extension of this hypothesis suggests that a developing fetus adapts to the nutritional status it experiences in utero to optimize its survival and anticipates a comparable postnatal nutritional status, so the consequence of a diet in childhood and adulthood that varies from this projection is a predisposition to adult disease. Hence, maternal under- or over-nutrition in the pre-pregnancy period, not uncommon in developed countries, can have a profound effect on obesity in subsequent generations.[1] These effects can alter the germline of subsequent generations, through both the paternal and maternal lineage. Retrospective epidemiologic studies in Sweden showed that the nutritional status of the grandfather from ages 8 to 12 years (known as the slow growth period) was the strongest predictor for both life span and tendency to develop diabetes in his grandsons, even after controlling for social circumstances and education.[28] It is sobering to contemplate, for example, that a woman's own health may be affected by the nutritional status of her grandmother during the grandmother's pregnancy with her mother, particularly during the critical stages when epigenetic reprogramming of the embryo's (mother's) germline occurred.

Effect of Environmental Exposures

The role of environmental exposures in the prenatal period has been well established for some substances such as tobacco smoke, but is still being explored for others. Exposure to tobacco smoke before and during pregnancy has been associated with birth defects such as orofacial clefts, premature birth, and intrauterine growth restriction, but also with childhood obesity and neurobehavioral problems such as attention-deficit/hyperactivity disorder and psychosis.[20,29] The biological basis for these findings is hypothesized to involve chronic fetal hypoxia, diminished placental blood flow, and carbon monoxide–induced fetal oxygen consumption.[30] However, recent data suggest that the variable susceptibility to tobacco exposure risks in fetuses may be related to differences in in-

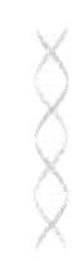

ducible genes that metabolize toxins such as nicotine and polycyclic aromatic hydrocarbons; both maternal and fetal polymorphisms in genes of the cytochrome P450 and glutathione-S-transferase systems are prone to differential methylation and may influence adverse fetal outcomes.[30]

Some environmental toxins have been shown to directly induce DNA mutations, while other substances are carcinogenic because of epigenetic effects. Many of these latter chemicals are known as endocrine disruptors, because they function as steroid receptor signaling agonists or antagonists and affect reproductive development and, in some cases, promote adult disease. One of the best examples of a known endocrine disruptor is diethylstilbestrol, a synthetic estrogen previously administered to women during pregnancy to prevent miscarriage, which resulted in higher rates of cervical and vaginal cancer in their exposed daughters and epididymal cysts in their exposed sons.[30] Another endocrine disruptor, the fungicide vinclozolin used by the wine industry, has been shown to disrupt DNA methylation in the developing rat testis. Exposure of pregnant female rats during the period of testis sex differentiation results in spermatogenic deficiencies in their male progeny with an increase in adult-onset prostate and kidney disease, tumors, and male infertility, findings that can be transmitted through the male germline and persist for 3 more generations.[31] Phthalates and bisphenol A (BPA) are potential endocrine disruptors commonly found in plastic containers and food packaging, and BPA in particular may increase the risk of prostate, breast, and other reproductive tract cancers at low doses previously assumed to be safe.[31]

Imprinting and X chromosome inactivation occur prenatally and have profound influences on development and disease. A description of these epigenetic processes is found on pages 21–29.

Mosaicism and Somatic Mutation

Mosaicism, in its basic definition, indicates a mixture of cells with different genetic compositions. Mosaicism can affect not only the germline but also somatic tissues, resulting in genetic diseases that may be difficult to diagnose. One of the best examples of a mosaic condition is McCune-Albright syndrome, in which somatic activating mutations in the *GNAS1* (guanine nucleotide binding protein [G protein], alpha-stimulating activity polypeptide-1) gene contribute to a spectrum of findings characterized by bony lesions known as polyostotic fibrous dysplasia, café au lait macules on the skin, and precocious puberty, among other endocrine disorders.[32] Although these mutations typically occur in the embryonic post-zygotic period, the spectrum of anomalies that develop during childhood is highly variable and dependent on the proportion and distribution of cells carrying the mutation in specific tissues of the body.[33] Presumably, a mutation that affected the entire embryo would be lethal during development.

Other conditions, such as Proteus syndrome and hypomelanosis of Ito, are also hypothesized to be due to mosaicism of an early embryonic change that would otherwise be lethal. The special situation of a mutation that affects the gametes and could be passed on to progeny is termed germline mosaicism. (See page 33 in this chapter.)

Childhood Period

Maternal Behavior

Studies suggest that maternal behavior in the postnatal period can also affect the response of their infants to stress, and this response persists into adulthood. Rat pups whose mothers exhibited increased levels of licking and grooming in the first 10 days of life showed reduced levels of cortisol production in response to stress as adults, an effect that correlated with differential patterns of methylation and histone acetylation at the glucocorticoid receptor promoters in the brains of the pups. These effects could be reversed by cross-fostering by mothers with reduced licking and grooming behaviors.[34] Although a direct correlation with human development is overly simplistic, the importance of early maternal-infant bonds and parental involvement has implications for children exposed to early life stressors. For example, physical or sexual abuse, persistent emotional neglect or family conflict, and deprivation in institutionalized settings such as orphanages can compromise growth, intellectual development, and emotional resilience and can increase the risk for adult obesity, depression, and anxiety disorders.[35] Individual differences in vulnerability to psychopathology throughout life are no doubt influenced by the complex interplay between genetic, environmental, and epigenetic factors that are not completely understood.

Microbiome

The intestinal microbiome is established primarily during infancy and shows particular correlates with certain aspects of child health. For example, a less diverse gut microbiome with high levels of *Bacteroides*, *Clostridium*, *Enterobacteriaceae*, and *Staphylococcus* species early in life has been associated with an increased risk of allergies, asthma, and atopic disease. Correlations with childhood obesity have also been identified, with members of the same household tending to show similar gut flora and body weight patterns.[36]

Adulthood and Aging

Adult Diseases Caused by Inherited Mutations

Some diseases of adulthood are caused by inherited mutations that do not manifest symptoms until later in life. Examples of genetic disorders with typical onset in adulthood but implications for children at risk to inherit causative mutations include Huntington disease (HD), Charcot-Marie-Tooth (CMT) disease, and hereditary breast and ovarian cancer (HBOC).

Huntington Disease

Huntington disease is an autosomal dominant triplet repeat disorder, characterized by CAG repeats within the coding portion of the gene that, when expanded beyond a critical threshold, results in selective neuronal death. In HD, the onset of symptoms for those with 36-55 CAG repeats is typically between 35 to 44 years of age, with progressive motor, cognitive, and psychiatric disturbances; typically, death ensues within 15 to 18 years of onset.[37] There is no treatment, but genetic testing is available. Many individuals inherit the triplet expansion from an affected parent, but the parent may not show symptoms before reproducing. The decision to pursue genetic testing in minors who may be at 50% chance of inheriting a progressive neurodegenerative disorder without a cure is a problematic one, and most geneticists would not advocate testing in minors unless the minor exhibited symptoms. (See Chapter 11.) There is a tendency for the triplet repeat to expand during transmission from an affected father, a phenomenon known as anticipation, and extreme expansions over 60 CAG repeats can cause onset of symptoms prior to age 21 and, in some cases, even younger, further complicating genetic testing decisions.

Charcot-Marie-Tooth Disease

Charcot-Marie-Tooth disease, a hereditary sensory-motor neuropathy, affects approximately 1:3,300 individuals, typically adults, although there can be significant variability with regard to age of onset and severity of symptoms. Initial symptoms include foot drop, with development of distal muscle weakness and atrophy, mild to moderate sensory loss, reduced tendon reflexes, weakened grip, and high-arched feet. Although most cases are autosomal dominant, some X-linked and autosomal recessive forms exist, complicating the options for genetic testing, as more than 40 causative genes and genetic loci exist.[38] One of the most common causes of CMT, accounting for up to 40% of cases, is the duplication of chromosome 17 involving the *PMP22* (peripheral myelin protein 22) gene.[38] Genetic testing for this microduplication is available. However, detection of this genomic duplication can be identified by routine cytogenomic microarray analysis ordered for diagnostic evaluation in a child with global developmental delay, for example, and would complicate genetic counseling for a family in which this chromosome difference was identified presymptomatically in a child being evaluated for other indications. For this reason, some diagnostic laboratories do not report incidental findings on microarray studies that are not relevant to the purpose of the test.

Hereditary Breast and Ovarian Cancer

A third example of an inherited adult disorder is a cancer predisposition syndrome, BRCA, which can be caused by dominant mutations in the *BRCA1* or *BRCA2* genes that carry a cumulative risk of developing breast and/or ovarian cancer by age 70 of approximately 85%.[39] Up to 10% of breast cancer patients have a genetic predisposition, and each of these 2 genes contributes to approximately 2.5% of cases. Genetic testing is a reasonable option for women with a positive family history of ovarian cancer, early-onset breast cancer (prior to the age of 50 years), or male breast cancer. Identification of a causative *BRCA1* mutation in a woman with breast cancer influences treatment approaches and medical surveillance for other associated risks, such as ovarian cancer. For healthy daughters of individuals with a *BRCA* gene mutation and a 50% risk of inheriting the mutation, the decision to undergo genetic testing is a personal one that is best made in adulthood. Individuals who carry a disease-associated mutation and have not yet developed cancer have several options for screening and primary prevention, including annual breast cancer screening by mammography and breast magnetic resonance imaging starting in the mid-20s, annual pelvic examinations for ovarian cancer, and consideration of prophylactic mastectomy or oophorectomy after reproduction has been completed.[39] Identification of a familial cancer predisposition syndrome has significant implications for at-risk first-degree relatives and affects family planning decision-making.

Cancer, Epigenetics, and Mutations

The development of cancer is influenced by the accumulation of mutations in critical genes. Although most pediatric cancers are presumed to arise from acquired somatic mutations, the presence of a cancer predisposition syndrome can result in early-onset, bilateral, multiple, independent tumors. In patients with retinoblastoma, malignant tumors of the retina typically arise before the age of 5 years because of cancer-causing mutations in both copies of the *RB1* tumor suppressor gene (the "2 hit" Knudson hypothesis of cancer causation). Approximately 40% of affected children have bilateral tumors with a mean age of diagnosis of 15 months, and these children are more likely to harbor an inherited germline mutation in the *RB1* gene (Figure 2-6A). Children heterozygous for a cancer-predisposing mutation in one *RB1* allele also have an increased risk of developing radiation-induced secondary cancers and other non-ocular tumors such as osteosarcomas.[40] In contrast, about 60% of affected children have a unilateral tumor with a mean age of diagnosis of 24 months and are more likely to have an acquired (somatic) mutation in each of the 2 *RB1* genes in the retinal cell that develops the tumor (Figure 2-6B).

DNA Changes and Tumor Development

Epigenetic alterations, particularly DNA methylation, are well-known to contribute to cancer development. During tumor development, methylation is usually globally decreased, with selective hypermethylation of CpG sites

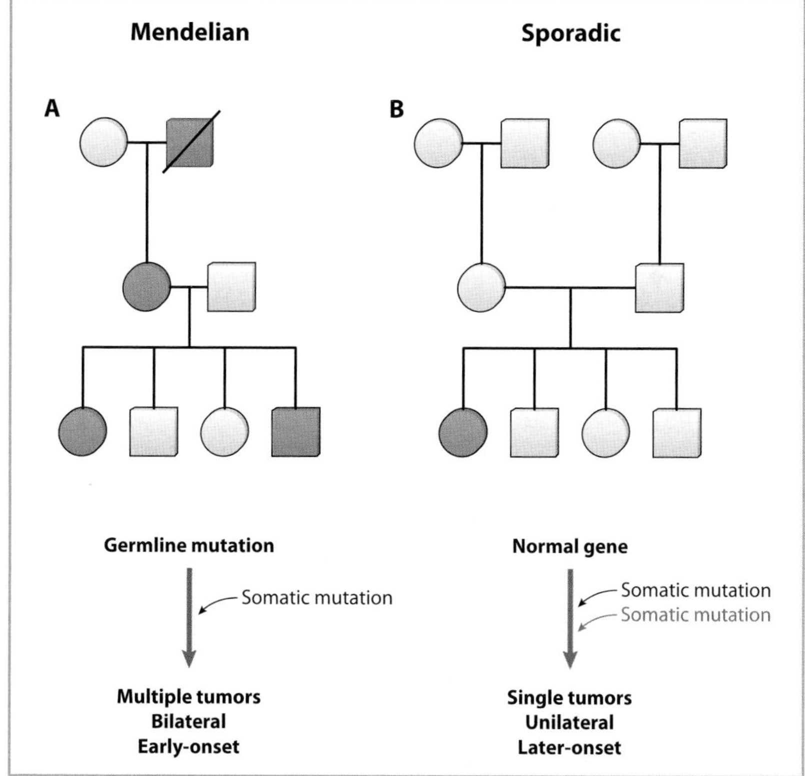

Figure 2-6. The Knudson 2-hit hypothesis and differences between (A) inherited cancer predisposition syndromes and (B) somatic cancer development.

within the promoters of tumor suppressor genes, silencing these genes and promoting tumor progression.[5] Human bladder cancers exhibit increased promoter methylation of critical tumor suppressor genes, which is highly associated with known bladder carcinogens, such as cigarette smoking, arsenic exposure, and other occupational hazards.[41] Inflammation may also play a role in tumor progression via changes in histone modification and chromatin remodeling. A complex series of accumulated mutations in oncogenes and tumor suppressor genes, acquired chromosome abnormalities, epigenetic changes involving methylation, histone modification and microRNAs, alterations in gene expression, host inflammatory responses, and other factors can all affect cancer development.[5]

Pharmacogenomics and Aging

The level of expression and activity of drug-metabolizing enzymes (such as the cytochrome P450 enzymes important in metabolism of many classes of medications) and receptors that are important for drug action (such as opioid receptors) are known to vary between individuals and influence drug responsiveness. Some individuals may be either fast or slow metabolizers of specific medications, which in the latter case can result in significant toxicity. With increasing age, the general efficiency of drug metabolism tends to decrease, resulting in increased sensitivity to many pharmacotherapeutic agents, but these effects are also tempered by genetic factors, environmental exposures, sex, and race. In the burgeoning field of pediatric pharmacogenomics, emerging evidence suggests that genetic and epigenetic factors as well as the developmental stage of the individual contribute to alterations in drug response. For example, young infants with particular cytochrome P450 enzyme polymorphisms are at increased risk of hepatotoxicity from valproic acid because of the relative immaturity of the drug-metabolizing system in the postnatal period.[42]

Twin Studies and Environmental Factors

The influence of the environment on epigenetic modifications and later-onset disease is demonstrated in studies of twin pairs. Monozygotic (MZ) twins are derived from the same egg and sperm and thus assumed to be identical with regard to DNA sequence and genetic makeup, whereas dizygotic (DZ) twins are derived from 2 separate zygotes. Classical genetic studies have compared the rates of complex traits and diseases in MZ versus DZ twins in order to calculate the heritability of traits and provide

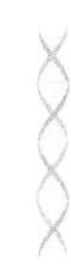

an indirect measure of the contribution of environmental factors, since it is assumed that the prenatal and postnatal environment is similar for twins.[43] For example, the calculated heritability coefficients for psychiatric disorders such as schizophrenia, bipolar disorder, and depression are relatively high, suggesting significant genetic contributions; however, the concordance rates for schizophrenia in MZ twin pairs are only 41% to 65%.[44] Further extension of these studies examining MZ twins reared apart versus those reared together has revealed high concordance rates for certain personality traits, suggesting that environment has relatively little impact on some aspects of phenotype.[44] However, these approaches are decidedly simplistic, because even MZ twins diverge on significant physical traits and disease susceptibilities. For example, epigenetic factors have been shown to play a role in differential skewing of X-chromosome inactivation in female MZ twin pairs discordant for X-linked traits such as fragile X syndrome and Duchenne muscular dystrophy and in genomic imprinting differences for MZ twins discordant for conditions such as Beckwith-Wiedemann syndrome.[44]

Perhaps the most striking example of epigenetic differences is derived from studies of the methylation and histone acetylation patterns in a variety of tissues in a large cohort of MZ twins of different ages. Twin pairs at 3 years of age had very low levels of DNA methylation and virtually identical gene expression patterns, while 50-year-old twins exhibited higher but more divergent levels of methylation across different tissue types.[45] These changes in methylation patterns associated with aging appeared to be more pronounced in twins that had different lifestyles and had spent less time living together, suggesting that epigenetic changes could account for differences in frequency and onset of adult diseases in MZ twins.

Many diseases of adulthood are related to acquired gene mutations rather than inherited mutations. Environmental influences and lifestyle choices can contribute to somatic mutations in tissues that are sensitive to specific genetic alterations. It is likely that most adult diseases are caused by a complex combination of inherited genetic polymorphisms that confer a certain risk profile, environmental triggers, lifestyle choices, and acquired mutations in critical tissues, with no single factor playing a dominant role.

Telomere Shortening

Aging is a complex process associated with the accumulation of cellular injury mediated by DNA damage. Theories to explain sources of DNA damage include oxidative stress related to formation of reactive oxygen species, defective DNA repair pathways for damaged bases and double-strand breaks, loss of telomere stability, defects in assembly of the spindle during mitosis leading to chromosomal aneuploidy, and disruption of the nuclear lamina.[46] Clues to some of these mechanisms have emerged from premature aging syndromes such as Werner syndrome and Hutchinson-Gilford progeria, in which children demonstrate accelerated changes of normal aging, such as hair loss, atherosclerosis, and degenerative joint disease. Hypermethylation of specific genes has also been identified in tissues of aging individuals and may be influenced by oxidative stress. The contribution of aging to an increase in the occurrence of autosomal dominant disorders is reflected in the higher frequency of new mutations in the male germline seen with advanced paternal age (as described previously). Telomeres are particularly interesting mediators of aging, as they are composed of long DNA repeats and protein complexes that protect the ends of chromosomes from being detected as double-strand breaks and hence being degraded during cell division.[47] Although some maintenance of telomeres is accomplished by telomerase, a reverse transcriptase that adds telomere repeats after each cell division to help maintain their length, progressive telomere shortening occurs in many cells, ultimately contributing to senescence and cell death. There is evidence that epigenetic regulation of telomeres impacts their function and homeostasis, thus reinforcing the role of genetic and epigenetic factors in the process of aging.[47]

Key Points

- The DNA sequence of a human is inadequate to explain the complexity of human phenotypes and development of disease.
- Epigenetic factors such as DNA methylation and histone modification alter gene expression and chromatin structure without affecting the genotype of an individual.
- Some specific pediatric disorders and syndromes are due to errors in epigenetic regulation at genes that are imprinted, or expressed selectively from either the maternally or paternally derived copy; examples include Prader-Willi and Angelman syndromes.
- The complex interplay of genetic and epigenetic elements, coupled with stochastic events and environmental factors such as diet and toxic exposures, play an important role in determining the phenotype of the individual and the health outcomes of children and adults.

- There are critical periods of susceptibility when genetic, epigenetic, and environmental factors affect the development of a person throughout the life span.
- Nutritional and environmental factors during the periconceptional and prenatal period can result decades later in long-term health effects such as diabetes, obesity, heart disease, and predisposition to psychiatric disease in an adult; some of these disease tendencies can be stably transmitted to subsequent generations, presumably through epigenetic reprogramming.
- Most DNA does not encode proteins but rather ncRNA species that play a critical role in gene expression and may serve as targets for some disease processes.
- Some diseases of children and adults are inherited as dominant genetic mutations, whereas others may be due to somatic or acquired genetic and epigenetic changes.
- Many cancers are examples of an accumulation of deleterious events, which may include a mutation in a dominant cancer predisposition gene, acquired chromosomal abnormalities, epigenetic changes, environmental factors, and inflammatory responses.
- The progressive shortening of telomeres at the ends of chromosomes contributes to the aging process, which is related to the accumulation of cellular injury mediated by DNA damage from a variety of mechanisms.

References

1. Gluckman PD, Hanson MA, Buklijas T, et al. Epigenetic mechanisms that underpin metabolic and cardiovascular diseases. *Nat Rev Endocrinol.* 2009;5(7):401–408
2. Reik W, Walter J. Genomic imprinting: parental influence on the genome. *Nat Rev Genet.* 2001;2(1):21–32
3. Reik W. Stability and flexibility of epigenetic gene regulation in mammalian development. *Nature.* 2007;447(7143):425–432
4. Luedi PP, Dietrich FS, Weidman JR, et al. Computational and experimental identification of novel human imprinted genes. *Genome Res.* 2007;17(12):1723–1730
5. Barros SP, Offenbacher S. Epigenetics: connecting environment and genotype to phenotype and disease. *J Dent Res.* 2009;88(5):400–408
6. Morison IM, Ramsay JP, Spencer HG. A census of mammalian imprinting. *Trends Genet.* 2005;21(8):457–465
7. Hitchins MP, Moore GE. Genomic imprinting in fetal growth and development. *Expert Rev Mol Med.* 2002;4(11):1–19
8. Navarro P, Avner P. When X-inactivation meets pluripotency: an intimate rendezvous. *FEBS Lett.* 2009;583(11):1721–1727
9. Chow J, Heard E. X inactivation and the complexities of silencing a sex chromosome. *Curr Opin Cell Biol.* 2009;21(3):359–366

10. Dupont C, Armant DR, Brenner CA. Epigenetics: definition, mechanisms and clinical perspective. *Semin Reprod Med.* 2009;27(5):351–357
11. Orstavik KH. X chromosome inactivation in clinical practice. *Hum Genet.* 2009;126(3):363–373
12. Lander ES, Linton LM, Birren B, et al. Initial sequencing and analysis of the human genome. *Nature.* 2001;409(6822):860–921
13. Brosnan CA, Voinnet O. The long and the short of noncoding RNAs. *Curr Opin Cell Biol.* 2009;21(3):416–425
14. Rinn JL, Kertesz M, Wang JK, et al. Functional demarcation of active and silent chromatin domains in human HOX loci by noncoding RNAs. *Cell.* 2007;129(7): 1311–1323
15. Shrey K, Suchit A, Nishant M, et al. RNA interference: emerging diagnostics and therapeutics tool. *Biochem Biophys Res Commun.* 2009;386(2):273–277
16. Arnett AL, Chamberlain JR, Chamberlain JS. Therapy for neuromuscular disorders. *Curr Opin Genet Dev.* 2009;19(3):290–297
17. Barker DJ, Winter PD, Osmond C, et al. Weight in infancy and death from ischaemic heart disease. *Lancet.* 1989;2(8663):577–580
18. Arnheim N, Calabrese P. Understanding what determines the frequency and pattern of human germline mutations. *Nat Rev Genet.* 2009;10(7):478–488
19. Edwards MJ, Wenstrup RJ, Byers PH, et al. Recurrence of lethal osteogenesis imperfecta due to parental mosaicism for a mutation in the *COL1A2* gene of type I collagen. The mosaic parent exhibits phenotypic features of a mild form of the disease. *Hum Mutat.* 1992;1(1):47–54
20. Manipalviratn S, DeCherney A, Segars J. Imprinting disorders and assisted reproductive technology. *Fertil Steril.* 2009;91(2):305–315
21. Reddy UM, Wapner RJ, Rebar RW, et al. Infertility, assisted reproductive technology, and adverse pregnancy outcomes: executive summary of a National Institute of Child Health and Human Development workshop. *Obstet Gynecol.* 2007;109(4):967–977
22. Ravelli GP, Stein ZA, Susser MW. Obesity in young men after famine exposure in utero and early infancy. *N Engl J Med.* 1976;295(7):349–353
23. Heijmans BT, Tobi EW, Stein AD, et al. Persistent epigenetic differences associated with prenatal exposure to famine in humans. *Proc Natl Acad Sci U S A.* 2008;105(44): 17046–17049
24. Hoek HW, Brown AS, Susser E. The Dutch famine and schizophrenia spectrum disorders. *Soc Psychiatry Psychiatr Epidemiol.* 1998;33(8):373–379
25. St Clair D, Xu M, Wang P, et al. Rates of adult schizophrenia following prenatal exposure to the Chinese famine of 1959–1961. *JAMA.* 2005;294(5):557–562
26. Swanson JM, Entringer S, Buss C, et al. Developmental origins of health and disease: environmental exposures. *Semin Reprod Med.* 2009;27(5):391–402
27. Nafee TM, Farrell WE, Carroll WD, et al. Epigenetic control of fetal gene expression. *BJOG.* 2008;115(2):158–168
28. Kaati G, Bygren LO, Pembrey M, et al. Transgenerational response to nutrition, early life circumstances and longevity. *Eur J Hum Genet.* 2007;15(7):784–790
29. Zammit S, Thomas K, Thompson A, et al. Maternal tobacco, cannabis and alcohol use during pregnancy and risk of adolescent psychotic symptoms in offspring. *Br J Psychiatry.* 2009;195(4):2294–2300
30. Suter MA, Aagaard-Tillery KM. Environmental influences on epigenetic profiles. *Semin Reprod Med.* 2009;27(5):380–390

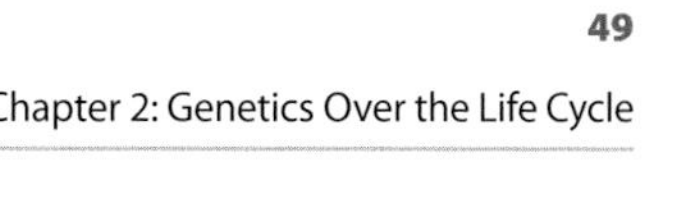

31. Guerrero-Bosagna CM, Skinner MK. Epigenetic transgenerational effects of endocrine disruptors on male reproduction. *Semin Reprod Med.* 2009;27(5):403–408
32. Happle R. The McCune-Albright syndrome: a lethal gene surviving by mosaicism. *Clin Genet.* 1986;29(4):321–324
33. Lumbroso S, Paris F, Sultan C. Activating Gs alpha mutations: analysis of 113 patients with signs of McCune-Albright syndrome—a European Collaborative Study. *J Clin Endocrinol Metab.* 2004;89(5):2107–2113
34. Weaver IC, Cervoni N, Champagne FA, et al. Epigenetic programming by maternal behavior. *Nat Neurosci.* 2004(8):847–854
35. Cirulli F, Francia N, Berry A, et al. Early life stress as a risk factor for mental health: role of neurotrophins from rodents to non-human primates. *Neurosci Biobehav Rev.* 2009(4):573–585
36. Vael C, Desager K. The importance of the development of the intestinal microbiota in infancy. *Curr Opin Pediatr.* 2009;21(6):794–800
37. Gatchel JR, Zoghbi HY. Diseases of unstable repeat expansion: mechanisms and common principles. *Nat Rev Genet.* 2005;6(10):743–755
38. Bird TD. Charcot-Marie-Tooth hereditary neuropathy overview. In: GeneReviews at GeneTests: Medical Genetics Information Resource (database online). http://www.genetests.org. Accessed January 31, 2010
39. Petrucelli N, Daly MB, Bars Culver JO, et al. *BRCA1* and *BRCA2* hereditary breast/ovarian cancer. In: GeneReviews at GeneTests: Medical Genetics Information Resource (database online). http://www.genetests.org. Accessed January 31, 2010
40. Lohmann DR, Gallie BL. Retinoblastoma: revisiting the model prototype of inherited cancer. *Am J Med Genet C Semin Med Genet.* 2004;129C(1):23–28
41. Marsit CJ, Karagas MR, Schned A, et al. Carcinogen exposure and epigenetic silencing in bladder cancer. *Ann N Y Acad Sci.* 2006;1076:810–821
42. Neville KA, Becker ML, Goldman JL, Kearns GL. Developmental pharmacogenomics. *Pediatr Anesthesia.* 2011;21:255–265
43. Hall JG. Twinning. *Lancet.* 2003;362(9385):735–743
44. Haque FN, Gottesman, II, Wong AH. Not really identical: epigenetic differences in monozygotic twins and implications for twin studies in psychiatry. *Am J Med Genet C Semin Med Genet.* 2009;151C(2):136–141
45. Fraga MF, Ballestar E, Paz MF, et al. Epigenetic differences arise during the lifetime of monozygotic twins. *Proc Natl Acad Sci U S A.* 2005;102(30):10604–10609
46. Sinclair DA, Oberdoerffer P. The ageing epigenome: damaged beyond repair? *Ageing Res Rev.* 2009;8(3):189–198
47. Schoeftner S, Blasco MA. A 'higher order' of telomere regulation: telomere heterochromatin and telomeric RNAs. *EMBO J.* 2009;28(16):2323–2336

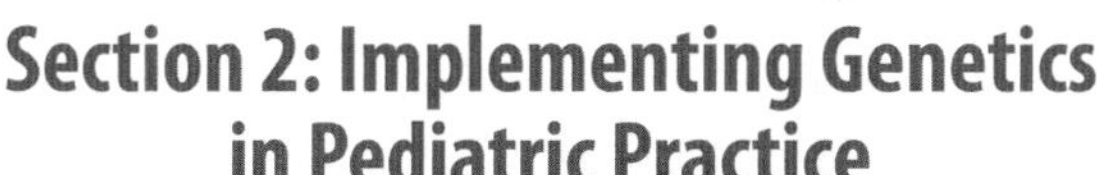

Section 2: Implementing Genetics in Pediatric Practice

Chapter 3

Integrating Genetics in Primary Care

Tracy L. Trotter, MD
Robert A. Saul, MD

Introduction

Primary care medicine combines the treatment of acute illness with disease prevention and anticipatory guidance. With the recent expansion of genetic science and its translation to clinical medicine, primary care physicians (PCPs) must increasingly integrate genetics into their daily practices. It is conceivable that virtually all medical decisions will someday be informed at least, in part, by genomics, yet it will be impossible to have a medical geneticist involved in each decision. While the explosion of genetic/genomic information is occurring at an unprecedented rate, the translation of that information into evidence-based clinical tools is moving considerably more slowly. We have seen some practical applications become available much sooner than expected, as well as some expected applications lag behind due to the unexpected complexity in applying the science of genetics to the practice of medicine. Detailed genetic information is now critical to the delivery of effective health care for everyone.[1] Increased public awareness of genetic and genomic information and the availability of direct-to-consumer DNA-based testing have led patients and families to demand genetic information and advice from their PCPs. Therefore, PCPs must become more knowledgeable about advances in genetics to meet these new challenges in an effective and responsive manner.

A Brief History of Genetics in Medicine

Since Sir Archibald Garrod's description of alkaptonuria in 1908,[2] physicians have understood that rare diseases can be genetically transmitted; however, tests for genetic diseases were still decades away. In 1956, after the full complement of human chromosomes was determined to be 46, cytogenetics for diagnosis became part of primary care practice.[3] Later that decade, trisomy of the 21st chromosome was found to be the cause of Down syndrome.[4] Testing for phenylketonuria in newborns became a standard procedure in primary care practices in the 1960s.[5] As a result, PCPs have ordered genetic testing for virtually every newborn and provided follow-up for patients with genetic disorders over the last 5 decades. The number of congenital conditions in newborn screening programs has greatly increased since the 1960s, and public health support for early diagnosis and treatment of genetic diseases is robust.[6]

The 1970s and 1980s saw the rise of molecular genetics. This led to the complete sequencing of the human genome in 2001[7] and, subsequently, the exponential growth in genetic knowledge and genetic tests.[8–11] It is now essential that PCPs stay abreast of the continually expanding array of genetic tests. Identifying patients whose symptoms, physical findings, or family history indicate a need for genetic testing, and determining how to use the results to improve disease prevention and treat existing disease, is an ever-increasing challenge for PCPs.[12] In this age of genetics, primary care is evolving from treating diseases to treating individuals with inherited and acquired risks for disease.

Thinking Genetically

To take full advantage of the genetic information available today, PCPs must make a mental shift to "thinking genetically," a term coined by Hayflick and Eiff.[13] They defined thinking genetically as considering genetics a possibility in every patient encounter. While the genetic component is not always critical or even important, it should always be considered so appropriate action can be taken when it is needed. For example, a PCP should think genetically with siblings of a child with asthma and eczema, because the siblings are more likely to develop atopic disease than children without that family history. Similarly, physicians should understand that the risk of recurrence of multifactorial disorders, such as congenital heart disease, isolated cleft lip, or spina bifida, is increased if one family member is affected. Primary care physicians should also know how to counsel families about genetic risk when a single-gene disorder, such as cystic fibrosis, sickle cell disease, or neurofibromatosis, is diagnosed in a family member.

Thinking genetically for every diagnosis may take a conscious effort at first. Many PCPs still view genetic issues as rare presentations, though most PCPs care for children with a variety of genetic abnormalities and already assume a number of roles for these patients—from evaluation and diagnosis, to interpretation of genetic testing, appropriate referrals, and management (or comanagement). Many PCPs have not yet embraced the concept that genetic factors likely play a role in most diseases and disorders.

Evaluation and Diagnosis

Although individual genetic disorders are rare, collectively genetic disorders constitute a significant proportion of pediatric and adult illness.[14] The presentation of genetic conditions is diverse, so PCPs must be alert for genetic clues. Using a methodical approach to "thinking genetically" (ie, considering genetic etiologies in the differential diagnosis of conditions encountered in primary care) is helpful.[15] Chapters 6 through 9 cover appropriate approaches to evaluating and diagnosing genetic disorders.

Methodology

The red flags concept is an aid for increasing genetic thinking developed by the Genetics in Primary Care Faculty Development Initiative (GPC),[16] whose goal was to increase the number of primary care faculty qualified to teach genetics.[15] The GPC defined a red flag as any clinical finding discovered in the history, physical examination, or laboratory studies that suggests the presence of a genetically influenced disease and that may require further action, such as intervention, counseling, referral, screening, or follow-up. A small number of broad categories were developed along with the mnemonic device, F GENES, for family genes (Box 3-1).[15]

Box 3-1. Red Flags to Genetic Conditions[a]

Use F GENES as a mnemonic device to recall the situations listed below that may require further action, including intervention, follow-up, counseling, or referral.

- **F** Family history. Multiple affected siblings or individuals in multiple generations. A lack of family history does NOT rule out genetic causes.
- **G** Groups of congenital anomalies. Two or more anomalies are much more likely to indicate the presence of a syndrome with genetic implications.
- **E** Extreme or exceptional presentation of common conditions. Early onset of disease, unusual gender, or severe reaction to infectious or metabolic stress.
- **N** Neurodevelopmental delay or degeneration.
- **E** Extreme or exceptional pathology. Rare tumors or other pathology, or multiple primary cancers in one or more tissue types, for example.
- **S** Surprising laboratory values. Abnormal laboratory values in an otherwise healthy individual or extreme values for a typical clinical situation.

[a]From Whelan AJ, Ball S, Best L, et al. Genetic red flags: clues to thinking genetically in medical practices. *Prim Care Clin Office Pract*. 2004;31:497–508, with permission from Elsevier.

Diagnostic Tools

Collecting an accurate family history is the first step in identifying patients or families for whom genetic testing or intervention would be beneficial.[17] A family history describes the genetic relationships and medical history of a family. It is the most traditional diagnostic tool in clinical genetics, and when represented as a diagram with standard symbols and terms, is referred to as a pedigree.[18] The family history is the most cost-effective approach to identifying individuals at risk for common disorders with a genetic etiology. It is also used for complex common conditions for which a genetic cause is unknown. As testing for the genetic factors of human disease becomes more common, the family history will become not just a tool for providing appropriate care for specific diseases, but also a tool for public health and preventive medicine.[19] The family history is truly the first genetic screen and a crucial element in risk assessment. See Chapter 5 for detailed information and history-taking tools for the PCP.

In addition to the family history, a PCP can determine whether genetic testing or referral is required with careful reproductive, environmental, and medical histories, and a complete physical examination.

The Shift From Genetics to Genomics

To keep pace with advances in screening (Chapter 17), testing (Chapters 10–12), and pharmacogenomics (Chapter 20), and accurately interpret and communicate genetic risk assessment to their patients, PCPs must become conversant in the language of genetics. They must also learn about the genetic aspects of complex common diseases, such as coronary heart disease, asthma, and diabetes, and the normal genetic variations in drug metabolism and immune response. Medical genetics has gradually shifted from genetics to genomics.

Guttmacher and Collins' primer on genomic medicine[20] defined genetics as "the study of single genes and their effects" and genomics as "the study not just of single genes, but of the functions and interactions of all the genes in the genome." Medical genetics has traditionally focused on conditions caused by mutations in single genes (eg, sickle cell disease), whole chromosomes (eg, Down syndrome), or those associated with birth defects and developmental disabilities.[21] Medical genomics focuses on the interaction of genetic and environmental factors (eg, how variation at one or multiple gene loci interacts with diet, drugs, infectious agents, chemicals, physical agents, and behavioral factors).

Multidisciplinary research is delineating the value of genomic information in improving health outcomes and preventing human diseases. Genomics will soon provide PCPs with more information than traditional genetics about the increased risk for various diseases. Therefore, PCPs must increase their skills in interpreting and communicating complex, probabilistic genetic information.

Both the individual genetic code that predisposes a patient to common diseases and the epigenetic mechanisms that control gene expressions will soon become available for diagnostic purposes during the prenatal period or infancy. While it is not clear how the concepts of epigenetics will affect primary care, it is clear they will have a substantial impact. Primary care physicians will have the first opportunity to actively intercede in the progression of these disorders, thus translating genomics into practice, policy, and communities.[22]

Genetic Testing and Communicating Risk

Genetic tests encompass the evaluation of DNA, RNA, chromosomes, proteins, and certain metabolites to detect heritable disease-related genotypes, mutations, phenotypes, or karyotypes for clinical purposes. While genetic testing is not a new tool, physicians must remain sensitive to the unique ethical, legal, and social implications of genetic testing in children. (See Chapters 10, 11, and 15.)

To prepare for the influx of genetic information in the coming years, PCPs should begin to develop a strategy for incorporating new genetic testing into patient care. It will become as necessary to be facile in interpreting genetic predictive information as it is with any other medical information. Genetic testing can be used for a range of reasons, including diagnosis in symptomatic or asymptomatic patients, risk assessment, reproductive decision-making, and population screening. Knowing when to order genetic testing and how to interpret the results is complex and has specific risks and benefits, especially for pediatric patients. Identifying the correct test and appropriate testing laboratory can also be challenging, although Web-based resources such as GeneTests can help facilitate these tasks. The PCP also must decide when to refer patients for medical genetic consultation. By combining "thinking genetically" with diagnostic and management skills, the PCP can provide patients with a cost-effective route to appropriate genetics professionals when necessary. Primary care physicians can test their ability to "think genetically"(Box 3-2).[23]

Box 3-2. Questions Primary Care Physicians (PCPs) Should Be Able to Answer When "Thinking Genetically"[a]

- What are the 3 types of genetic tests?
  - Biochemical
  - Cytogenetic
  - Molecular analysis
- How is genetic testing used in patient care?
  - Medical
    - Diagnostic (primary or confirmatory)
    - Predictive (to initiate treatment)
  - Personal decision-making
    - Carrier testing
    - Preimplantation genetic diagnosis
    - Prenatal diagnosis
    - Predictive (no medical intervention available)
- Who needs to be tested?
  - Neonates, infants, and children
  - Family members of affected patients
- Why should patients be tested?
  - To influence medical management
  - To benefit multiple family members
- When should patients be referred for genetic consultation?
  - When the PCP's knowledge base and comfort level has been exceeded
  - For a potential treatment of a genetic condition
  - The family needs an expert or second opinion
  - To counsel the patient or family on inheritance and recurrence risk
- Where can help and information be found?
  - Numerous sources available (Appendix A)

[a]Adapted from Pagon R, Trotter TL. Genetic testing: when to test and when to refer. *Paediatr Child Health*. 2007;17(9):367–370.

Pharmacogenomic Tests

Pharmacogenomic tests are a special category of predictive genetic tests for gene variants, usually in drug-metabolizing enzymes, and can predict an individual's response to a drug or class of drugs. Results of pharmacogenomic tests allow physicians to write personalized drug prescriptions for individual patients, which may reduce adverse reactions and increase the efficacy of drug treatment.[24] A few pharmacogenomic tests are currently available, and several more are undergoing prospective evaluation to ensure that they provide a health outcome benefit. (See Chapter 20.)

Direct-to-Consumer Genetic Tests

In recent years, there has been a boom in direct-to-consumer (DTC) genetic testing products and services being sold over the Internet and locally. These tests provide genetic test results directly to the consumer without the benefit of a professional interpretation by a qualified health care provider.[25] Without professional interpretation, DTC testing can lead to misuse of the tests, misinterpretation of the results, and misguided follow-up or attempted treatment.[26] (See Chapters 11 and 19.) Consumers confused about their test results are turning to their PCP for interpretation and clarification. Physicians must be prepared to consult with patients about their DTC genetic test results and know how to seek further information and consultation as needed.

Management and Coordination of Care

After patients receive a genetic diagnosis, their ongoing care typically falls to the PCP. The American Academy of Pediatrics developed the medical home model of care to ensure that care is accessible, continuous, comprehensive, family-centered, coordinated, compassionate, and culturally effective, and meets preventive, primary, and tertiary needs. (See Chapter 4.) In 2007 this model was adopted by major primary care organizations as the patient-centered medical home.

For children and youth with special health care needs (CYSHCN), care coordination is an essential component of the medical home model that links children and their families with appropriate services and resources.[27] Patients with genetic diagnoses frequently have several medical providers involved in their care; therefore, their care must be coordinated or integrated across the health care system (eg, subspecialty care, hospitals, home health agencies, and public health) and the patient's community (eg, family, public, and private community-based services). The complexity of the health care network for CYSHCN highlights the importance of effective communication between the PCP, subspecialty physicians, and the family.

A key element of the medical home model of care is a comprehensive assessment of needs and strengths developed in conjunction with the patient's family. The assessment should include a thorough review of medical and nonmedical needs. Information obtained from the assessment and the resulting care plan will support effective collaboration within the medical system and among community partners. In addition to the general care (or action care) plan, the medical team should develop an emergency care

Box 3-3. Role of the Primary Care Physician in Genetic Medicine[a]

1. Identify individuals who may benefit from genetic services, including those with genetic disorders and those at increased risk of transmitting a genetic disorder.
2. Recognize historical and physical features of common genetic conditions.
3. Monitor the health of individuals with a genetic disorder, in collaboration with an appropriate subspecialist.
4. Provide basic genetics information to patients and their families to foster understanding and informed decision-making.
5. Provide a medical home for individuals who need complex genetics services.
6. Recognize the special psychosocial issues for a family affected by a genetic disorder or susceptibility.
7. Know how to access the full range of genetics services that patients might benefit from.
8. Refer patients that need additional genetics services, as appropriate.
9. Facilitate the use of genetics services.

[a]Adapted from Hayflick SJ, Eiff MP. Role of primary care providers in the delivery of genetic services. *Community Genet.* 1998;1:18–22.

plan that is portable and immediately available to personnel working with CYSHCN in hospital emergency departments, office and clinic settings, community settings (school, child care, athletic venues), and even in the family home.[28] This tool often has a substantial genetic component or needs significant input from the genetic subspecialist.

Key Point

- Medical genetics is rapidly expanding, and an increasingly wide range of genetic tests is available. Primary care physicians are in an ideal position to evaluate and treat patients with genetic diseases. There are many potential roles for PCPs in genetic medicine that are critical to the health and well-being of children (Box 3-3).[13]

References

1. Guttmacher AE, Collins FS, Carmona RH. The family history: more important than ever. *N Engl J Med.* 2004;351:2333–2336
2. Garrod AE. The Croonian lectures on inborn errors of metabolism; lecture II: alkaptonuria. *Lancet.* 1908;2:73–79
3. Tjio J, Levan A. The chromosome number of man. *Heriditas.* 1956;42:1–6

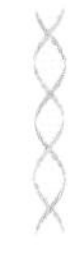

4. Lejeune J, Gautier M, Turpin R. Etude des chromosomes somatiques de neuf enfants mongoliens. *Comptes Rendue des l'Academie des Sciences Paris*. 1959;248:1721–1722
5. Guthrie R, Susi A. A simple phenylalanine method for detecting phenylketonuria in large populations of newborn infants. *Pediatrics*. 1963;32:338–343
6. American Academy of Pediatrics Newborn Screening Authoring Committee. Newborn screening expands: recommendations for pediatrics and medical homes—implications for the system. *Pediatrics*. 2008;121(1):192–217
7. International Human Genome Sequencing Consortium. Initial sequencing and analysis of the human genome. *Nature*. 2001;409:860–921
8. Holtzman NA, Watson MS. Promoting safe and effective genetic testing in the United States. Final report of the Task Force on Genetic Testing. *J Child Fam Nurs*. 1999;2: 388–390
9. Moore CA, Khoury MJ, Bradley LA. From genetics to genomics: using gene-based medicine to prevent disease and promote health in children. *Semin Perinatol*. 2005;29:135–143
10. American Academy of Pediatrics Committee on Genetics. Molecular genetic testing in pediatric practice: a subject review. *Pediatrics*. 2000;106:1494–1497
11. Pagon RA, Pinsky L, Beahler CC. Online medical genetics resources: a US perspective. *Br Med J*. 2001;322:1035–1037
12. Burke W. Genetic testing in primary care. *Annu Rev Genomics Hum Genet*. 2004;5:1–14
13. Hayflick S, Eiff M. Role of primary care providers in the delivery of genetics services. *Community Genet*. 1998;1:18–22
14. McCandless SE, Brunger JW, Cassidy SB. The burden of genetic disease on inpatient care in a children's hospital. *Am J Hum Genet*. 2004;74(1):121–127
15. Whelan AJ, Ball S, Best L, et al. Genetic red flags: clues to thinking genetically in medical practice. *Prim Care Clin Office Pract*. 2004;31:497–508
16. Burke W, Acheson L, Botkin J, et al. Genetics in primary care: a USA Faculty Development Initiative. *Community Genet*. 2002;5:138–146
17. Trotter TL, Martin HM. Family history in pediatric primary care. *Pediatrics*. 2007;120: S60–S65
18. Bennett RL. *The Practical Guide to the Genetic Family History*. New York, NY: Wiley Liss; 1999
19. Yoon P, Scheuner M, Faucett A, et al. Can family history be used as a tool for public health and preventive medicine? *Genet Med*. 2002;4(4):303–310
20. Guttmacher AE, Collins FS. Genomic medicine: a primer. *N Engl J Med*. 2002;347: 1512–1520
21. Hobbs CA, Cleves MA, Simmons CJ. Genetic epidemiology and congenital malformations: from the chromosome to the crib. *Arch Pediatr Adolesc Med*. 2002;156:315–320
22. Cheng TL, Cohn RD, Dover GJ. The genetics revolution and primary care pediatrics. *JAMA*. 2008;299(4):451–453
23. Pagon R, Trotter TL. Genetic testing: when to test and when to refer. *Paediatr Child Health*. 2007;17(9),367–370
24. Weinshilboum R. Inheritance and drug response. *N Engl J Med*. 2003;348:529–537
25. Gollust SE, Wilfond BS, Hull SC. Direct-to-consumer sales of genetic services on the Internet. *Genet Med*. 2003;5:332–337
26. Haga SB, Khoury MJ, Burke W. Genomic profiling to promote a healthy life style: not ready for prime time. *Nat Genet*. 2003;34:347–350

27. American Academy of Pediatrics Council on Children With Disabilities. Care coordination in the medical home: integrating health and related systems of care for children with special health care needs. *Pediatrics*. 2005;116(5);1238–1244
28. Antonelli R, Stille C, Freeman L. Enhancing collaboration between primary and subspecialty care providers for children and youth with special health care needs. Washington, DC: Georgetown University Center for Child and Human Development; 2005

Chapter 4

Genetics Services and Children With Special Health Care Needs

Nancy J. Mendelsohn, MD
Tamison Jewett, MD

Introduction

The *integration* of genetics services into the care of children with special health care needs (CSHCN) is essential in providing comprehensive, co-ordinated care for children and families with inherited disorders and birth defects. The medical geneticist's practice is not focused on the skills or infrastructure needed to provide primary care. Similarly, it is impractical to expect the primary care physician (PCP) to offer state-of-the-art care for uncommon or rare disorders. Efforts to provide up-to-date, comprehensive, coordinated care for children with complex diseases have included disease-specific clinics, multidisciplinary specialty clinics, and the medical home approach. The availability and use of multidisciplinary specialty clinics for different inherited disorders is inconsistent across the country. Access to genetics care may be limited by location and the small number of existing clinicians. For some disorders, such as hemophilia and cystic fibrosis, there are disease-specific, effective, national networks of specialty clinics that exist and reach large proportions of individuals with these conditions. Fewer such centers are available for children with other disorders. Genetic disorders as a whole are common but individually are uncommon or rare, and the PCP rarely has the background or facilities to manage most of these conditions. Models of comanagement are essential for promoting ongoing communication and coordination between primary care and other specialists and subspecialists, particularly during the transition from pediatric to adult care.[1]

Most CSHCN are comanaged by primary care providers and subspecialists. The coordination of medical care for a child with a genetic disease has historically been based on the specialty clinic or the center of excellence model for the care of most children with rare disorders. This care model sometimes led to the exclusion of the PCP. As we change and improve paradigms for care, identifying the roles of PCP and geneticist for patients with complex needs improves medical care and decreases inefficiencies associated with older models.

The role of the PCP is not prescribed but evolves to suit the needs of the patient and family. A plan of care is central to the medical home. This is based on an accurate unifying diagnosis. The first step in the genetic referral process is identifying the need for a genetic consultation. Reasons to consider a genetics evaluation are discussed in Chapter 6.

Medical Home

Children with special health care needs are defined by the Department of Health and Human Services, Health Resources and Services Administration, Maternal and Child Health Bureau (MCHB) as "those who have or are at increased risk for a chronic physical, developmental, behavioral, or emotional condition and who also require health and related services of a type or amount beyond that required by children generally."[2]

Approximately 10.2 million children in the United States, or 14% of all US children, have special health care needs based on the MCHB definition. In March 2007 a consensus statement on patient-centered care medical home principles was developed and jointly endorsed by the American College of Physicians (ACP), American Academy of Family Physicians (AAFP), American Osteopathic Association, and American Academy of Pediatrics (AAP) in which the AAP emphasizes the critical pediatric medical home principles (Box 4-1).[3,4]

The basic tenet of a medical home in childhood is that there is a central relationship between the pediatrician, the patient, and the family. The pediatrician serves as the primary contact for all providers who care for the patient. The pediatrician is the director of the patient's care and not only develops, but also oversees the overarching care plan for each child with SHCN beginning in the prenatal care setting and extending through the transition plan to adulthood. Quality and safety are the central principles of the medical home, and a properly designed plan ensures that care is delivered in a safe and effective manner. Communication with the medical home provider is also vital to the patient and provider.[3,5]

Box 4-1. Principles of the Pediatric Medical Home[3,4]

- Family-centered, trusting, collaborative, working partnership with families, respecting their diversity, and recognizing that they are the constant in a child's life
- A community-based, family-centered, coordinated network designed to promote the healthy development and well-being of children and their families
- The provision of high-quality, developmentally appropriate health care services that continue uninterrupted as the individual moves along and within systems of services and from adolescence to adulthood
- Appropriate financing to support and sustain medical homes that promote system-wide quality care with optimal health outcomes, family satisfaction, and cost efficiency

The Genetics Referral

The initial referral to a medical geneticist should be discussed and explained to the patient and family by the PCP. Some families may be frightened or reluctant based solely on the word "genetic." Parents are concerned the visit may reveal that the child's developmental delays or unusual physical features come from one of them or that blame will be placed on them. Explaining the goals of the genetic evaluation before a visit is important. The major objective is to provide a unifying diagnosis for the child's differences. This allows the medical community to provide a coordinated management plan tailored to that diagnosis, which guides further medical evaluations, surveillance, and communication. Having a diagnosis also allows for an understanding of the natural history, which is critical to educational and lifestyle plans. While providing recurrence risk for first-degree relatives is a part of the outcome, it is not the central reason for referral. Families should be informed that most genetics evaluation includes a team of providers. Becoming familiar with the genetics services in the region will help prepare families for initial genetic consultations. The AAP publishes a fact sheet that explains the role of the medical geneticist.[6] The pediatrician's office is the central site for coordination of pertinent data and medical records. In addition to specifying the reason for consultation, at the time of referral for a genetics evaluation, providing relevant records is essential. Ideally, these should include prenatal records; copies of newborn screen results; length, weight, and head circumference growth charts; and copies of previous relevant genetic or other laboratory testing results.

Case Studies

A case study (Box 4-2) provides an example of the importance of the exchange of information from the PCP to the geneticist before the initial visit.

Most children with Angelman syndrome (78%) have abnormal parent-specific DNA methylation (see Chapter 2). This includes those children with a deletion, uniparental disomy, or an imprinting defect.[7]

The pediatrician provided the previous test results, and the medical geneticist recognized that testing for Angelman syndrome was incomplete. Further testing was needed to make a unifying diagnosis for this child and family.

Most CSHCN have more than 2 subspecialty providers. In the past, medical care traditionally occurred in silos, yet families need coordinated management of health care with communication among the providers. Improved coordination of care results in safer, higher-quality medical care. Comanagement is the goal for genetics patients. The role of the genetics provider is similar to that of all specialists and subspecialists. There is emphasis placed on family education regarding the specific diagnosis as well as provision of appropriate resource materials.

Another case study (Box 4-3) illustrates the importance of the integration of medical history, family history, physical examination, and laboratory testing before appropriate counseling can be given and information communicated to the PCP.

Box 4-2. Case Study—Developmental Delay

A 3-year-old boy is referred to the genetics clinic for evaluation of developmental delay. His parents report in vitro conception with a subsequently normal pregnancy. Growth parameters at birth were normal, including the head circumference. His growth continues to be normal with evolving microcephaly. Feeding in infancy was difficult. Developmental delays became apparent between 6 months and 1 year of age. Some examiners described his movements as tremulous. His parents describe him as a child with poor sleep habits who seems content and smiles frequently. The boy was seen and evaluated by a developmental pediatrician and a pediatric neurologist who report, "testing for Angelman syndrome was negative."

Careful review of previous testing provided by the pediatrician showed chromosome analysis and fluorescent in situ hybridization studies for 15q11.2-q13 to be normal (no evidence of deletion). After evaluating the child in the genetics clinic, DNA methylation studies were ordered that confirmed the diagnosis of Angelman syndrome, which was consistent with the child's clinical presentation.

Box 4-3. Case Study—Neurofibromatosis

A woman has been diagnosed as having neurofibromatosis type1 (NF1). Her primary care physician is her only medical provider. At the time of her son's birth, she requests testing for the infant. The pediatrician sends the baby's blood for molecular testing of the NF1 gene. The result reveals that there is a change found in the NF1 gene that is a "variant of unknown significance" (VOUS) that has not been previously reported to be associated with NF1. Genetic counseling is recommended. The baby is referred to the genetics clinic.

The family is seen, and a 3-generation pedigree is constructed. There are multiple persons in the extended family with features of NF1, including numerous café au lait spots (CALS), neurofibromas, and tibial pseudoarthrosis. The proband (the baby) has 2 older siblings, one with similar features to the mother and one who appears healthy at 12 years of age. No one other than the proband has had molecular testing.

The infant is examined (a Wood lamp is rarely used to identify CALS seen in NF1) and has 4 CALS but no axillary or inguinal freckling. The mother is examined. She has greater than 30 CALS as well as axillary and inguinal freckling, and several cutaneous neurofibromas scattered over her trunk. She meets the diagnostic criteria for NF1 (Table 9-9, page 211). In order to sort out her infant son's diagnostic status, it is recommended that the mother have testing of the NF1 gene.

The mother's test reveals a small deletion within the NF1 gene, which has been previously described and known to cause NF1. She does not have the VOUS described in the infant. The 2 older children in the family are tested in this case. The older child (with features of NF1) carries the same small deletion as his mother, confirming the diagnosis of NF1. The second carries the VOUS.

The family returns to the genetics clinic for follow-up and explanation of the genetic testing to date. It is explained to the mother that the 2 children with the VOUS in the NF1 gene do not have NF1 based on the clinical examination and family history. The older child is affected.

After a clinic visit, the genetics clinic that participates in a medical home model provides a summary of that visit to the pediatrician. This includes tests sent, referrals recommended, and a review of the information provided to the family. Ongoing communication of the genetics team with the family and PCP is an expectation.

The diagnosis of neurofibromatosis (NF) is based on well-established clinical stigmata. Genetic testing is often not necessary. If the mother is affected with NF1, however, molecular testing of the newborn infant might be indicated if the family wants to know right away if the child is affected (this should be done only after the family's gene mutation is known). The medical genetics team is best equipped to interpret molecular testing for physicians, patients, and families.

Given the complexities of care often needed for patients and their conditions, medical geneticists can provide more care or provide more management of the care in conjunction with the primary care provider. All of the issues should be well elucidated in a comanagement agreement.

In the event of the diagnosis of a life-shortening illness, the geneticist may suggest (or even have as part of their team) the involvement of palliative care specialists to help manage pain and other symptoms and to support the family and pediatrician.

Transition to Adult Care

New developments in medical practice and advances in our technological capabilities have ensured survival and improved outcomes for most CSHCN. It is estimated that 90% of children with SHCN now survive into adulthood.[8] Currently in the United States, more than 2 million children aged 10 to 18 years have impairment of function due to ongoing, disabling conditions.[9] This number represents a 100% increase since 1960 and underscores the need for effective transitions from pediatric to adult care.

The MCHB has established, as a core goal of the Healthy People 2010 challenge, the requirement that "all youth with special needs will receive the services necessary to make transitions to all aspects of adult life, including adult health care, work, and independence."[10] Successful transition efforts involve all parties concerned with the care and support of the patient, including the individual with SHCN, his or her parents and family, all members of the health care team, and community providers and programs.

Just as children are best served by physicians who are experienced in the care of a pediatric population, adults should be cared for by physicians experienced in adult medicine. Traditionally, some pediatricians have continued to provide care for adults with congenital disorders and special needs. Health care is optimal when every individual, regardless of age, receives services that are tailored to his or her medical and developmental needs.

After transition to adult care, individuals with syndromes and genetic conditions often continue to be served by medical geneticists. This occurs for at least 2 reasons: (1) medical genetics is a specialty that emphasizes knowledge of the natural history of genetic disorders across the life span, and (2) most primary adult care physicians do not have training or sufficient experience to serve this population. The medical geneticist often continues to be a partner in the health care of individuals with SHCN through the transition phase and into adulthood.

If a diagnosis is determined that could lead to a shortened life span with or without very complex medical problems, palliative care specialists may provide further assistance for the child and family through transition and continue to be of help in managing symptoms and assisting the child, the parents, and providers with developing advance directives and other end-of-life discussions.

Transition Planning

Primary care physicians should anticipate and initiate the health care transition when the child is 11 to 13 years of age (Table 4-1).[11,12] As children age they are given increasing responsibility for becoming an informed health care consumer. Health care transition can occur from a pediatric to an adult practice, or it can occur within a practice that cares for children and adults. Successful transition to adult care not only ensures appropriate medical care but promotes a healthy adult lifestyle. Through this process, the individual with SHCN is afforded the opportunities to become more self-aware, to recognize strengths and weaknesses, to declare preferences, and to strive for as much independence as possible in adult life.

Table 4-1. Activities and Skills Needed for Health Care Transition[a]

	Ages 11–13 (Begin)	Ages 14–16 (Update Progress)	Ages 17 and 18 (Final Steps)
Reintroduce the practice transition policy or introduce idea of transition to family if policy is not available	X		
Youth carries and presents insurance card and copays	X	X	X
Youth given choice in medical decisions/decision-making (assent to consent)	X	X	Youth makes all decisions and signs if capable
Youth prepares 3–5 questions for office visit (increasing ownership of medical condition)	X	X	X
Youth knows wellness baseline	X	X	X
Youth knows when to call health care provider for change in illness status; has an emergency plan		X	X

Table 4-1. Activities and Skills Needed for Health Care Transition[a] *(continued)*

	Ages 11–13 (Begin)	Ages 14–16 (Update Progress)	Ages 17 and 18 (Final Steps)
Complete a portable medical record with youth and family age 14		X	Prepare medical history for transition to new physician
Youth makes own doctor appointments and calls in own refills		X	X
Youth can describe his or her illness correctly (what it is, how it affects them) and knows medications and dosages		X	X
Youth seen alone for part of the visit	(X)	X	Youth seen alone at age 18 unless signed release for parents to be present
Youth seen without parents if legally able to make own medical decisions			Age 18
Send youth with list of questions to adult primary care physician for intro visit 2–3 years before transfer so youth learns what is expected by adult system and returns to pediatrics to sharpen skills		X	
One year before leaving home or transfer to adult provider, youth tests capability to handle his or her health care without parent involvement			X
Assess: insurance, supplemental security income, vocational rehabilitation			X
Gather disability documentation if needed		X	X

[a]From White PH. Destination known: planning the transition of youth with special needs to adult health care. *Adolesc Health Update.* 2009;21:3.

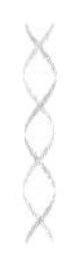

In 2002 a consensus statement regarding health care transitions for young adults with SHCN was approved as policy by the AAP, AAFP, and ACP-American Society of Internal Medicine.[11] This document prescribes 6 critical first steps to secure a favorable transition to adult health care (Box 4-4).

There are numerous impediments to successful transition. These include low expectations on the part of individuals with SHCN and their caregiv-

Box 4-4. Critical Steps in Transitioning Care

1. Ensure a medical home.

   The health care transition process is best managed by an identified health care professional (often an allied health professional) who works in concert with other existing and potential health care providers to bring a plan to fruition.

2. Identify individuals with the necessary knowledge and skills to provide developmentally appropriate health care throughout the transition.

   As part of this effort, it is critical to determine what competencies should and can be fostered in the child with special health care needs (SHCN). Who will be in charge of future health care decisions? If it is determined that the child/young adult requires significant oversight, it is important to think about power of attorney and legal guardianship issues before the child reaches age 18 years.

3. Prepare an up-to-date medical summary that is portable and easily maintained.

   This is critically important in ensuring that all involved health care professionals have access to the often complicated medical issues at hand.

4. Create a health care transition plan by age 14 years.

   This is a cooperative effort that includes the adolescent/young adult and family as well as others of their choice who play important roles in ongoing care. Consideration should be given to specific services needed, who will provide the services, and how the services will be financed. Differences between pediatric and adult care models (eg, family-centered vs individual-centered care) should be discussed to prepare the adolescent/young adult for his or her role as self-advocate. Important aspects of transition planning include emergency plan(s), educational goals, career goals, prescription for a healthy lifestyle, and decision-making regarding independent or assisted living.

5. Primary and preventive care should adhere to standardized guidelines with the understanding the individuals with SHCN may require more resources.

   Examples of these guidelines include *GAPS*[12] and *Bright Futures.*[13]

6. Ensure ongoing coverage of health care costs.

   Insurance coverage must be both affordable and uninterrupted and should compensate for transition planning and care coordination for individuals with SHCN.

ers, difficulty in identifying adult and specialty care providers, resistance to transition by the adolescent and/or family, lack of institutional support for planning, and lack of payment for services.[9] There may be cultural, language, and economic barriers. The more complex an individual's needs, the higher their risk for receiving suboptimal or discontinuous access to care. A case study (Box 4-5) highlights the importance of effective transition planning.

A recent AAP Periodic Survey of Fellows shows that fewer than 50% of respondents regularly offer services that facilitate transition to adult care for their adolescent patients with SHCN.[13] Participants included the following as major barriers to transition: lack of available family/internal medicine physicians, lack of adult specialists, lack of knowledge about community resources, and lack of skills in transition planning.

Box 4-5. Case Study—Down Syndrome and Transition to Adult Care

Doug, a 34-year-old man with Down syndrome, is brought to the genetics clinic by his mother due to concerns regarding his behavior. She says that he used to be "happy-go-lucky," but for the past several months, he has been argumentative and easily angered. He struck one of his siblings at a recent family gathering for no apparent reason, and for the past few weeks he has been difficult to engage, frequently talking to himself.

Doug underwent successful heart surgery for repair of an atrioventricular canal defect in childhood. Aside from being overweight, he is generally healthy, but he hasn't seen a doctor for 10 years. He completed high school with a certificate at age 21. He attended a sheltered workshop for several years, but his mother withdrew him from the program because he was arguing with the other participants. He now stays at home with her and mainly watches TV.

Physical examination is notable for an overweight man with physical features of Down syndrome who is agitated and talks to himself throughout the visit. He doesn't answer questions and barely acknowledges the examiner. In addition to concerns about obesity and delinquent health care surveillance, the geneticist is worried about mental illness, which is a comorbidity in up to 50% of adults with Down syndrome. She refers Doug to a psychiatrist with experience in managing adults with intellectual disability as an initial management step, with a referral to an internist or family practitioner.

Following the visit, the geneticist and genetic counselor made many calls to arrange for a psychiatry appointment for Doug. Finding a provider who would accept Doug as a patient was challenging because his health insurance is not accepted by many providers, and many providers are not comfortable treating a man with Down syndrome. Finally, Doug was seen by a psychiatrist about 100 miles from his hometown. Locating a primary care physician presented similar challenges.

Key Points

- Medical care for individuals with SHCN accounts for the majority of all health care expenditures in the United States and is often poorly planned and executed, underscoring the importance of a cohesive, well-designed approach to caring for these individuals.
- The "medical home" principle was conceived and developed to provide seamless, quality care across the life span; it is a partnership between physician, patient, and family or caregiver that acts in the patient's best interest.
- Genetic services are an integral part of this effort, with clinical geneticists offering care through the lifespan for individuals with SHCN.
- Clinical geneticists strive to make unifying diagnoses for patients, which serve to guide future management; they also provide much-needed information for caregivers, including education and resources.
- The clinical geneticist is not a replacement for the medical home, but instead augments the plan by providing specialty care and recommendations.
- Transition to adult care is a team effort that evolves over years and relies on input from all involved parties.
- Potential barriers to the successful completion and implementation of the transition plan should be recognized and addressed. A successful plan is agreed on by all team members, is able to be amended as needed, and can be successfully implemented while being cost-effective.

Resources

National Center for Medical Home Implementation
http://www.medicalhomeinfo.org/index.html

Healthy and Ready to Work National Center on Transitions
www.hrtw.org

Health Care Transitions Resources
http://hctransitions.ichp.edu/resources.html

Family Village: Transition and the Internet
http://familyvillage.wisc.edu/sp/trans.html

Adolescent Health Transition Project
http://depts.washington.edu/healthtr/index.html

References

1. Grosse SD, Schechter MS, Kulkarni R, Lloyd-Puryear MA, Strickland B, Trevathan E. Models of comprehensive multidisciplinary care for individuals in the United States with genetic disorders. *Pediatrics*. 2009;123(1):407–412

2. McPherson M, Arango P, Fox HB. A new definition of children with special health care needs. *Pediatrics*. 1998;102:137–140
3. American Academy of Family Physicians, American Academy of Pediatrics, American College of Physicians, American Osteopathic Association. Joint Principles of the patient-centered medical home. March 2007. http://www.medicalhomeinfo.org/Joint%20Statement.pdf
4. American Academy of Pediatrics. National Center for Medical Home Implementation Web site. http://www.medicalhomeinfo.org
5. Sia C, Tonniges TF, Osterhus E, Taba S. History of the medical home concept. *Pediatrics*. 2004;113(suppl):1473–1478
6. American Academy of Pediatrics. What is a Pediatric Geneticist? HealthyChildren.org Web site. http://www.healthychildren.org/English/family-life/health-management/pediatric-specialists/Pages/What-is-a-Pediatric-Geneticist.aspx
7. Dagli AI, Williams CA. Angelman syndrome. In: Pagon RA, Bird TD, Dolan CR, Stephens K, ed. *GeneReviews*. Seattle, WA: University of Washington, Seattle; 1998. http://www.ncbi.nlm.nih.gov/bookshelf/br.fcgi?book=gene&part=angelman
8. Burdo-Hartman WA, Patel DR. Medical home and transition planning for children and youth with special health care needs. *Pediatr Clin North Am*. 2008;55:1287–1297
9. Allen PJ, Vessey JA, Schapiro NA. *Primary Care of the Child with a Chronic Condition*. 5th ed. St Louis, MO: Mosby Elsevier; 2010:61–73
10. Healthy People 2010. HealthyPeople.gov Web site. www.healthypeople.gov
11. American Academy of Pediatrics, American Academy of Family Physicians, American College of Physicians-American Society of Internal Medicine. A consensus statement on health care transitions for young adults with special health care needs. *Pediatrics*. 2002;110;1304–1306
12. American Medical Association, Department of Adolescent Health. *Guidelines for Adolescent Preventive Health (GAPS): Clinical Evaluation and Management Handbook*. Chicago, IL: American Medical Association; 2000
13. American Academy of Pediatrics. *Periodic Survey #71. Pediatricians' Interest in Expanding Services and Making Practice Changes to Improve the Care of Adolescents*. http://www.aap.org/en-us/professional-resources/Research/Pages/PS71_

Chapter 5

Family History and Pedigree Construction

Howard M. Saal, MD
Emily Chen, MD, PhD

The Family History

The family history is an important tool for making diagnoses, medical management, and anticipatory guidance for all medical conditions, not just genetic disorders. The treatment of routine and complex childhood diseases is facilitated by knowledge of the family history and its potentially associated risk factors. The family history is also essential for genetic counseling, including discussion of reproductive planning and understanding recurrence risks, as well as informing other members of a patient's extended family about their medical and reproductive risks.

Understanding the potential recurrence of genetic disorders, such as birth defects, depends on knowing the occurrence of birth defects in the extended family. The incidence of birth defects is 3% and has remained stable over several decades[1]; however, their impact remains substantial. Birth defects are the leading cause of infant death and account for 20% of infant deaths.[2,3] In addition, many birth defects and genetic disorders may not be recognized until later infancy, childhood, or even adulthood. Approximately 12% of pediatric hospitalizations can be attributed to birth defects. Moreover, these children have longer hospitalizations, higher morbidity, and greater hospital costs,[4] and 71% of hospitalized children have an underlying disorder with a significant genetic component.[5]

Several factors are essential for recording an accurate family history, including knowledge of specific illnesses and medical conditions in family members, infertility, growth and development, and race and ethnicity.

Reasons for Obtaining a Family History

There are thousands of known genetic disorders, and it is not possible for any physician to be familiar with all of these conditions. The family history may uncover a familial pattern of birth defects, cognitive disabilities, malignancies, or other medical problems that may be hereditary. This information is frequently essential for early diagnosis, timely management and treatment, and appropriate referrals.

There are several reasons why the family history plays a major role in pediatric practice, including

- Identifying familial and hereditary disorders
- Determining inheritance patterns and recurrence risks for known and suspected genetic disorders
- Identifying patients and family members at risk for a genetic disorder
- Identifying patients and family members who are *not* at risk for a genetic disorder
- Providing information necessary for appropriate genetic counseling
- Providing an important adjunct to patient management of all childhood diseases, such as growth problems and asthma

Ideally a family history is recorded at the time of initial evaluation. This can include the prenatal visit. The family history should also be updated annually with each follow-up routine visit.[6]

Asking the Right Questions

The 5 questions to start the conversation about family health history, which are recommended by the American College of Medical Genetics and Genomics, are as follows:

1. Are there any health problems that are known to run in your family, or that close relatives have been told are genetic? If so, what are these conditions?
2. Is there anyone in the family who had cancer, heart disease, or other adult-onset health problem at an early age, such as between 20 and 50?
3. Does/did anyone in the family have intellectual disability, learning problems, or have to go to a special school?
4. Have there been any early deaths in the family, including stillbirths, infant deaths, multiple miscarriages, or shortened life span?
5. Have any relatives had extreme or unexpected reactions to medications or therapy?

It may help also to refer to the SCREEN mnemonic for family history collection and strategies for the clinician (Box 5-1).[6]

BOX 5-1. The SCREEN Mnemonic for Family History Collection[a]

SC	Some concerns	"Do you have any (some) concerns about diseases or conditions that run in your family?"
R	Reproduction	"Have there been any problems with pregnancy, infertility, or birth defects in your family?"
E	Early disease, death, or disability	"Have any members of your family become sick or died at an early age?"
E	Ethnicity	"How would you describe your ethnicity?" OR "Where were your parents born?"
N	Nongenetic	"Are there any other risk factors or nonmedical conditions that run in your family?"

[a]From Trotter TL, Martin HM. Family history in pediatric primary care. *Pediatrics*. 2007;120:S60–S65. http://pediatrics.aappublications.org/cgi/content/full/120/SUPPLEMENT_2/S60.

A family health history and the construction of the pedigree (see next section) requires good documentation of (1) correct diagnosis/disease, (2) age of onset, (3) age at death, (4) cause of death, (5) relationships between members, (6) ethnic origins of both sides of the family, and (7) consanguinity, if present.

Obtaining a family history can be time-consuming; however, the amount of information obtained is usually extremely helpful and can lead to identifying information helpful in diagnosis and treatment. The information in a family history also might reveal those individuals who are not at risk for a specific disorder. Involving families in gathering family history information can increase their direct involvement in their child's health care. An additional benefit may be that the family history may give some insight into some familial psychosocial issues, including information about family dynamics, concerns about mental health issues, and early deaths.

Ethnic and Racial Factors

Racial and ethnic origins of the patient and family are important to note because some specific genetic disorders may be seen in high frequency because of evolutionary forces and geographic and cultural isolation. Certain geographic, ethnic, and racial groups may be at relatively high risk for otherwise rare genetic disorders. Sickle cell disease is common in those of African and Mediterranean ancestry because heterozygous carriers of the sickle hemoglobin have some protection against malaria. Similarly, β-thalassemia in those of Mediterranean ancestry and α-thalassemia in Southeast Asians offer some resistance to malaria as well. Rare genetic disorders are seen in some ethnic groups as a result of geographic isolation. An example of this is Hermansky-Pudlak syndrome, an autosomal recessive disorder with oculocutaneous albinism, a platelet abnormality, and an abnormal fat protein compound, has a prevalence of 1 in 500,000 to 1 in 1 million in the world, but has a prevalence of 1 in 1,600 in northwest Puerto Rico.[7,8] A combination of geographic and cultural factors has contributed to the incidence of several hereditary disorders in individuals of Ashkenazi Jewish descent, including Tay-Sachs disease, hereditary breast and ovarian cancer, and Gaucher disease.[9] The ancestors of these individuals settled in small communities in Eastern Europe and, because of the geographic separation and cultural/religious issues, there were limited reproductive options. Therefore, the ethnic and racial backgrounds of patients provides an initial screen for specific disorders (as is done routinely in most states with newborn screening for cystic fibrosis and sickle cell disease) as well as a reason to discuss carrier testing with patients and their families. Table 5-1 lists examples of several major ethnic and racial groups and associated genetic disorders.

Table 5-1. Examples of Genetic Disorders Seen in Specific Ethnic and Racial Groups

Racial or Ethnic Group	Genetic Disorder	Inheritance
African American		
	Sickle cell disease	AR
	Glucose-6-phosphate dehydrogenase deficiency	XLR
Amish/Menonite[1,2]		
	Maple syrup urine disease	AR
	Chondroectodermal dysplasia (Ellis-van Creveld syndrome)	AR
	Cartilage-hair hypoplasia	AR
	McKusick-Kaufman syndrome	AR
	Limb girdle muscular dystrophy	AR
	Glutaric aciduria type I	AR
Ashkenazi Jewish[3]		
	Tay-Sachs disease	AR
	Canavan disease	AR
	Gaucher disease type 1	AR
	Hereditary breast/ovarian cancer	AD
	Sensorineural deafness	AR
	Familial dysautonomia	AR
	Mucolipidosis type IV	AR
	Niemann-Pick disease type A	AR

Racial or Ethnic Group	Genetic Disorder	Inheritance
Finnish[4]		
	Hereditary nephrosis	AR
	Cartilage-hair hypoplasia	AR
	Infantile neuronal ceroid lipofuscinosis	AR
	Mullibrey nanism	AR
French Canadian[5]		
	Leigh syndrome, French-Canadian type	AR
	Hereditary multiple intestinal atresias	AR
	Tyrosinemia type I	AR
	Tay-Sachs disease	AR
	Cystinosis	AR
	Pseudo–vitamin D deficiency rickets	AR
Mediterranean (Italian, Greek, North African)		
	β-thalassemia	AR
	Glucose-6-phosphate dehydrogenase deficiency	XLR
	Sickle cell disease	AR
Middle Eastern		
	β-thalassemia	AR
	Familial Mediterranean fever	AR
Portuguese		
	Machado-Joseph disease	AR
Puerto Rican[6]		
	Hermansky-Pudlak syndrome	AR
Southeast Asian		
	α-thalassemia	AR
	β-thalassemia	AR

Abbreviations: AD, autosomal dominant; AR, autosomal recessive; XLR, X-linked recessive.

Additional Family History Questions

The primary care physician (PCP) should elicit a history of conditions in the family in the categories of reproductive and prenatal history, early and unexpected death, cognitive and behavioral disorders, growth and stature, and sensory organ deficits (Table 5-2). Answers to questions regarding a history

Table 5-2. Conditions and Commonly Associated Diagnoses

Symptom	Possible Diagnosis
Reproductive and Prenatal History	
Recurrent pregnancy loss	– Familial balanced chromosome anomaly – Maternal uterine anomaly (eg, müllerian, renal tract, and cervicothoracic somite association; incompetent cervix) – Maternal thrombophilia
Infertility in males	– Klinefelter syndrome – Cystic fibrosis – Pituitary abnormalities and hypogonadotrophic hypogonadism
Infertility in females	– Turner syndrome – Androgen insensitivity syndrome – Congenital adrenal hypoplasia – Uterine anomalies – Pituitary abnormalities and hypogonadotrophic hypogonadism
Early and Unexpected Death	
Infant death	– Biochemical (metabolic) disorders – Congenital anomalies – Chromosome disorders – Neuromuscular disorders – Abnormal airway and Pierre Robin sequence – Sudden infant death syndrome – Medium-chain acyl-CoA dehydrogenase deficiency
Late childhood and early adult death	– Heart disease: cardiomyopathy, arrhythmia, myocardial infarction – Cancer: colorectal, thyroid, pheochromocytomas – Suicide: depression, bipolar disorder
Cognitive and Behavior Disorders	
Cognitive disability	– Chromosome disorders – Fragile X syndrome – Hydrocephalus – Structural brain anomalies – Microcephaly – Lysosomal storage disease – Biochemical (metabolic) disorders – Autism spectrum disorder
Behavior disorders	– Schizophrenia – Bipolar disorder – Learning disability – Attention-deficit/hyperactivity disorder

Symptom	Possible Diagnosis
Growth and Stature	
Short stature	– Constitutional delay (often familial) – Familial short stature – Skeletal dysplasia – Intrauterine growth restriction – Growth hormone deficiency – Turner syndrome – Chromosome disorder – Fetal alcohol syndrome – Russell-Silver syndrome
Overgrowth or tall stature	– Beckwith-Wiedemann syndrome – Marfan syndrome – Sotos syndrome – Klinefelter syndrome
Sensory Organ Deficits	
Deafness and hearing loss	– Conductive deafness – Sensorineural deafness – Townes-Brock syndrome – Branchio-oto-renal syndrome – Stickler syndrome – Tumors associated with deafness (vestibular schwannoma in neurofibromatosis 2)
Blindness and vision loss	– Albinism – High myopia – Retinal detachment – Retinitis pigmentosa – Microphthalmia – Peters anomaly – Colobomas
High myopia and retinal detachment	– Stickler syndrome
Ocular albinism	– Herman-Pudlak syndrome
Myopia and lens detachment	– Marfan syndrome
Cleft lip and/or cleft palate	– Deletion 22q11.2 syndrome – Stickler syndrome – Van der Woude syndrome
Seizures and epilepsy	– Tuberous sclerosis – Structural brain anomalies – Neurofibromatosis

of conditions in these categories can provide a great deal of insight into diagnosing and understanding birth defects and genetic disorders. For example, a history of recurrent pregnancy loss may indicate a parental chromosome translocation or a maternal thrombophilia, such as factor V Leiden.

Heritable factors and birth defects are among the most common causes of infant mortality, accounting for more than one-third of infant deaths.[10] Hence a familial history of death in infancy and early childhood should be documented. In addition, although injuries, homicide, and suicide are the major causes of death in young adults,[11] malignant neoplasms, heart disease, and congenital anomalies rank in the top 10 causes of mortality. Genetic factors play a major role in early onset malignancies, heart anomalies, and even suicide, since schizophrenia, depression, and bipolar disorder are known to have significant known genetic predisposition. Malignancies not routinely seen in older children and young adults may indicate cancer predisposition syndromes, such as familial polyposis and colon cancer, multiple endocrine neoplasia type 2 and medullary thyroid carcinoma and pheochromocytomas, Li-Fraumeni syndrome and soft tissue tumors, and breast cancer and sarcomas.

It is widely accepted that developmental and cognitive disabilities often have genetic etiologies. Comprehensive family history with pedigree analysis can often expedite the diagnostic evaluation by documenting a family history with inheritance pattern. In addition, certain genetic disorders are associated with mental illness. Schizophrenia and bipolar disorder are seen frequently in individuals with deletion 22q11.2 syndrome.[12]

Short stature may occur because of endocrine or genetic factors. On the other hand, overgrowth is often related to genetic disorders. Tall stature may be associated with connective tissue disorders such as Marfan syndrome, which requires careful screening and management. It is often helpful to document parental and sibling heights (percentiles) as well as birth weights on the pedigree.

Approximately 50% of all non-syndromic deafness has a genetic etiology.[13] Similarly, vision loss has multiple etiologies. In addition to retinopathy of prematurity or accidents, genetic disorders can cause vision loss throughout childhood and early adulthood. Stickler syndrome can cause high myopia and retinal detachment. Marfan syndrome is associated with myopia and lens dislocations. Most forms of albinism are associated with nystagmus and vision loss, and there are some albinism disorders that cause primarily ocular albinism (eg, Hermansky-Pudlak syndrome, which is prevalent in Puerto Rico).

Constructing a Pedigree

The most helpful method for recording a family history is the pedigree. Many health care record models use a checklist for recording family history. These are commonly found in electronic medical records (EMRs). Checklists can be comprehensive, but by being primarily a list of family health issues, it is not amenable to identifying patterns of disorders.

Pedigrees have the advantage of being a visual record of the family history and allow for identification of patterns of occurrence of medical issues in a family, often giving clues to inheritance and therefore risk analysis. Also, a visual tool may help parents remember information that may not be readily acknowledged by answering yes and no to a checklist. Clinical geneticists and genetic counselors construct at least a 3-generation pedigree using standard symbols[14] (Figure 5-1). Males are designated by squares and females by circles. If gender is not known, then a diamond is used. Deceased individuals are represented by a circle, square, or diamond with a diagonal line drawn through the symbol. Miscarriages are represented by triangles, and stillbirths are represented by squares, circles, or diamonds with a diagonal line and the designation of "SB" below the figure. The symbols representing affected individuals (or pregnancies) are designated by filling in the symbol, a portion of the symbol, cross-hatching or other shadings, or cross-hatching with the specific designation being noted in a key

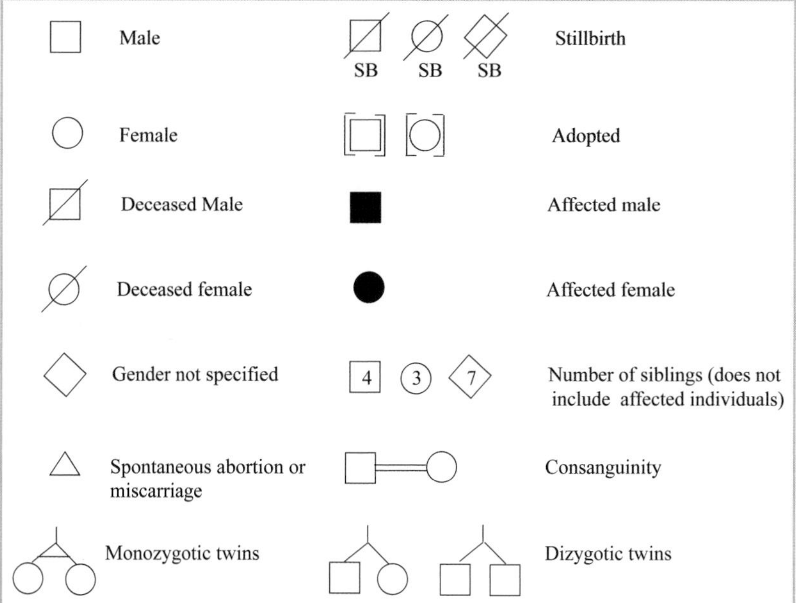

Figure 5-1. A representative sample of symbols used in pedigree construction.

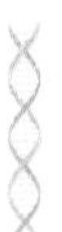

on the pedigree. The proband (usually the patient) is usually denoted by an arrow. In a relationship, the male partner is typically placed on the left and the female partner on the right. Additional information, which can be written on the pedigree under each symbol, should include age or date of birth, age of death, age of diagnosis (especially for adult diseases, including malignancies), expected date of delivery for pregnancies, and gestational age for miscarriages or stillbirths. Consanguinity and twinning can also be denoted with appropriate connecting lines.

See Figure 5-2 for a stepwise look at pedigree creation, briefly described as the following steps:

- **Step 1—Begin with core family.**
  When constructing a pedigree, it is best to start with the patient (usually the proband) and parents. In order of birth, siblings and other pregnancies that may have resulted in miscarriage or stillbirth are added.
- **Step 2—Add aunts and uncles.**
  At the same level of parents, their siblings (the aunts and uncles of the proband) are filled in.
- **Step 3—Add cousins.**
  The offspring of the aunts and uncles (the cousins of the proband) should be entered at the same level of the proband to be consistent with generational relationships, including similar information regarding results of all pregnancies, including live births and pregnancy loss.
- **Step 4—Add grandparents and their siblings.**
  The next step is to go up one generation and add the grandparents, great aunts and uncles and, as indicated, their offspring. The result will be a 3-generation pedigree. If the great grandparents are added, a 4-generation pedigree will be constructed.
- **Step 5—Identify the individuals in a pedigree.**
  To consistently name the individuals in a pedigree, the generations are noted in Roman numerals, with the first numeral as the most distant, and specific individuals in Arabic numbers from left to right. For example, the proband in Figure 5-2 is III-4. Particular disorders to include in the pedigree are birth defects (eg, cleft lip, cleft palate, spina bifida), unusual physical features (eg, lip pits, lots of café au lait spots, polydactyly, loss of the sense of smell or anosmia, short stature for the family), respiratory diseases, organ abnormalities, heart disease (including congenital), cancers, early or sudden deaths, hypertension, infertility, multiple miscarriages, premature ovarian failure, intellectual disability, obesity, skeletal abnormalities, stroke, vision impairment, or hearing impairment. There may be a higher genetic risk if the age of onset of a medical condition is at an extraordinarily young age.

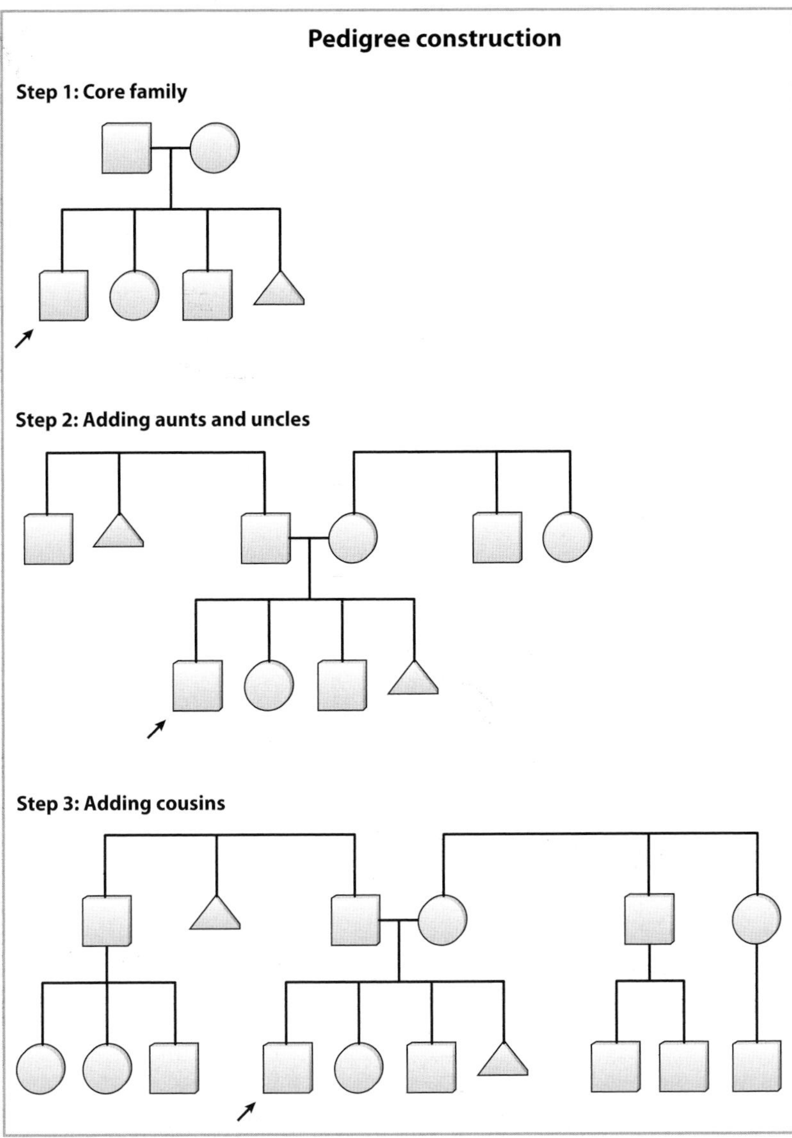

Figure 5-2. Sample pedigree construction. This 3-generation pedigree shows steps for information gathering. **Step 1**—gathering the information for the core family (the proband identified by arrow, the siblings and the parents [the small triangle indicates a spontaneous abortion]); **Step 2**—adding aunts and uncles of the proband (the siblings of the parents); **Step 3**—adding the cousins of the proband.

Continued

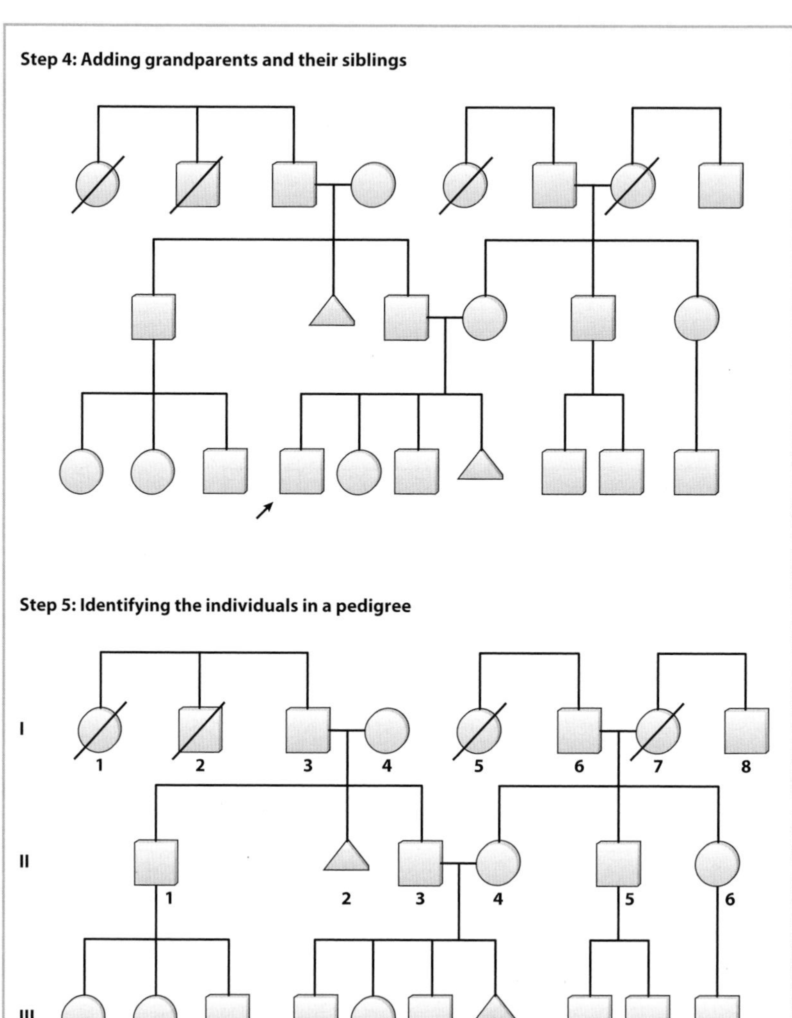

Figure 5-2, continued. Sample pedigree construction. This 3-generation pedigree shows steps for information gathering. **Step 4**—adding the grandparents of the proband and their siblings; **Step 5**—identifying the individuals in the pedigree by generation (Roman numerals I, II, and III) and by individual (Arabic numerals).

Other Tools to Collect Family History

According to a survey by the Centers for Disease Control and Prevention, although 96.3% of Americans considered knowledge of family history important to their personal health, only about 30% have ever tried to actively gather and organize their families' health histories.[15] An observational study of PCPs indicated that family histories were discussed about half the time at new visits and 22% of the time during follow-up visits.[16] Each year since 2004, the Surgeon General has declared Thanksgiving to be National Family History Day. Over the holiday or at other times when families gather, the Surgeon General encourages Americans to talk about, and to write down, the health problems that seem to run in their family. Pediatricians should encourage all of their patient families to use this online tool,[17] which initially only takes 15 to 20 minutes, and can be downloaded to the family's computer when completed. Family history should be recorded by parents and relatives prior to seeing the pediatrician, either initiated online or drawn out on paper to be scanned into the EMR for easy access to other providers. The pediatrician should have access to a pedigree for each family in the EMR.

Here are some guidelines for pediatricians to help families obtain a complete pedigree.

1. All members of 3 generations should be included.
2. The pediatrician should ask family members to obtain medical records to clarify diagnoses and disease course.
3. The family history can be obtained over multiple pediatric visits.
4. The family history may shift in emphasis depending on the age of the child.

Alternatively, a preconception/prenatal or adolescent/adult family history questionnaire is available from the March of Dimes[18] to be filled out ahead of a visit. See Appendix A for samples.

Barriers to Obtaining a Family History

Barriers for families include lack of time, incomplete records, inaccessible family members, adoption, incorrect or vague diagnoses, denial, guilt, family members not talking to each other, blame, multiple family members who care for a child, poor follow-through on questions asked about the family history, and fear of discrimination and stigmatization. Barriers for pediatricians are lack of time and prioritization, and lack of payment for family history collection.

Interpreting the Family History

Because genes and proteins (or enzymes) are involved in all disease processes, pediatricians should not ask "Is this a genetic disease?" Rather, "What roles do genes play in the expression of this disease?" The pediatrician, with the help of a geneticist or genetic counselor, can define and refine diseases, risks, and modes of inheritance. Modes of inheritance, which should be considered while constructing a pedigree, are autosomal dominant, autosomal recessive, X-linked recessive or dominant, chromosomal, mitochondrial, multifactorial, and other rare modes such as uniparental disomy. (See Chapter 1.) Good resources for determining the known mode(s) of inheritance of a condition can be obtained from GeneTests (www.genetests.org) or Online Mendelian Inheritance in Man (www.ncbi.nlm.nih.gov/omim/), or assumed based on the relationships between affected members of the family. Parental or other family member studies (molecular or chromosomal) may need to be done to sort out the inheritance. Some genetic conditions, such as polycystic kidney disease, osteogenesis imperfecta, or Charcot-Marie-Tooth disease, can be either autosomal dominant or recessive, or X-linked (for Charcot-Marie-Tooth disease), depending on the gene involved. Pediatricians need to be mindful of the variable expression, non-penetrance (when usually a dominant condition can appear to skip generations) or decreased penetrance, and unusual patterns of inheritance of genetic disorders. If questions arise about drawing a family pedigree, or interpreting the relevance of a family history, geneticists and genetic counselors should be consulted.

The result of the pedigree construction is a graphic depiction of the family medical history over 3 or 4 generations. Often patterns of illness, neurodevelopmental abnormalities, early death, malignancies, or pregnancy and fertility issues become apparent. It should be emphasized that once abnormalities are found, the PCP should keep asking questions. More questions often yield more information that may identify associations or clinical information that aids diagnosis.

In autosomal dominant conditions, one will often see affected individuals in consecutive generations (Figure 5-3). Autosomal recessive disorders are often rare and are usually seen in a single sibship; although, for some disorders, affected individuals may be seen in more than one generation for disorders that may be seen more commonly in certain racial or ethnic groups, such as sickle cell disease in Africans and African Americans, and cystic fibrosis, usually more common in Caucasians of northern European

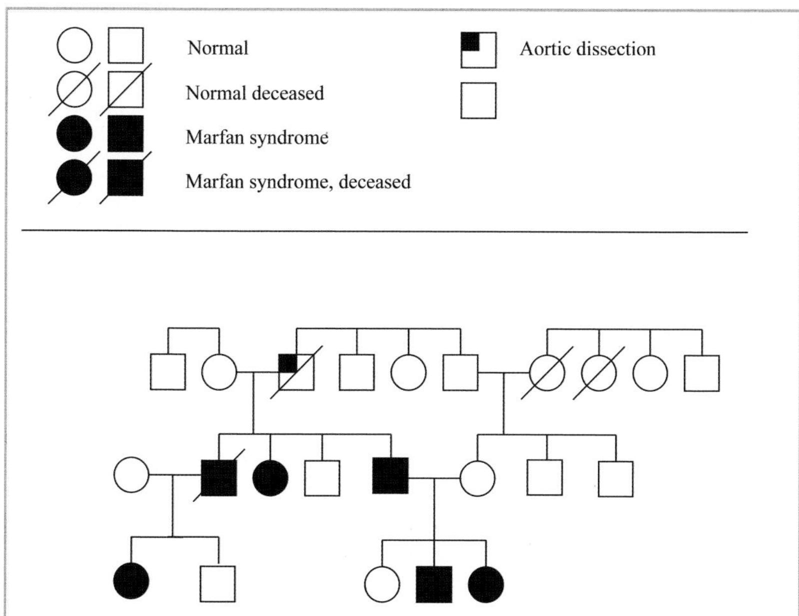

Figure 5-3. A partial pedigree of a family and multiple individuals (male and female) affected with Marfan syndrome. This pedigree demonstrates autosomal dominant inheritance with male-to-male transmission.

ancestry (Figure 5-4). Consanguinity also increases risks for autosomal recessive disorders, since related reproductive partners are more likely to have more genes in common, including those for rare recessive disorders (Figure 5-5). If a pedigree shows that only males are affected, and this can be seen in consecutive generations, one should consider X-linked recessive disorders, such as Duchenne muscular dystrophy, hemophilia, or fragile X syndrome (Figure 5-6). Chromosome disorders may present in many ways in a family. Many chromosome disorders will be de novo, and the pedigree will show no unusual patterns. However, in families with balanced chromosome translocations, the pedigree may show multiple miscarriages, infants born with multiple anomalies, or infant death (Figure 5-7).

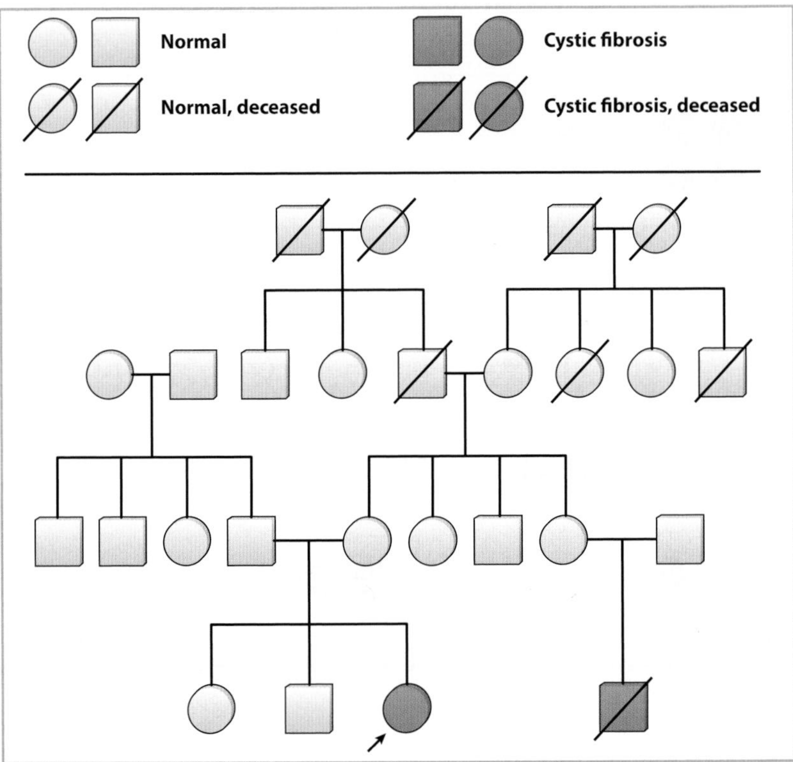

Figure 5-4. A partial pedigree of a family and 2 cousins affected with cystic fibrosis. This pedigree demonstrates autosomal recessive inheritance.

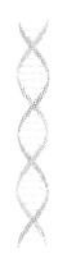

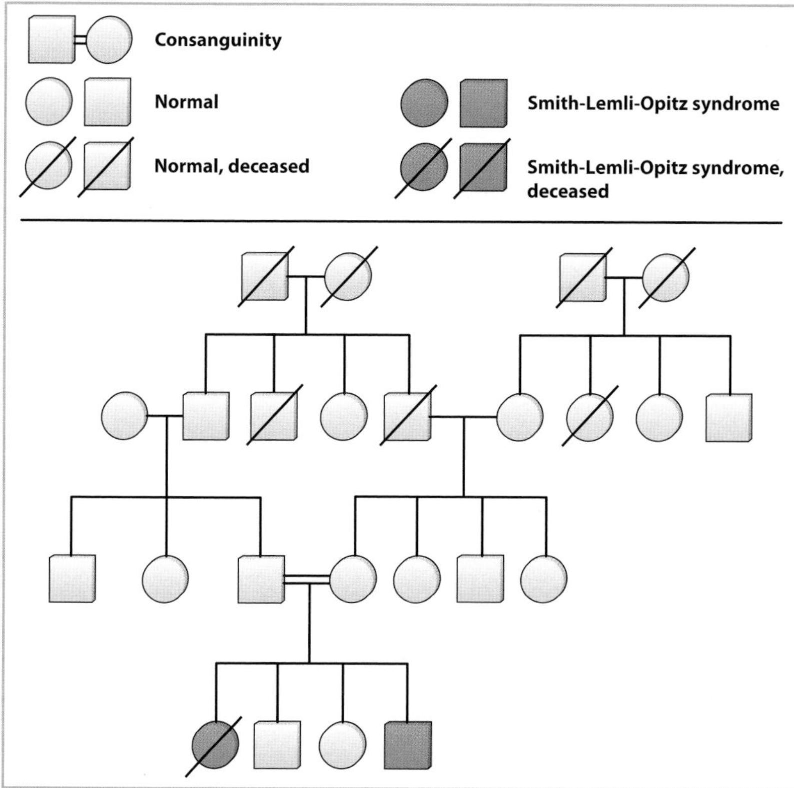

Figure 5-5. A partial pedigree of a family and 2 siblings affected with Smith-Lemli-Opitz syndrome. This pedigree demonstrates autosomal recessive inheritance and, in addition, consanguinity.

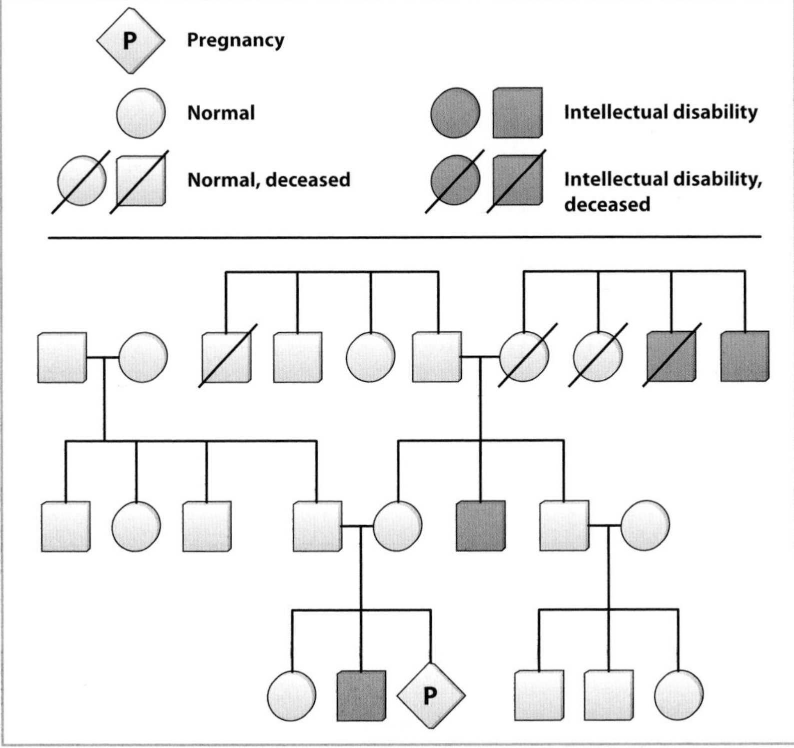

Figure 5-6. A partial pedigree of a family and multiple males affected with fragile X syndrome. The pedigree demonstrates X-linked inheritance and a current pregnancy for a known carrier.

Key Points

- The family history and pedigree are essential to the diagnosis and management of birth defects and genetic disorders.
- The family history and pedigree enhance the management of any child.
- Information gathered in the family history can be useful for anticipatory guidance, health and developmental screening, and prediction of reproductive risks.
- Use of the family history and pedigree analysis is a low-technology way to offer high-technology medicine.
- Several excellent online and print resources that can be very helpful in obtaining family histories and constructing pedigrees are listed at the end of this chapter.

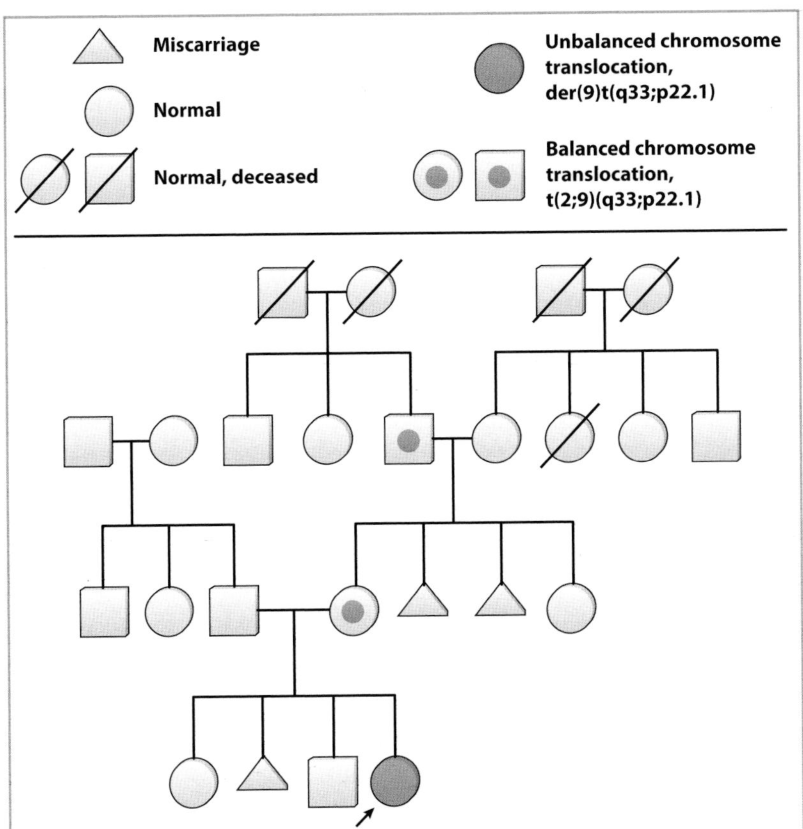

Figure 5-7. A partial pedigree of a family with a balanced chromosome rearrangement and a female proband with an unbalanced rearrangement. This pedigree demonstrates multiple miscarriages (spontaneous abortions), often seen in multiple generations with chromosome rearrangements.

Resources

Family Medical History in Disease Prevention, American Medical Association
http://www.ama-assn.org/ama1/pub/upload/mm/464/family_history02.pdf

Family Tree, The National Society of Genetic Counselors
www.nsgc.org/consumer/familytree/index.cfm

The Genetic Alliance
www.geneticalliance.org/fhh

My Family Health Portrait Tool, US Department of Health and Human Services through the Surgeons General's Family Health History Initiative
www.hhs.gov/familyhistory/

National Coalition for Health Professional Education in Genetics, Family History Tool
www.nchpeg.org/index.php?option=com_content&view=article&id=61&Itemid=74

References

1. Centers for Disease Control and Prevention. Update on overall prevalence of major birth defects—Atlanta, Georgia, 1978–2005. *MMWR Morb Mortal Wkly Rep.* 2008;57(01):1–5
2. Kochanek KD, Xu J, Murphy SL, Minino AM, Kung H-C. Deaths: preliminary data for 2009. *Nat Vital Stat Rep.* 2011;50(4):1–95
3. Petrini J, Damus K, Russell R, Psochman K, Davidoff MJ, Mattison D. Contributions of birth defects to infant mortality in the United States. *Teratology.* 2002;66(suppl 1):S3–S6
4. Yoon Pw, Olney RS, Khoury MJ, Sappenfield WM, Chavez GF, Taylor D. Contributions of birth defects to and genetic diseases to pediatric hospitalizations. A population-based study. *Arch Pediatr Adolesc Med.* 1997;151:1096–1103
5. McCandless SE, Brunger JW, Cassidy SB. The burden of genetic diseases on inpatient care in a children's hospital. *Am J Hum Genet.* 2004;74(1):121–127
6. Trotter TL, Martin HMT. Family history in pediatric primary care. *Pediatrics.* 2007;120:S60–S65
7. Santiago Borrero PJ, Rodriguez-Perez Y, Renta JY, Izquierdo NJ, et al. Genetic testing for oculocutaneous albinism type 1 and 2 and Hermansky-Pudlak syndrome type 1 and 3 mutations in Puerto Rico. *J Invest Dermatol.* 2006;126(1):85–90
8. Nazarian R, Huizing M, Helip-Wooley A, Starcevic M, Gahl WA, Dell'Angelica EC. An immunoblotting assay to facilitate the molecular diagnosis of Hermansky-Pudlak syndrome. *Mol Genet Metab.* 2008;93(2):134–144
9. Charrow J. Ashkenazi Jewish genetic disorders. *Fam Cancer.* 2004;3(3–4):201–206
10. Stevenson DA, Carey JC. Contribution of malformations and genetic disorders to mortality in a children's hospital. *Am J Med Genet A.* 2004;126A(4):393–397
11. Centers for Disease Control and Prevention. *Life Expectancy Hits Record High Gender Gap Narrows.* http://www.cdc.gov/nchs/pressroom/05facts/lifeexpectancy.htm. Accessed April 12, 2012
12. Bassett AS, Chow EW, Husted J, et al. Clinical features of 78 adults with 22q11 deletion syndrome. *Am J Med Genet A.* 2005;138(4):307–313
13. Morton CC, Nance WE. Newborn hearing screening—a silent revolution. *N Engl J Med.* 2006;354(20):2151–2164
14. Bennett RL, French KS, Resta RG, Doyle DL. Standardized human pedigree nomenclature: update and assessment of the recommendations of the National Society of Genetic Counselors. *J Genet Couns.* 2008;17(5):424–433
15. Centers for Disease Control and Prevention. Awareness of family health history as a risk factor for disease—United States, 2004. *MMWR Morb Mortal Wkly Rep.* 2004;53(44):1044–1047
16. Acheson LS, Wiesner GL, Zyzanski SJ, Goodwin MA, Stange KC. Family history-taking in community family practice: implications for genetic screening. *Genet Med.* 2000;2:180–185
17. US Department of Health and Human Services. Surgeon General's Family Health History. HHS.gov Web site. http://www.hhs.gov/familyhistory. Accessed April 12, 2012
18. March of Dimes. Your family health history. March of Dimes Web site. http://www.marchofdimes.com/pregancy/trying_healthhistory.html. Accessed April 12, 2012

Chapter 6

Reasons to Consider a Genetics Evaluation

John B. Moeschler, MD, MS

Introduction

This chapter outlines the clinical circumstances that call for referral to a medical geneticist (Box 6-1), but does not address newborns with congenital malformations or medical conditions requiring immediate hospital specialty consultations (eg, congenital hypotonia), nor those children with acute onset of symptoms requiring hospital admission, such as stupor or coma.

The medical home best coordinates health care for all children, including those children with special health care needs.[1,2] It is there that interactions among pediatricians, families, and medical genetics specialists gather to improve the health care processes and health outcomes for children. McGrath et al[3] observed that as income and education attainment decrease, barriers to genetics services rise. The presence of a medical home is the single most important factor in facilitating access to genetics services. The presence of insurance, particularly private or a combination of private and public insurance, is also an important factor in access to genetics subspecialty care. The medical genetics evaluation process is outlined in Box 6-2, and what families and the primary care physician can expect from the clinical genetics evaluation is outlined in Box 6-3.

Box 6-1. Reasons to Refer to a Geneticist

- **Disorders of Development**
  - Global developmental delay—significant delay in ≥2 of
    - Gross or fine motor skills
    - Speech and language
    - Cognition
    - Social/personal skills
    - Activities of daily living
  - Positive autism spectrum disorder screen
- **Disorders of Growth**
  - Short stature (significant, with developmental delay, or with dysmorphology)
  - Somatic overgrowth
  - Excessive growth velocity
- **Structural or Morphological Variations**
  - Major anomaly
- **Minor Anomaly (See Chapter 8.)**

Box 6-2. The Medical Genetics Diagnostic Evaluation Process for Developmental Delays or Intellectual Disability

- Clinical history
- Family history
- Physical examination (particularly for presence of minor anomalies)
- Neurologic examination
- Specific confirmatory genetic tests for suspected syndromes
- Chromosome microarray
- Fragile X molecular genetic testing
- Metabolic screening in all children with delay and intellectual disability
- Targeted brain magnetic resonance imaging

Adapted from Moeschler JB, Shevell MI; American Academy of Pediatrics Committee on Genetics. Clinical genetic evaluation of the child with mental retardation or developmental delays. *Pediatrics*. 2006;117:2304–2316.

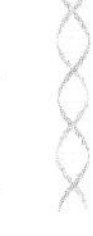

Box 6-3. What Families Might Expect From the Clinical Genetics Evaluation

- **Before the Visit**
  - Request for child's medical charts; neurodevelopment test results; copies of magnetic resonance imaging (MRI), computed tomography (CT), or other imaging studies
  - Request to bring photographs of child and family members
  - Asked about the family history
  - Asked to set aside sufficient time for prolonged consultation
- **At the Visit**
  - Clarification of the purpose of the visit
  - Review of the child's medical history and neurodevelopmental status
  - Review of family history (≥3 generations)
  - Completion of physical and neurologic examinations
  - Discussion of geneticist's initial impressions
- **After the Visit**
  - Clinical photographs
  - Laboratory studies (blood and/or urine tests)
  - Arrangements for MRI or CT studies
  - Arrangements for other consultations (neurology, developmental pediatrics, ophthalmology, etc)
  - Arrangements for ongoing communication and follow-up visits

Adapted from Moeschler JB, Shevell MI; American Academy of Pediatrics Committee on Genetics. Clinical genetic evaluation of the child with mental retardation or developmental delays. *Pediatrics.* 2006;117:2304–2316.

Noteworthy Clinical Symptoms or Signs

Three categories of presenting symptoms or signs in children that should prompt a referral to a medical geneticist are

1. Disorders of development
2. Disorders of growth
3. Structural or morphological variations (congenital anomalies)

Children With Disorders of Development

Definitions

Global developmental delay is defined as significant delay in 2 or more developmental domains—gross or fine motor, speech/language, cognitive, social/personal, and activities of daily living—and is thought to predict a future diagnosis of intellectual disability.[4,5] Such delays require accurate documentation using norm-referenced and age-appropriate standardized measures of development administered by qualified specialists. The term global developmental delay is usually reserved for younger children (ie, typically <5 years), whereas the term intellectual disability is usually applied to older children when IQ testing is valid and reliable.[6] Children with developmental delays are those with delays in the attainment of developmental milestones at the expected age. The term implies deficits in learning and adaptation, suggesting that the delays are significant and predict later disability. Delays in development, however, especially those that are mild, may be transient and lack predictive reliability for intellectual disability. Schaefer and Bodensteiner[7] wrote that a *clinical* diagnosis is that which "can be translated into useful clinical information for the family, including providing information about prognosis, recurrence risks, and preferred modes of available therapy." Van Karnebeek et al[8] defined *etiologic* diagnosis as "sufficient literature evidence…to make a causal relationship of the disorder with mental retardation [sic] likely, and if it met the Schaefer-Bodensteiner definition." The *clinical* diagnosis and *etiologic* diagnosis differ subtly but significantly. For example, the clinical diagnosis of mild intellectual disability with agenesis of the corpus callosum describes the phenotype and fits the Schaefer and Bodensteiner criteria but differs from the etiologic diagnosis of FG syndrome due to the recurrent R961W mutation in the *MED12* gene. The purpose of the referral to a medical geneticist is to address the *etiologic* diagnosis in order to improve health care and health outcomes.

Global Developmental Delay and Intellectual Disability

Early treatment of developmental delays optimizes developmental outcomes.[9] Screening identifies those patients at risk for significant developmental disabilities or autism spectrum disorders (ASDs). The primary care physician then typically refers the screen positive child to a child development clinical team led by a specialist, such as a developmental-behavioral pediatrician or neurodevelopmental pediatrician. This team typically confirms or rules out the presence of a developmental or intellectual disability.[9]

All children with documented global developmental delays or any degree of intellectual disability of uncertain etiology should be referred to a medical geneticist for diagnostic evaluation.

For the medical home physician, for patients, and for their families, there are specific benefits to establishing an etiologic diagnosis, including the following[6]:

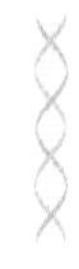

- Clarification of etiology, prognosis, genetic mechanism(s), recurrence risks, and treatment options
- Avoidance of unnecessary tests
- Information regarding management or surveillance and family support
- Access to research and treatment protocols
- The opportunity for comanagement of appropriate patients in the context of a medical home to ensure the best health and social outcomes for the child

The causes of global developmental delay are highly heterogeneous. Estimates of the etiologic yield in children with global developmental delay or intellectual disability are highly variable (from 10%–81% depending on the study) with a genetic etiology proved or suspected in the majority. The most often quoted yield for the diagnostic genetics evaluation ranges from 40% to 60%,[10] with the variability attributed to differences in a variety of factors, including sample population characteristics, severity of delay in the children studied, extent of diagnostic investigations, and technological advances over time, especially with respect to genetics and neuroimaging techniques.

The diagnostic evaluation guidelines published by the American College of Medical Genetics and Genomics,[10] the American Academy of Pediatrics (AAP),[5] and the American Academy of Neurology Child Neurology Society[4] generally agree on the evaluation process for children with global developmental delay or idiopathic intellectual disability. In a systematic review of the literature, van Karnebeek et al[8] reported a very high yield from the dysmorphological examination, ranging from 39% to 81% (Table 6-1). They reported the following methods: cytogenetics 9.5%, fragile X studies 2.0% (cytogenetic fragile X study yield of 5.4%), metabolic studies 1%, neurologic examination 42.9%, and neuroimaging studies 30% for abnormalities and 1.3% for an etiology. Approximately 5% of cases of global developmental delay are etiologically determined by clinically applied high-resolution standard karyotype and another 5% by fluorescent in situ hybridization (FISH) for subtelomere rearrangements.

There appears to be an additional 10% diagnostic yield from microarray comparative genomic hybridization (CGH) diagnostic studies of patients who have idiopathic intellectual disability and who have had normal karyotype and normal FISH for subtelomere abnormalities.[11,12] This is a significant advance for the diagnostic evaluation of children with global

Table 6-1. Clinical Use of Genetic Tests or Physical Examination for Global Developmental Delay or Intellectual Disability[a]

Clinical Test or Physical Examination	Diagnostic Rate (%)
History and physical exam	39–81
Neurologic exam	42
Microarray	20
Cytogenetics	9.5
Fluorescent in situ hybridization subtelomere study	5
Fragile X molecular study	2.0
Neuroimaging studies	1.3
Metabolic studies[b]	1

[a] Adapted from Van Karnebeek CDH, Janswiejer MCE, Leenders AGE, et al. Diagnostic investigations in individuals with mental retardation: a systematic literature review of their usefulness. *Eur J Human Genet.* 2005;13:2–65; Moeschler JB. Genetic evaluation of intellectual disability. *Semin Pediatr Neurol.* 2008;15:2–9; van Karnebeek CD, Stockler S. Treatable inborn errors of metabolism causing intellectual disability: a systematic literature review. *Mol Genet Metab.* 2012;105(3):368–381.
[b] Blood for amino acids, total homocysteine; urine for organic acids, creatine metabolites, glycosaminoglycans, oligosaccharides, purines, and pyrimidines.

developmental delay or intellectual disability, and may aid in the discovery of new syndromes and new genes that cause disability. The microarray CGH techniques will identify well-known syndromes such as Williams syndrome, velocardiofacial syndrome, and Angelman syndrome in those patients who would be positive on FISH testing and also will identify those patients with subtelomere imbalances identified on the FISH testing. It has also identified new syndromes not seen on standard karyotype or with FISH techniques. Consequently, all patients with global developmental delays or intellectual disability of unknown etiology should have microarray CGH diagnostic testing.[12] Recently a systematic review of the literature identified 51 inborn errors of metabolism that present with global developmental delay or intellectual disability, are identified by diagnostic tests that are readily available, and are amenable to medical treatment addressing the pathophysiology. Although the rate of diagnosis of inborn errors of metabolism seems to be low in this population, there seems to be improved outcomes resulting from medical treatments at relatively low cost for the testing.

Autism Spectrum Disorders

The AAP advocates the medical home as the site of surveillance and screening for ASDs among children aged 18 to 24 months.[13] The goal is to provide early support and services for those with an ASD in an effort to optimize outcomes. Autism spectrum disorders can be divided between those of no known cause (idiopathic) and those with an identifiable cause (secondary).[13,14] From 2% to 25% of ASD patients have an identifiable etiology after comprehensive medical genetics evaluation (ie, secondary ASD).[13,15,16] The benefits of an etiologic diagnosis for ASD build on the benefits of having a genetics evaluation in general (Box 6-4). All patients with a diagnosis of ASD require a comprehensive diagnostic evaluation, and in approximately 80% of patients that effort will not result with a known diagnosis. Nevertheless, there is benefit for the family and medical home in knowing that there is no medical treatment in addition to that provided by the medical home, special education professionals, and behavioral health specialists. The single most important test for a cause for ASD is the expertise of the medical home physician and the medical geneticist in taking a detailed, comprehensive history and physical examination.[8,17]

Significant dysmorphology (ie, minor anomalies not present in parents) is present in 25% of individuals with autism.[18] Macrocephaly (head circumference >98th percentile) is present in approximately 30% of children with autism[19]; microcephaly (head circumference <2nd percentile) occurs in 5% to 15% of children with ASD.[18–20] Seizures develop in approximately 25% of children with autism; more have nonspecific electroencephalogram changes.[21] The diagnostic evaluation process is based on the findings on history and physical examination with special attention paid to the neurologic

Box 6-4. Benefits of Medical Genetics Evaluation

- **For Patient**
  - Improved health outcomes
  - Improved health care and surveillance
  - Improved understanding of condition
  - Improved educational planning
  - End of unwarranted medical testing and treatments
- **For Families**
  - Understanding that comes from genetic counseling, including family planning discussion
  - Health care changes (for some)
  - Diagnostic testing for other family members, if warranted
  - Understanding of condition
  - Social support and peer networking

and dysmorphology findings (Box 6-5). Most medical geneticists have a stepwise or tiered approach to the evaluation based on history and examination[22] (Table 6-2 and 6-3).

Disorders of Growth

The primary care physician should consider referring patients with growth disorders, including either short stature or somatic overgrowth, because a genetic syndrome or condition should be considered. The purpose of the genetics evaluation of children with disordered growth is to provide an accurate diagnosis and information to the patient and family regarding natural history, prognosis, available treatment, genetic basis, and recurrence risk.[23]

Box 6-5. Key Findings on History and Examination in the Patient With Autism Spectrum Disorder

- **Positive family history in first-degree relatives or X-linked pattern**
- **Regressive course in development**
- **Macrocephaly**
- **Microcephaly**
- **Dysmorphology**
- **Skin findings**
  - Café au lait macules
  - Hypomelanotic macules
    - Or other cutaneous findings of tuberous sclerosis; penile freckling (with macrocephaly) in PTEN gene–related disorders
- **Abnormal somatic growth**
  - Short stature
  - Somatic overgrowth
- **Other**
  - Tone or coordination abnormalities
  - Delayed motor milestones
  - Gastrointestinal symptoms
  - Allergic history
  - Seizure disorder
  - Organomegaly
  - Signs of storage disorders ("coarse features")

Table 6-2. Diagnostic Studies in Autism Spectrum Disorder Based on Key Findings

Key Finding	Key Considerations
X-linked pedigree	• Fragile X testing • Urine guanidinoacetate and creatine for disorders of creatine synthesis and/or transport • X-linked intellectual disability genetic testing and *NLNG3, NLGN4, NRXN1* gene testing
Affected siblings	• None (see X-linked; nonspecific) • Rare autosomal recessive gene: *HOXA1*
Female gender	• Consider Rett syndrome genetic testing (*MECP2, CDKL5*)
Macrocephaly	• Sotos syndrome genetic testing • *PTEN*-associated disorders (Riley-Ruvalcaba-Bannayan syndrome), particularly in males with genital freckling • Consider brain MRI
Microcephaly	• Brain MRI • 7-dehydrocholestrol for Smith-Lemli-Opitz syndrome • Other "common metabolic tests"[a]
Dysmorphology	• Testing for specific suspected syndrome • Chromosome microarray
Short stature	• Testing for specific suspected syndrome • Chromosome microarray • Other common metabolic tests
Somatic overgrowth	• Fragile X testing • Sotos syndrome • *PTEN*-associated disorders testing
Dermatologic findings	• Neurofibromatosis, type 1 • Tuberous sclerosis • *PTEN*-associated conditions
Motor delays, tone and coordination disorders	• Metabolic screening • Brain MRI, MRS • Mitochondrial disorders
Seizure disorder	• Neurology consultation • Landau-Kleffner syndrome (overnight sleep EEG) • Metabolic testing[a]
Coarse features, organomegaly	• Metabolic testing[b]

Abbreviations: CGH, comparative genomic hybridization; EEG, electroencephalogram; MRI, magnetic resonance imaging; MRS, magnetic resonance spectroscopy.

[a] Blood for amino acids, ammonia, lactate, acylcarnitine profile, total homocysteine level, carbohydrate-deficient transferrin for congenital disorders of glycosylation; urine organic acids, creatine metabolites, glycosaminoglycans, oligosaccharides, purines, pyrimidines.

[b] Based on clinical signs and symptoms.

Table 6-3. Suggested Diagnostic Testing for Those With Autism Spectrum Disorder and No Key Findings[a]

Tiered Approach to the Diagnostic Evaluation	
Tier 1	History, dysmorphology exam, Wood lamp for TSC signs— • If specific signs, proceed to targeted testing to confirm or rule out Rule out hearing loss, congenital rubella, when appropriate. Metabolic testing • Urine organic acids, mucopolysaccharides • Serum lactate, ammonia, amino acids, acylcarnitine profile Fragile X testing Chromosome microarray
Tier 2	Brain MRI EEG Rett syndrome testing (*MECP2, CDKL5*) in girls 15q methylation for Angelman/Prader-Willi syndrome
Tier 3	Serum and urine uric acid levels • If increased production, HGPRT and PRPP synthetase superactivity testing • If decreased production, purine and pyrmidine panel Rare genetic conditions • *HOX1A, SHANK3, NRXN1, NLGN3, NLGN4* • *PTEN*, if macrocephaly present

Abbreviations: CGH, comparative genomic hybridization; EEG, electroencephalogram; HGPRT, hypoxanthine-guanine phosphoribosyltransferase; MRI, magnetic resonance imaging; PRPP, phosphoribosyl pyrophosphate; TSC, tuberous sclerosis.

[a] Adapted from Schaefer GB, Lutz RE. Diagnostic yield in the clinical genetics evaluation of autism spectrum disorders. *Genet Med.* 2006;8(9):549–556; Mendelsohn N, Schaefer GB. Genetic evaluation of autism. *Semin Pediatr Neurol.* 2008;15:27–31; Lintas C, Persico AM. Autistic phenotypes and genetic testing: state-of-the-art for the clinical geneticist. *J Med Genet.* 2009;46;1–8.

Short Stature

Short stature is a common condition managed within the medical home and often comanaged with a pediatric endocrinologist. Those patients with disproportionate short stature, major or minor anomalies (dysmorphology), or developmental delays in association with the short stature are the specific patients who most need a medical genetics referral (Box 6-6 and 6-7). Lam et al[24] reviewed a series of patients referred for short stature and reported that nearly half of the patients were considered to have either constitutional delay of growth or familial short stature. The most common genetic condition was from a chromosome abnormality, primarily Turner syndrome. In 3% of cases, a diagnosis of a recognized syndrome was made, and in nearly 2% a previously unrecognized endocrine cause was identified.

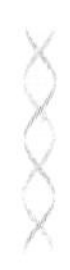

Box 6-6. Referring a Child With Short Stature

If a child has significant disproportionate short stature or if the following findings are present in a child with short stature, a referral to a geneticist is recommended.

- Presence of familial short stature in siblings, parents (X-linked pattern)
- Developmental delays
- Dysmorphology or major anomalies
- Special health care needs

Box 6-7. Evaluation of Short Stature, Proportionate and Disproportionate (Suggested Testing Modalities in Parentheses)

- **Proportionate**
  - Major and/or minor anomalies present
    - Recognizable syndromes including Turner syndrome (chromosome microarray and/or karyotype)
  - Major and/or minor anomalies absent
    - Constitutional delay (longitudinal follow-up)
    - Familial short stature (family data and longitudinal follow-up)
    - Endocrinopathy (endocrinologic evaluation)
    - Genetic short stature (*SHOX* gene mutation)
  - Developmental delay present
    - Recognizable syndromes (chromosome microarray)
- **Disproportionate**
  - Skeletal dysplasias (skeletal radiographs; diagnostic genetic testing)

For example, in the evaluation of a young girl with short stature the primary care pediatrician often will obtain a standard karyotype to rule out Turner syndrome. If Turner syndrome is the diagnosis, then comanagement among the primary care physician, medical geneticist, and pediatric endocrinologist optimizes the health care and outcomes. The evaluation process for the child with short stature is often dictated by local circumstances, including availability of consulting pediatric endocrinologists and medical geneticists, and the skills and interests of the primary care physician. In addition, many pediatric endocrinologists are especially skilled in recognizing and treating common genetic conditions presenting as short stature.

Tall Stature (Somatic Overgrowth)

Pediatrics has tended to focus more on short stature and its causes when, at least theoretically, the numbers of children with tall stature is equal to that of those with short stature. Tall stature is defined as height 2 standard deviations or more above the mean for age. An overgrowth disorder must also be suspected in children growing outside their target range (based on gender-corrected mid-parental height), or children with excessive growth velocity.[25] The study of overgrowth syndromes is rather recent compared with that of short stature.[26] While in short stature some international agreement has been reached on its diagnostic classification,[27] this is not the case for tall stature. It is common to classify tall stature as primary growth disorder, secondary growth disorder, and idiopathic tall stature.[28] Primary growth disorders are genetic conditions often with intrinsic defect in bone and/or connective tissue, growth is frequently disproportionate, and dysmorphic features are common. Secondary overgrowth refers to those conditions with endocrinopathies, many of which are genetic. Idiopathic tall stature particularly includes the group of constitutional or familial tall stature: normal variants in which one or both parents are tall, mean birth length is at or above the 75th percentile, and tall stature becomes evident at 3 to 4 years of age.[28] Idiopathic tall stature is the most common cause of tall stature.

The purpose of the comprehensive evaluation of the child with overgrowth is to ensure that the proper treatment is instituted and maintained. As with any diagnosis, the natural history can be discussed, including the need for surveillance for complications or special health care needs associated with the diagnosis. When appropriate, genetic counseling for the family and patient is important. The presence of an accurate diagnosis can assist with minimizing unnecessary medical testing and procedures. For those children with suspected idiopathic or constitutional tall stature or who have an accelerated growth rate, it is best to refer to a pediatric endocrinologist as a first step. Referral to a medical geneticist might best be done first for the patient with tall stature and presence of developmental delays or disability, major or minor malformations present (or dysmorphic features), positive family history of similar growth pattern, disproportionate growth, or presence of suspected syndrome (eg, Marfan syndrome) (Box 6-8). The presence of certain signs and symptoms allows the pediatrician to determine a possible genetic diagnosis (Table 6-4) and indicates that a referral to a medical geneticist may facilitate diagnosis and treatment. In addition, there are many endocrine disorders that are inherited or a part of a genetic syndrome that can be suspected on the basis of the medical history and dysmorphology examination (Table 6-5).

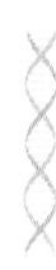

Box 6-8. Referring a Child With Tall Stature (Overgrowth)

If a child has significant disproportionate tall stature or if the following findings are present in a child with tall stature, a referral to a geneticist is recommended.

- Developmental delays or differences
- Dysmorphology (major or minor anomalies)
- Suspected syndrome (eg, Marfan syndrome)
- Family history of tall stature

Table 6-4. Common Overgrowth Syndromes by Symptom or Sign

Symptom or Sign	Syndrome	Gene or Karyotype
Developmental delay	Fragile X syndrome	*FMR1*
	Klinefelter syndrome	47,XXY
	Phelan-McDermid syndrome	22q13.3 deletion
	47,XXX "syndrome"	47,XXX
	Mosaic trisomy 8	+8 mosaicism
	Sotos syndrome	*NSD1*
	PTEN hamartoma tumor syndrome	*PTEN*
Dysmorphology	Beckwith-Wiedemann syndrome	11p15 uniparental disomy, *CDKN1C*, H19
	Sotos syndrome	*NSD1*
	Simpson-Golabi-Behmel syndrome	*GPC3*, *GPC4*
	Weaver syndrome	*NSD1*
	Perlman syndrome	
	Nevo syndrome (Ehlers-Danlos syndrome, kyphoscoliotic type)	*PLOD1*
	Marshall-Smith syndrome	
Disproportionate growth	Marfan syndrome	*FBN1*
	Klinefelter syndrome	47,XXY
	Homocystinuria	CBS
Other syndromes to consider	San Filippo syndrome (mucopolysaccharidosis, type IIIA, B, C, D)	Several genes
	Sclerosteosis	*SOST*

Table 6-5. Inherited Endocrinopathies by Symptoms[a]

Symptoms	Endocrinopathy	Genetic Syndromes	Gene(s)
Gigantism, acromegaly	↑ Growth hormone	McCune-Albright	*GNAS1*
		Carney complex, type 1	*PRKAR1A*
		Multiple endocrine neoplasia, type 1	*MEN1*
Precocious puberty	↑ Sex hormones (androgens, estrogens)	McCune Albright syndrome	*GNAS1*
		Congenital adrenal hyperplasia	*CYP11B1*
Hyperthyroidism	↑ Thyroid hormone	McCune-Albright syndrome	*GNAS1*
		PTEN hamartoma tumor syndrome	*PTEN*
Hypogonadism	Sex hormone resistance or ↓	XY gonadal dysgenesis	*DHH* *AR*
		Androgen insensitivity syndrome	*FGFR1*
		Kallman syndrome	
Hyperinsulism	Insulin ↑ or resistance	Beckwith-Wiedemann syndrome	*CDKN1C*, *H19*
		Simpson-Golabi-Behmel syndrome	*GPC3*, *GCP4*
Hyperglucocorticoidism	ACTH resistance	Familial glucocorticoid deficiency	*MC2-R*

Abbreviations: ↑, increased or elevated; ↓, decreased or reduced; ACTH, adrenocorticotropic hormone.
[a] Selected; after Kant et al 2005.

The Child With Major or Minor Anomalies (Dysmorphic Features)

There are occasions in pediatric primary care when the careful physical examination of a child finds minor physical anomalies in the absence of other concerns—no developmental or growth abnormalities. The question arises then about how to approach this best on behalf of the child and family. If the minor anomaly is noted by the pediatrician and the parent is unconcerned, the pediatrician should explore this lack of concern, and explain the finding or refer to a medical geneticist who can do so. Often the question is put to the medical geneticist—"Should I refer my patient

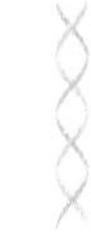

with [minor anomaly] to you?" or "I have a patient who is dysmorphic [sic]. Should I refer her to you?" How this is addressed is often based on the local relationships between the medical home and consulting medical geneticist. The purpose of the medical genetic consultation in this setting is to address whether the findings noted by the pediatrician might indicate a genetic condition, place the child at risk for special health care needs, or explain known existing conditions or needs. In addition, there are minor findings that might be considered insignificant in the individual child but are a minimal expression of an inherited malformation and have implications for parental genetic counseling. Several associated problems to consider are shown in Box 6-9. For example, a bifid uvula in a child with multiple ear infections might be a minimal expression of a cleft palate syndrome or a chromosome deletion disorder such as 22q11 deletion (or velocardiofacial syndrome). It is the role of the pediatrician to identify patients with minor anomalies (see Chapter 8) who warrant referral to the medical geneticist.

Recently a group of specialists in dysmorphology published a series of 6 articles that "initiated the standardization of terms to describe human morphology."[29] These authors chose to begin with developing a common terminology for the cranium, the face and its features, and the hands and feet—the parts of the body that are often used in dysmorphology to describe patients and delineate syndromes. Syndromes are typically diagnosed by various combinations of features and, therefore, differential diagnoses of single features are of limited use. There are textbooks (eg, Jones[30]) and databases (eg, London Dysmorphology Databases[31]; POSSUM Web version[32]) of medical dysmorphology for this information. It is the role of the pediatrician to identify those patients with minor anomalies (see Chapter 8) and determine whether they have additional features that warrant referral to the medical geneticist. If such patients have any of these factors, a referral to a medical geneticist should strongly be considered.

Box 6-9. Referral of Patients With Dysmorphic Features

Refer if the following are present:

- Developmental delays
- Abnormal growth
- Organ dysfunction or chronic illness
- Concern that genetic syndrome might be present

Key Points

The medical home and the consulting medical genetics team working together can optimize the health care and outcomes for those patients who present with

- Developmental delays, intellectual disability
- Autism spectrum disorders
- Disorders of growth (short stature and tall stature)
- Dysmorphic features

Care is best when there is a tight link between the medical home and consulting medical geneticist, and when there is explicit understanding of the roles of each in the comanagement of patients with genetic conditions.

References

1. Antonelli R, Antonelli D. Providing a medical home: the cost of care coordination services in a community-based, general pediatric practice. *Pediatrics.* 2004;S113(5S):1522–1528
2. Cooley WC, McAllister JW. Building medical homes: improvement strategies in primary care for children with special health care needs. *Pediatrics.* 2004;113(5S):1499–1506
3. McGrath RJ, Laflamme DJ, Schwartz AP, et al. Access to genetic counseling for children with autism, Down syndrome, and intellectual disabilities. *Pediatrics.* 2009;124S:449
4. Shevell M, Ashwal S, Donley D, et al. Practice parameter evaluation of the child with global developmental delay—report of the Quality Standards Subcommittee of the American Academy of Neurology and the Practice Committee of the Child Neurology Society. *Neurology.* 2003;60:367–380
5. Moeschler JB, Shevell MI; American Academy of Pediatrics Committee on Genetics. Clinical genetic evaluation of the child with mental retardation or developmental delays. *Pediatrics.* 2006;117:2304–2316
6. Moeschler JB. Genetic evaluation of intellectual disability. *Semin Pediatr Neurol.* 2008;15:2–9
7. Schaefer GB, Bodensteiner JB. Evaluation of the child with idiopathic mental retardation. *Pediatr Clin North Am.* 1992;39:929–943
8. van Karnebeek CDH, Jansweijer MCE, Leenders AGE, et al. Diagnostic investigations in individuals with mental retardation: a systematic literature review of their usefulness. *Eur J Human Genet.* 2005;13:2–65
9. American Academy of Pediatrics Council on Children With Disabilities, Section on Developmental Behavioral Pediatrics, Bright Futures Steering Committee, Medical Home Initiatives for Children With Special Needs Project Advisory Committee. Identifying infants and young children with developmental disorders in the medical home: an algorithm for developmental surveillance and screening. *Pediatrics.* 2006;118:405–420
10. Curry CJ, Stevenson RE, Aughton D, et al. Evaluation of mental retardation: recommendations of a consensus conference—American College of Medical Genetics. *Am J Med Genet.* 1997;72:468–477
11. Manning M, Hudgins L; Professional Practice and Guidelines Committee of the American College of Medical Genetics. Array-based technology and recommendations

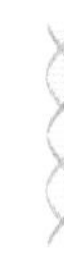

for utilization in medical genetics practice for detection of chromosomal abnormalities. *Genetic Med.* 2010;12(11):742–745

12. Miller DT, Adam MP, Aradhya S, et al. Consensus statement: chromosomal microarray is a first-tier clinical diagnostic test for individuals with developmental disabilities or congenital anomalies. *Am J Hum Genet.* 2010;14;86(5):749–764
13. Johnson CP, Myers SM; American Academy of Pediatrics Council on Children With Disabilities. Identification and evaluation of children with autism spectrum disorders. *Pediatrics.* 2007;120(5):1183–1215
14. Filipek PA, Accardo PJ, Ashwal S, et al. Practice parameter: screening and diagnosis of autism: report of the Quality Standards Subcommittee of the American Academy of Neurology and the Child Neurology Society. *Neurology.* 2000;55:468–479
15. Battaglia A, Carey JC. Etiologic yield of autistic spectrum disorders: a prospective study. *Am J Med Genet C Semin Med Genet.* 2006;142:3–7
16. Schaefer GB, Lutz RE. Diagnostic yield in the clinical genetics evaluation of autism spectrum disorders. *Genet Med.* 2006;8(9):549–556
17. Mendelsohn N, Schaefer GB. Genetic evaluation of autism. *Semin Pediatr Neurol.* 2008;15:27–31
18. Miles JH, Hillman RE. Value of a clinical morphology examination in autism. *Am J Med Genet.* 2000;91:245–253
19. Miles JH, Hadden LL, Takahashi TN, et al. Head circumference is an independent clinical finding associated with autism. *Am J Med Genet.* 2000;95:339–350
20. Fombonne E, Roge B, Claverie J, et al. Microcephaly and macrocephaly in autism. *J Autism Dev Disord.* 1999;29:113–119
21. Tuchman R, Rapin I. Epilepsy in autism. *Lancet Neurol.* 2002;1:352–358
22. Schaefer GB, Mendelsohn NJ; Professional Practice and Guidelines Committee. Clinical genetics evaluation in identifying the etiology of autism spectrum disorders. *Genet Med.* 2008;10(4):301–305. Erratum in: *Genet Med.* 2008;10(6):464
23. Seaver LH, Irons M. ACMG practice guideline: genetic evaluation of short stature. American College of Medical Genetics (ACMG) Professional Practice and Guidelines Committee. *Genet Med.* 2009;11(6):465–470. Erratum in: *Genet Med.* 2009;11(10):765
24. Lam WFF, Hau WLK, Lam TSS. Evaluation of referrals for genetic investigation of short stature in Hong Kong. *Chin Med J.* 2002;115:94:607–611
25. Kant SG, Wit JM, Breuning MH. Genetic analysis of short stature. *Horm Res.* 2003;60:157–165
26. Cohen MM Jr. Overgrowth syndromes: an update. *Adv Pediatr.* 1999;46:441–491
27. Ranke MB. Towards a consensus on the definition of idiopathic short stature. *Horm Res.* 1996;45(suppl 2):64–66
28. Drop SL, Greggio N, Cappa M, et al. International Workshop on Management of Puberty for Optimum Auxological Results. Current concepts in tall stature and overgrowth syndromes. *J Pediatr Endocrinol Metab.* 2001;14(suppl 2):975–984
29. Allanson JE, Biesecker LG, Carey JC, et al. Elements of morphology: introduction. *Am J Med Genet.* 2009;149A(1):2–5
30. Jones KL. *Smith's Recognizable Patterns of Human Malformation.* 6th ed. Philadelphia, PA: Elsevier Saunders; 2005
31. London Medical Databases. http://www.lmdatabases.com/index.html. Accessed January 6, 2010
32. POSSUM Web. http://www.possum.net.au/. Accessed January 6, 2010

Chapter 7

Recognizing Inborn Errors of Metabolism

Carol L. Greene, MD

Introduction

Inborn errors of metabolism (IEM) collectively affect more than 1 per 1,000 individuals, by conservative estimates. These errors can present at any age and affect any organ system. Failure to suspect and diagnose the inborn errors leads to lost opportunities for intervention, possibly resulting in harm to the child and family. Appropriately integrating approaches to diagnosing IEM in pediatric practice yields some of the highest benefits in medicine (Box 7-1).

Understanding basic principles, presentations, and approaches to IEM will increase the likelihood of prompt recognition, diagnosis, and appropriate management for your patient and their families.

Defining IEM: Basic Principles, Types, and Pathophysiology

Inborn errors in metabolism are conditions in which a change in a gene alters function of a protein with enzyme, transport, or other activity, causing alteration in a metabolic pathway that leads to clinical consequences. A block in a pathway can lead to the increase of a compound normally present but toxic in excess (eg, ammonia or methylmalonic acid), inadequate levels of some essential metabolic product (eg, glucose, or ATP for energy), or production via an alternative pathway of a toxic compound that is not normally present (Figure 7-1).

Box 7-1. Case Report

A baby is brought to the primary care physician (PCP) at the age of 3 months, with reports of irritability and frequent spit-up. A diagnosis of reflux is made, and treatment measures are somewhat helpful. Weight gain slows over the next few months. At 9 months the PCP notes inadequate developmental progress. Further evaluation over the next 8 months involves multiple invasive studies, and eventually a combination of urine and blood studies reveals a diagnosis of methylmalonic acidemia. The condition is autosomal recessive; therefore, the 2-month-old sibling should be tested. Results reveal the infant is also affected.

Some children with methylmalonic acidemia respond to B_{12} therapy. Fortunately, the now 17-month-old patient is responsive to treatment that prevents further brain damage. However, the patient will have permanent brain damage that could have been prevented if the diagnosis had been made at 4 months of age. The 2-month-old sibling benefits from earlier treatment.

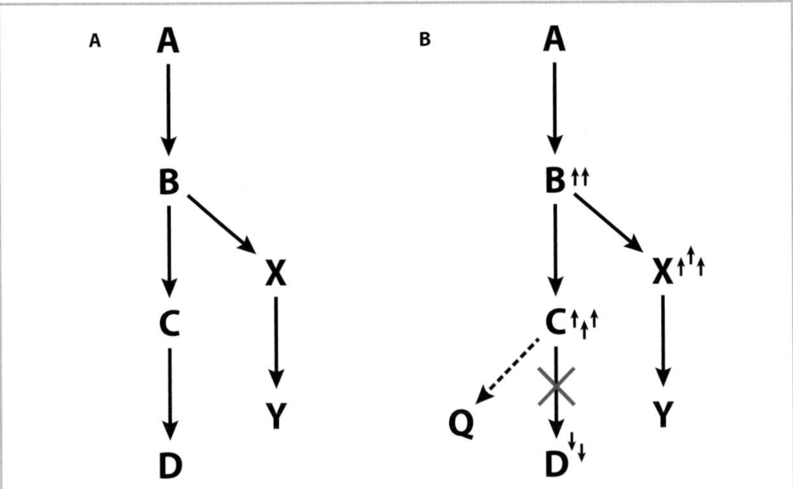

Figure 7-1. A. Normal pathway. Relative activity of various enzymes may be constant or may vary (eg, fasting vs fed for biochemistry of energy). **B.** Inborn error with altered levels of metabolites and activation of alternate path to metabolite (Q) not normally seen.

Some categories of IEM are identified by the types of molecules involved and some by the organelle into which certain metabolism is compartmentalized. Some involve small molecules and some involve very large molecules. In many categories there is more than one kind of pathophysiology. The primary metabolic defects range from simple catalytic failure of an enzyme, failure of post-translational modification of multiple enzymes and other proteins, failure to transport enzyme to appropriate metabolic compartment, failure of production or activation of a cofactor essential for enzyme activity, or complete failure to build a cellular compartment.

Any system of categorization is imperfect. For example, pyruvate carboxylase deficiency is here categorized as an inborn error of mitochondrial energy metabolism. However, pyruvate carboxylase deficiency may also be part of multiple carboxylase deficiency or biotinidase deficiency, and in that case is found together with abnormalities of other enzymes that are clearly inborn errors of organic acid metabolism. Other important examples are the disorders of cobalamin (B_{12}) metabolism that can cause either altered metabolism of methylmalonic acid (organic acidemia) or homocysteine (amino acidopathy) or both, depending on the step in the cobalamin pathway that is altered. Maple syrup urine disease (MSUD) can be classified as an amino acid disorder or organic acidemia depending on what aspect of the biochemistry is considered. No attempt is made to categorize certain biochemical conditions, such as glucose transporter defect (a cause of seizures) and α-1-antitrypsin deficiency (cause of liver disease in children) that do not fit into any biochemical model of categorization, but they are included as appropriate in the recommendations for evaluation of clinical presentation. However, certain biochemical conditions that are traditionally covered elsewhere are not included here, such as the inborn errors of steroid metabolism (eg, congenital adrenal hyperplasia) and the albinisms, though some of the latter conditions are lysosomal disorders and others are abnormalities of metabolism of tyrosine. Table 7-1 provides a practical classification for consideration of pathophysiology and presentation and for use in directing first steps in consideration of the differential diagnosis and evaluation. Inheritance is typically autosomal recessive (with some X-linked and a few autosomal dominant conditions) and maternal inheritance for some cases of mitochondrial disease.

When to Suspect IEM

The primary care physician (PCP) routinely evaluates for IEM in every healthy baby through newborn screening. (See Chapter 17.) Newborn screening is designed solely to identify neonates who need evaluation for specific conditions, and a normal newborn screen does not conclusively

Table 7-1. Categories of Inborn Errors of Metabolism

Category—Definition, Biochemistry, Genetics	Key Characteristics and Examples
Aminoacidopathies	
Involves abnormal levels of amino acids with the amino group still attached; includes primary catalytic defects, cofactor defects, transport defects. (Note: MSUD may be categorized here since amino acid levels are elevated in blood.) Almost all are autosomal recessive.	Usually not acidotic (except MSUD, or with the renal tubular acidosis of tyrosinemia). Typically but not always affects CNS (eg, PKU, glycine encephalopathy), may affect other organs (eg, liver and renal tubules in tyrosinemia type 1). Episodic, static or progressive. Homocystinuria may present with stroke or clotting, with or without intellectual disability. Diagnosis with PAA, sometimes UAA, sometimes confirm by enzyme assay and/or DNA. Special presentation—When the mother has PKU or hyperphenylalaninemia, she may be normal and unaware of diagnosis but have babies with microcephaly and intellectual disability; this has nearly 100% recurrence risk and adverse outcome is preventable with treatment of mother; diagnose it by plasma amino acids in mother.
Organic Acidemias	
Involves metabolites of amino acids after amino group removed and other compounds with C, H, and O (fatty acids and lactate/energy in separate categories). Essentially all are autosomal recessive.	Usually but not always acidotic, anorexia/vomiting; episodic altered consciousness; may include bone marrow depression or other end-organ failure. Diagnosis with urine organic acids; blood acylcarnitine profile may be helpful, enzyme assays or DNA for confirmation when available.
Urea Cycle Defects	
Involves the urea cycle, typically with altered levels of the amino acids in the urea cycle. Most are autosomal recessive but the most common is X-linked.	Altered mental status, decreased appetite or intractable or recurrent emesis including "cyclic vomiting," migraine, ataxia, and often with protein aversion. Typically not acidotic unless in shock; respiratory alkalosis is common. Diagnosis by PAA, in some cases confirmed with enzyme assays and/or DNA.
Fatty Acid Oxidation and Carnitine Metabolism Disorders	
Involves the oxidation of fatty acids to ketones and the transport of fatty acids into the mitochondrion for oxidation. Essentially all are autosomal recessive.	Classic presentation is Reye syndrome or SIDS in an infant or toddler, but more commonly the presentation is excessive irritability or lethargy with ordinary childhood illness or extended fasting. The hallmark is hypoketosis, but some ketones are usually present, and hypoglycemia is only sometimes present. Also may present with liver failure, FTT, cardiomyopathy, and/or rhabdomyolysis; retinopathy and bone marrow failure may occur. Diagnose with acylcarnitine profile, but that may be normal when well, and diagnose some conditions with carnitine levels. Some diagnosis may be confirmed with enzyme assays and/or DNA.

Category—Definition, Biochemistry, Genetics	Key Characteristics and Examples
Mitochondrial (Energy) Metabolism and Disorders of Lactate and Pyruvate	
Includes oxidative phosphorylation defects of the mitochondrial respiratory chain, defects of the Krebs cycle and of PDH and pyruvate carboxylase. May be due to defects of single enzymes, of transport into the mitochondria (of enzymes or substrate), of cofactor synthesis (eg, coenzyme Q), of multiple enzymes due to mutations in mitochondrial DNA (mDNA), or of mDNA repair or synthesis. X-linked inheritance (PDH deficiency and some creatine disorders), autosomal dominant inheritance, and maternal inheritance due to mDNA mutations occur; but most conditions are autosomal recessive.	Any presentation, any age, with variability in biochemical findings and clinical presentation. Examples include dysmorphic features with brain dysgenesis or porencephalic cysts; the normally formed neonate with overwhelming acidosis; Leigh syndrome (an infantile or childhood onset brain stem neurodegenerative disease); isolated organ failure of heart, liver, renal, diabetes, exocrine pancreas; bone marrow, retina, or others; and combinations (eg, Pearson syndrome [bone marrow and exocrine pancreatic failure]); or multisystem failure. Other classic pediatric conditions are MELAS, MERRF, and Alpers syndrome (progressive seizures and liver failure). Diagnostic testing depends on presentation; usually begin with PAA and UOA, lactate and pyruvate, and ACP, but in some cases first diagnostic testing is DNA in blood or biopsy of muscle or liver for histochemistry or enzyme assays. It is well described that enzyme assays or DNA can be normal in cases with proven disease.
Carbohydrate Disorders	
Involving metabolism of sugars (with glycogen storage disorders separated out); examples are galactosemia and the disorders of fructose metabolism. Essentially all are autosomal recessive.	Typically presenting with liver disease and/or hypoglycemia and acidosis, often with renal tubular disease. Cataracts may be seen in galactosemia at presentation in some cases and develop in untreated cases. Diagnosis based on enzyme assay or DNA.
Glycogen Storage Disorders	
The various disorders of glycogen synthesis and degradation. When glycogen is not normally branched, there is adverse effect on liver. Most are autosomal recessive and some are X-linked.	Typically including hepatomegaly, 2 major presentations are seen, with hypoglycemia (eg, GSD type 1) or with muscle weakness with or without cardiomyopathy and rhabdomyolysis (Pompe disease, McArdle disease). Some conditions lead to liver failure or liver tumors. However, glycogen synthase deficiency is "GSD type 0" and presents as ketotic hypoglycemia with a small liver. Diagnosis by histology, enzyme assay, DNA for some conditions.

Table 7-1. Categories of Inborn Errors of Metabolism *(continued)*

Category—Definition, Biochemistry, Genetics	Key Characteristics and Examples
Porphyrias	
Disorders of metabolism of the porphyrins in synthesis or degradation of hemoglobins. AIP is autosomal dominant, others are recessive or X-linked.	Most cases present in late childhood or adolescence, with or without skin findings, but some types present in the neonate. CNS is typically spared but AIP and hepatic coproporphyria can present with psychotic episodes, recurrent abdominal pain, and peripheral neuropathy, often diagnosed as psychosomatic disease. Diagnosis biochemistry, enzyme assay, DNA for some conditions
Lysosomal Storage Diseases	
Disorders due to alteration of function of individual enzymes responsible for breaking down large cell wall molecules (mucopolysaccharides, glycolipids, sphingolipids) within the lysosome, or of import into the lysosome affecting multiple pathways. Most are autosomal recessive, and Hunter syndrome and Fabry disease are X-linked.	Progressive disorders that until recently were untreatable. Some affect the CNS only (Krabbe disease), while others also have organomegaly (Tay Sachs), dysmorphic features, and skeletal changes (the mucopolysaccharidoses, except for Sanfilippo syndrome that affects primarily CNS). Cystinosis affects bone by causing renal tubular disease. Hepatosplenomegaly of Gaucher disease leads to preventable anemia and thrombocytopenia. Fabry disease is especially underdiagnosed, and untreated it causes renal failure (typically in early or mid-adulthood), cardiomyopathy, strokes, and pain from peripheral neuropathy; enzyme infusion prevents permanent damage. Diagnose by biochemistry (eg, urine MPS or oligosaccharides in some), enzyme assay, DNA for some conditions, and carrier testing available for some conditions.
Peroxisomal Disorders	
Disorders of individual enzymes in the peroxisome involved in various pathways, including very-long-chain fatty acid oxidation and plasmalogen synthesis, or defects of peroxisome development leading to multiple pathway dysfunction.	A wide variety of presentations, including the neurodegenerative condition adrenoleukodystrophy or isolated primary adrenal failure. May present as a dysmorphic syndrome, Zellweger syndrome, with Down syndrome–like face, hypotonia, liver and renal cysts, and progressive neurodegenerative disease. Most have alteration of either very-long-chain fatty acids, plasmalogens, or pipecolic acid and some have stippled epiphyses on plain film. Diagnose with histology, biochemistry; DNA in some conditions.
Disorders of Purines and Pyrimidines	
Disorders of synthesis or degradation, includes disorders of uric acid metabolism. Autosomal recessive or X-linked.	Variable presentation, mostly affecting the CNS and/or the bone marrow (eg, severe combined immunodeficiency). Includes Lesch-Nyhan disease, with self-mutilation; the same enzyme defect in milder cases causes gout. Diagnose with biochemistry; DNA in some conditions.

Category—Definition, Biochemistry, Genetics	Key Characteristics and Examples
Neurotransmitter Disorders (and Other Conditions Evident Only on Analysis of CSF)	
These are conditions in which critical neuro-active molecules are not properly synthesized or metabolized. Includes a number of conditions in which cofactor metabolism is the primary problem, including B_6-responsive seizures and disorders of pterin metabolism. Most are autosomal recessive.	By definition, these are conditions that affect function of the nervous system, central and/or peripheral. Typical presentations include seizures, irritability, or other altered mental status, and abnormalities of tone and development. Indirect evidence may be present (eg, low prolactin in blood resulting from low dopamine, or response to pyridoxine trial), but in general, collection and handling of spinal fluid requires special precautions for diagnosis. Diagnosis by biochemistry of spinal fluid, some can be confirmed with enzyme assay, DNA.
Disorders of Metals and Micronutrients	
Conditions that involve altered metabolism of metals, and some micronutrients including iron, copper, and molybdenum; they can involve excess storage or inability to incorporate metal into enzymes, for which it is a critical component. Recessive or X-linked and in some forms of hemochromatosis complex with asymptomatic homozygotes and symptomatic heterozygotes.	Disorders of copper include Menkes disease (neonatal seizures with unusual hair) and Wilson disease (progressive CNS and/or liver disease). Disorders of iron in pediatrics include neonatal hemochromatosis, presenting with liver disease, or rare late childhood presentation of classic hemochromatosis, causing initial nonspecific symptoms resulting in arthritis and/or single or multi-organ failure (typically liver, heart, and/or diabetes). This list does not attempt to consider the primary disorders of molybdenum, zinc, and other micronutrients. Diagnose with metal levels, other biochemistry, histology, and histochemistry; DNA in some conditions.
Disorders of Connective Tissue (Collagen, Fibrillin, Elastin)	
Not to be mistaken for the term "connective tissue disorder" meaning autoimmune disorders, these are typically disorders of structural proteins that affect the integrity of the connective tissue of selected or all organs. Recessive, dominant, or X-linked.	Usually considered in general genetics. Abnormal collagen may primarily affect bones causing osteogenesis imperfecta (with or without dental and hearing problems) or may affect joints and skin, with some causing rupture of vessels or hollow organs. Fibrillin mutations cause Marfan syndrome, and elastin mutations cause Williams syndrome. Diagnose by clinical evaluation, in some cases confirm by DNA or by biochemistry of the altered molecule in tissue.

Table 7-1. Categories of Inborn Errors of Metabolism *(continued)*

Category—Definition, Biochemistry, Genetics	Key Characteristics and Examples
Carbohydrate-Deficient Glycoprotein Disorders	
Disorders that involve multiple biochemical pathways because the primary disorder is a failure of one or more enzymes that attach carbohydrate moieties to proteins (including enzymes) required for correct structure and function. Most are autosomal recessive.	As a group, there are now more than 30 conditions identified with highly varied presentation, including conditions with dysmorphic features and malformations evident in the neonate, and others that present only much later; the classic "type 1A" has cerebellar hypoplasia. Often with involvement of the CNS and peripheral nervous system, and includes some primary muscular dystrophies. Some have acute episodes of metabolic crisis or organ failure and many have FTT. Diagnose by examination in blood for altered pattern of carbohydrates attached to various proteins, some can be confirmed by DNA.
Channelopathies	
Altered transport of ions across cell walls, including especially calcium. The classic disorder of transport, cystic fibrosis, is not typically considered an inborn error of metabolism but does fit the category. Recessive, dominant, or X-linked.	Leaving aside cystic fibrosis, the 2 major presentations of conditions in this category are neurologic (progressive ataxias, seizures, including heritable febrile seizures or progressive seizure disorders) or cardiac arrhythmias (including classic long QT syndrome). Typically without acidosis or altered organ function except for the primary presentation. Diagnosis clinical, confirmed in some cases by DNA.
Disorders of Cholesterol and Other Sterol Metabolism (Primarily Synthesis)	
Alteration in the synthesis of cholesterol and other sterols, pathophsyiology may be due to inadequate amounts of an essential metabolite, or interference from the abnormal metabolites. Typically autosomal recessive.	Presenting with FTT and neurologic disease, this category includes a previously well-described autosomal recessive dysmorphic syndrome (Smith-Lemli-Opitz syndrome). These disorders typically include feeding disturbance and hypotonia, and may have skin pigment abnormalities. Diagnosis by biochemistry; cholesterol may be low, but diagnosis depends on demonstration of abnormal patterns of sterols, some may be confirmed with DNA.

Abbreviations: ACP, acylcarnitine profile; AIP, acute intermittent porphyria; CNS, central nervous system; FTT, failure to thrive; GSD, glycogen storage disorder; MELAS, mitochondrial encephalomyopathy, lactic acidosis, and stroke-like episodes; MERRF, myoclonic epilepsy, ragged red fibers; MPS, mucopolysaccharidoses; MSUD, maple syrup urine disease; PAA, plasma amino acids; PDH, pyruvate dehydrogenase; PKU, phenylketonuria; SIDS, sudden infant death syndrome; UAA, urine amino acids; UOA, urine organic acids.

exclude IEM. Physicians should maintain a high index of suspicion for an IEM, because even expanded newborn screening detects only a fraction of known IEM.

Another critical point to remember in considering a diagnosis of an IEM is that finding evidence of one condition, such as infection, does not exclude the presence of an IEM. For example, the child with a fatty acid oxidation disorder may present with acute metabolic crisis as a result of an otitis or respiratory syncytial virus (RSV); the child may be easily diagnosed with the otitis or the RSV, but neither typically will cause or should be assumed to explain altered mental status and abnormal liver function. Even documentation of shaken baby syndrome or other non-accidental trauma does not exclude diagnosis of IEM, as infants with underlying medical or developmental problems are at increased risk of abuse. In addition, some IEMs present with signs easily mistaken for non-accidental trauma, such as the retinal and brain hemorrhages seen in glutaric acidemia type I.

An IEM can cause virtually any symptom or sign, and can present at any age. These diseases may be static, or may cause intermittent or progressive signs and symptoms. They may present commonly with intellectual disability, failure to thrive, and symptoms of septicemia. Symptoms that should particularly raise suspicion of an IEM are listed in Box 7-2.

History and Physical Examination

When taking the history, be sure to ask about tolerance of exercise and of typically mild childhood illnesses. Poor tolerance to exercise or to typical mild childhood illnesses can be an important clue to consider IEM. Also ask if there is any association of symptoms with changes in diet, or if there are any unusual diet cravings or aversions. In addition to noting the presence of any symptoms listed in the red flag symptoms (Box 7-2), be aware that IEM is more likely when there are problems in more than one organ or system, even if there appears to be a simple explanation for the problems.

The physical signs that should particularly raise suspicion of an IEM include those listed in Box 7-3. Measure head circumference even in the older child or adolescent, and examine for unusual texture of hair or unusual rashes. Pay careful attention to movement. The PCP should pay careful attention

Box 7-2. Symptoms That Raise Suspicion of an Inborn Error of Metabolism

- Altered consciousness, especially recurrent episodes of mental status abnormal out of proportion to physical health (eg, lethargy without hypoxia, shock, or meningitis); this includes altered behavior such as episodic irritability or inattention
- Seizures in the first day of life, intractable seizures
- Ataxia, especially recurrent, and any other movement disorder, especially dystonia
- Exercise intolerance with pain or fatigue that interferes with reasonable activity
- Regression in neurologic function, development, or behavior, including regressive autism
- Unusual diet preferences or avoidances (eg, avoidance of protein or of certain sugars), and especially when intermittent or progressive symptoms or signs follow a diet change (eg, from breast milk to formula, or introduction of sugars)
- Specific odors (maple syrup, "sweaty feet," "cat's urine," "mousy," rotten fish) suggest specific disorders, and the fruity smell of ketosis occurs in a number of conditions
- Recurrent or persistent pain, including headaches, abdominal pain, pain in extremities
- Sun aversion or sensitivity, heat intolerance
- Family history of consanguinity or of a relative with any symptom or sign seen in inborn errors of metabolism (Be aware that since most of the conditions are autosomal recessive, waiting for positive family history guarantees you will miss the opportunity to diagnose the index case in most families.)

Box 7-3. Physical Signs That Raise Suspicion of an Inborn Error of Metabolism

- Unusual tone—hypertonia in the neonate or hypotonia after 1 year (and certainly after 2 years) of age, and mixed tone
- Movement disorders (watch carefully over at least a few minutes to see if the baby can be still for more than seconds)
- Areflexia
- Decreased muscle mass or muscle quality
- Organomegaly
- Micro- or macrocephaly
- Odors
- Cataracts and retinopathy
- Coarse features
- Widening of joints, kyphosis, joint contractures
- Coarse or otherwise unusual hair, unusually thick skin, unusual rashes, including sun sensitivity

to the eyes—assessing for cloudiness or haziness—and consider an ophthalmologic evaluation to assess for the presence of these signs in the lens, cornea, or retina.

A short list of results of routine investigations, including laboratory studies that should particularly raise suspicion of an IEM, include those listed in Box 7-4. Basic laboratory testing for IEM can be accomplished with little added cost for the patient with acute or chronic neurodevelopmental or health problems by starting with complete blood cell count (CBC), electrolytes, liver enzymes, and urinalysis in almost all cases, and proper use of blood amino acids, urine organic acid studies, and acylcarnitine profile, as well as total and free carnitine and properly collected ammonia and lactate levels where appropriate.

In assessing for an IEM, the anion gap and the mean corpuscular volume (MCV) may provide important clues for metabolic acidosis and unexpected anemia, respectively. Consider whether urine ketones are appropriate for

Box 7-4. Results That Raise Suspicion of an Inborn Error of Metabolism

- Acidosis out of proportion to clinical status, especially but not exclusively high anion gap acidosis
- Alkalosis (suspect hyperammonemia)
- Low blood urea nitrogen (may indicate inability to make urea via the urea cycle)
- Hyperammonemia (can only be seen if ammonia is measured)
- Inappropriate ketosis—ketones positive in the neonate or the non-fasting older child, or ketones less than 80 mg/dL (large) in the infant or child who has extended fast or hypoglycemia
- Single or multiple failure of bone marrow cell lines and macrocytosis (seen in disorders of energy metabolism, B_{12} and folate metabolism, and purine/pyrimidine disorders)
- Liver dysfunction
- Pancreatitis
- Cardiomyopathy, especially hypertrophic and arrhythmogenic right ventricular dysplasia
- Hypsarrhythmia in neonate, triphasic waves, or any elecroencephalogram described as having abnormal background
- White matter disease, including stroke and periventricular leukomalacia in the absence of clear history of asphyxia or clot
- Routine x-ray with rickets with normal vitamin D, or stippled epiphyses or dysostosis

the child's medical status. Some test results depend on the status of the patient, so biochemical samples collected while acutely symptomatic may be diagnostic while samples for the same study collected in between episodes may be normal. This is especially true for some disorders of organic acids, amino acids, urea cycle, mitochondrial conditions, fatty acid oxidation, and some porphyrias. Therefore, diagnostic samples should be collected promptly on presentation of a symptomatic child. Normal results can only exclude a diagnosis if the sample was collected under appropriate circumstances. Artifacts of sample collection are particularly problematic for some tests, most particularly lactate and ammonia. See Table 7-2 for details.

Table 7-2. Routine Metabolic Testing

Electrolytes	Be sure to calculate anion gap (elevated in organic acidemias) and remember that RTA can be a result of IEM.
CBC	Be sure to examine MCV and remember that anemia (especially macrocytic) and/or hypoplasia of any cell line can be due to IEM.
Glucose	Hypoglycemia in a previously healthy toddler or older child with normal growth could be due to acute onset endocrine disease (eg, from tumor), but IEMs (especially due to disorders of fatty acid metabolism) are more common. MCADD alone affects approximately 1/10,000 white infants. Normal glucose does not exclude IEM, and it is critical to note that except for management of some glycogen storage diseases, the glucose level does not guide management. In particular, patients with MCADD have died with normal glucose levels.
Liver functions	Especially consider IEM if there is evidence of liver dysfunction without evidence for inflammation; consider IEM in cholestasis, and remember that PT is a true "liver function." Abnormal PT and hyperammonemia before complete liver failure is highly suggestive of IEM.
UA	Ketones and pH are both relevant to IEM. Ketones should be negative in the first days of life and in anyone who is not fasting/catabolic. Certain metabolites of IEM (eg, methylmalonic acid, propionic acid, and others) are keto-acids and will give positive "ketones" on UA, providing a clue to IEM. In addition, after the first days of life, the state of fasting/catabolism should lead to ketosis in the biochemically normal individual, so negative or inappropriately low ketones should be a clue to IEM, in particular disorders of fatty acid oxidation. Urine pH in association with electrolytes may be clue to RTA that can be due to a number of IEMs.

Ammonia Typically green top tube (do NOT use ammonia heparin tube), free-flowing and placed on ice and hand-carry to lab. However, each institution's lab has specific instructions.	Hyperammonemia is not evident on physical examination. Most accurate if collected without a tourniquet and couriered immediately to lab on ice as levels rise in the test tube until the sample is spun. Levels near or above 200 µmol/L (sometimes 150 µmol/L) cause brain cell dysfunction and may cause cerebral edema; brain damage is universal and typically irreversible after 3 days of ammonia greater than 200 µmol/L. Urea cycle defects may cause levels in the thousands of micromoles per liter. Hyperammonemia is an emergency; dialysis may be needed urgently, and specific drugs are available for "chemical dialysis." While ideally collected properly, if an inappropriately collected level is normal it excludes hyperammonemia as cause of coma, if it is markedly elevated it is unlikely to be artifact, and if it is mildly elevated an immediate repeat sample collected properly should clarify the situation, as ammonia does not change rapidly without specific therapy. The level of ammonia will not necessarily distinguish urea cycle defects from organic acidemias, although the latter are more often associated with metabolic acidosis and an elevated anion gap.
Lactate (and pyruvate) Ideally, special tube that hydrolyzes all protein, free-flowing and places on ice and hand-carry to lab. However, each lab has specific instructions.	Exquisitely sensitive to conditions of the patient and of the sample collection; lactate levels can change in minutes with changes in blood pressure and perfusion and with changes in IV glucose. Normal values are available for fasting and resting individuals. Nevertheless, lactate levels are useful in the emergency setting, and elevations out of proportion to clinical status may provide a clue to a wide variety of IEMs. Lactate to pyruvate ratio is altered in some patients with mitochondrial disease, in the same direction as the alteration of the ratio in hypoxia or hypoperfusion. Lactate levels should always be collected and handled properly.
Amino acids (PAA) Typically written PAA for plasma amino acids (green top), but some labs prefer serum (red or tiger top).	Labs that perform the test will have preference for either plasma or serum; however, if your sample is not of the preferred type, contact the biochemical lab directly as they will typically be able to analyze the sample. Lab will also typically be able to perform test on a sample smaller than that routinely requested for adults. Testing may also be done in some labs on filter paper. Amino acids can also be tested in other body fluids, most commonly urine and CSF, but in metabolic autopsy testing can be done on vitreous of the eye or on renal papilla. Amino acids are conserved (reabsorbed) in the kidney so that blood analysis is useful for most conditions, but urine amino acid analysis is key to diagnosis of conditions in which dysfunction of renal absorption of amino acids is the disorder.
OAs Typically written UOA for urine OA; typically a random sample.	Typically measured in urine as most organic acids are toxic compounds that are poorly reabsorbed by the renal tubule, but some labs can perform limited testing on blood in anuric patients. Labs can typically perform testing on small samples. For acutely ill patients, ideally collected at presentation before any therapies that affect metabolism.

Table 7-2. Routine Metabolic Testing *(continued)*

ACP Most laboratories request green top for plasma, some prefer serum (red or tiger top), and some can analyze filter paper.	This is an analysis of markers that indicate what compounds are bound to carnitine. This is NOT the same as a "carnitine profile." This is the preferred test for diagnosis of most disorders of fatty acid oxidation and is useful in many organic acidemias. For acutely ill patients, ideally collected at presentation before any therapies that affect metabolism. Often analyzed using the same methods that are used in newborn screening, but normal newborn screen does not substitute for ACP analysis in the symptomatic patient.
Carnitine total and free Most laboratories request green top for plasma, some prefer serum (red or tiger top), and some can analyze filer paper.	This is a measurement of the levels of free carnitine (that which is available for transport of fatty acids into the mitochondria) and of bound carnitine. It is NOT the same as ACP. It is particularly useful for diagnosis of disorders of carnitine transport, and is secondarily abnormal in many fatty acid oxidation disorders, OAs, and some nutritional states.
Neurotransmitters Typically CSF; requires special handling.	Some NTs can be measured in blood or urine, but certain conditions can only be identified by analysis of CSF. There is a rostro-caudal gradient of levels of the neurotransmitters in the CSF, and therefore in order to be interpretable, the laboratory requires that the sample for NTs be collected in special tubes available from the laboratory, and that the NT sample collection begin with the first drop of fluid—before measurement of pressure or collection of fluid for culture (the "special" tubes are also needed to prevent oxidation of some metabolites). CSF for NT therefore requires anticipation of collection and collaboration with appropriate specialists and with the local and the reference laboratories.
UMPS Spot urine typically requested, first morning sample is preferred but not required.	This is the test for MPS. In Hurler or Hunter syndrome and other dysmorphic conditions it can help to guide specific choice of enzyme or DNA testing. More controversial is the use of the test for screening patients with nonspecific developmental disability, including autism. However, the condition Sanfilippo syndrome is an MPS that has no coarse features for the first decade or more, and no skeletal problems; it presents as a nonspecific developmental disability and classic autism and is currently fatal; genetic counseling is indicated for effected families. Ideally if sending UMPS, send to a laboratory that will fractionate the mucopolysaccharides if the screen is positive, to avoid family stress by requesting follow-up sample.

Abbreviations: ACP, acylcarnitine profile; CBC, complete blood cell count; CSF, cerebrospinal fluid; IEM, inborn error of metabolism; IV, intravenous; MCADD, medium chain acyl-CoA; MCV, mean corpuscular volume; MPS, mucopolysaccharidoses; NT, neurotransmitter; OA, organic acid; PAA, plasma amino acids; PT, prothrombin time; RTA, renal tubular acidosis; UA, urinalysis ; UMPS, urine mucopolsaccharidoses.

Clinical Scenarios

Acutely Ill Patient (Shock, Possible Septicemia, Altered Mental Status)

Inborn errors of the amino acids, organic acids, urea cycle, fatty acid oxidation, mitochondrial metabolism, and several others may cause severe symptoms with a gradual or sudden onset. When altered mental status is apparent or when acid-base status is out of proportion to the physical findings, or when there is a history of prior episodes with the diagnosis of dehydration with intercurrent illnesses, suspect IEM. Inborn error of metabolism should certainly be considered when poisoning is suspected, unless a specific ingestion is known or suspected based on history or characteristic symptoms. Poisons can be created by intrinsic metabolic processes as well as ingested. Finding infection or non-accidental trauma does not exclude IEM. Be sure to examine ammonia level and liver functions to avoid missing important clues to diagnosis. Checking plasma ammonia is especially important in any neonate suspected of sepsis, because expanded newborn screening does not yet detect all urea cycle defects. Moreover, neonates may become symptomatic even before results of newborn screening are available.

While evaluation begins, remove all protein and lipids from the nutritional management, and all sugars except glucose. Provide adequate glucose to stop catabolism, which requires a glucose infusion rate (GIR) of 10 mg/kg/minute in the neonate and 6 mg/kg/minute in the older child. The purpose of this GIR is to prevent catabolism and is not driven by blood glucose level. If a patient with IEM has elevated blood glucose, insulin should be used to move glucose into cells. Since a very small fraction of IEM will worsen with these GIRs, all patients suspected of being in metabolic crisis should receive intravenous glucose initially unless a diagnosis known to require a low (<4 mg/kg/minute) GIR is known. Patients known to require an unusually low GIR should be carrying an emergency letter with instructions. Measure ammonia, and consider measuring lactate and pyruvate. If diagnosis is not already known, specific diagnostic testing for IEM in this setting begins with plasma amino acids (PAA), urine organic acids (UOA), acylcarnitine profile (ACP), and any other studies as indicated by presentation (Tables 7-1 and 7-2).

Child With Dysmorphic Features and Malformations

The classic dysmorphic syndromes due to IEM are Smith-Lemli-Opitz caused by a failure of cholesterol synthesis (classical presentation—small size, feeding disorders, characteristic facial features with cleft soft palate, heart defect, pyloric stenosis, syndactyly of toes 2 and 3, extra-axial polydactyly, hypospadias) and Zellweger syndrome caused by a failure of biogenesis of peroxisomes (cerebro-hepato-renal syndrome with characteristic facial features, including high forehead and flat face, liver and renal cysts, and extremely low tone). Other conditions involve brain malformations, especially the disorders of mitochondrial energy metabolism and the congenital disorders of glycosylation. Further, many of the mucopolysaccharidoses have characteristic coarse features of the face and progressive skeletal dystrophy. However, it should never be forgotten that patients with some chromosomal abnormalities are at increased risk for IEM. For example, patients with contiguous gene deletions may have only one carrier parent for an IEM if the gene is in the deleted region. Patients with uniparental isodisomy are homozygous for all genes on the affected chromosome, and are therefore affected with an IEM if the parent providing that chromosome was a carrier. Diagnostic evaluation is guided by physical examination.

Child With Failure to Thrive, With or Without Vomiting

Most patients with failure to thrive (FTT) do not have IEM, but many patients with IEM present with FTT. The PCP should consider IEM particularly if vomiting persists despite management of reflux, and certainly if there is any alteration of the patient's neurodevelopment. Brain growth and neurodevelopment for children with nutritional FTT are usually preserved unless the malnutrition is severe. Be certain to examine acid-base status, and remember that vomiting causes alkalosis, never acidosis, unless the patient is vomiting bile and/or has developed poor perfusion. Check liver functions and CBC, and examine the MCV in the CBC to avoid missing clues that further studies should be undertaken for IEM. Begin evaluation for IEM with PAA, UOA, ACP, and total and free carnitine.

Child With Abnormal Neurologic System

(Early Hypertonia, Late Hypotonia, Episodic or Progressive Ataxia or Other Movement Disorder, Atypical or Unresponsive Seizures, or Episodic Altered Consciousness)

Almost any category of IEM can cause an abnormal neurologic presentation. Careful attention to history can yield clues and lead to early diagnosis and treatment. Examine acid-base status and liver function. Assess for macrocytosis and collect PAA, UOA, and ACP. Measure blood ammonia in patients with acutely altered mental status or acute ataxia. Examination by ophthalmology for evidence of cataracts or retinopathy may provide clues to a specific IEM. When collecting cerebrospinal fluid (CSF), examine lactate and amino acids and consider planning in advance for special handling for the collection of a sample for measuring neurotransmitters and other metabolites for IEM. For evaluation of IEM as a cause of seizures, collect blood glucose and PAA immediately before the lumbar puncture so that ratio of CSF to plasma glucose and glycine can be evaluated. When planning magnetic resonance imaging (MRI), also ask for magnetic resonance spectroscopy to examine lactate for clues of inborn errors of energy metabolism.

Child With Intellectual Disability and Autism

(Especially With Slowing Development, Developmental Plateau, and Regression)

Regression should always be thoroughly evaluated immediately for IEM as a possible cause, both to identify those who will benefit from therapy and because many of the conditions are IEM, including some that are both fatal and autosomal recessive. For example, a boy with regression of development may need evaluation for X-linked adrenoleukodystrophy. However, at the initial presentation of a child with mental developmental disability or autism, it is not always clear whether the patient will be stable or improve, and/or will develop increased problems. History and examination can help to distinguish those in need of more aggressive evaluation (eg, those with hypotonia). There are no physical findings that exclude the presence of acidosis, liver disease, or macrocytosis, so basic studies of electrolytes, liver health, and CBC should be considered for all children presenting with intellectual disability, unless a clear cause for all presentation is known. Recommendations for use of more specific studies for IEM in absence of regression or other clues on history or examination (such as hypotonia) are variable. Addition of routine testing for IEM in children with developmental disability and otherwise normal history and examination has had little study, and is generally agreed to be low yield. However, testing of blood amino acids and urine mucopolysaccharidoses (MPS) is not costly, and the impact of making the diagnosis can be extremely high; therefore, many experts in IEM typically urge that all patients with intellectual disability or autism should be considered for the evaluation of PAA (for phenylketoneuria [PKU] and homocystinuria that can have been missed by newborn screen—some cases of PKU in particular are indistinguishable from autism) and urine MPS (for Sanfilippo syndrome that presents without abnormal physical features at onset and may be indistinguishable from classic autism).

Child With Single or Multi-Organ Failure

Renal failure from Fabry disease, liver failure from tyrosinemia, cardiomyopathy from fatty acid oxidation, or Pompe disease are potentially reversible. Other conditions are less responsive to therapy, such as the liver or bone marrow failure in those children with mitochondrial disease, but awareness of diagnosis can help with management. For example, it is necessary when possible to avoid valproic acid when treating children with seizures from IEM. Be aware that an infection may be the trigger leading to presentation of an IEM, and that some IEMs include immune deficiency that can increase the risk of infections. The evaluation for IEM in a child with single or multi-organ failure typically includes testing for those IEMs known to cause the specific presentation (eg, search for organic acidopathy as a cause of pancreatitis or tyrosinemia as a cause of liver failure), but in general includes evaluation of PAA, UOA, ACP, and carnitine (total and free) in addition to any other disease-specific testing.

A Child With Stroke or Clotting Disturbance

One of the standard presentations of classic homocystinuria due to cystathionine β-synthase deficiency is thrombotic stroke. Up to half the patients with classic homocystinuria and most with variant types are expected to be missed by newborn screening. While some patients may have marfanoid habitus or history of developmental disability, many others have no signs or symptoms of the presence of an IEM as the cause of stroke. Total homocysteine, PAA, and UOA should be included with studies for other genetic causes of stroke. When evaluating these children, consider the possibility that the child has experienced a stroke-like episode due to MELAS syndrome (mitochondrial encephalomyopathy, lactic acidosis, and stroke-like episodes) at initial presentation, and also include Fabry disease and congenital disorders of glycosylation in the differential diagnosis.

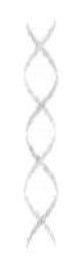

Special Considerations in the Biochemical Evaluation for IEM

Table 7-2 summarizes routine or common biochemical testing for the primary care or nongenetics pediatric specialist in the evaluation of a child with a suspected IEM. Begin with more general metabolic tests, and use additional specific tests as indicated by presentation and results of initial testing. Plans for special studies, such as enzyme assays and DNA testing, can be developed with the genetics team, but initial testing should typically be initiated before consultation.

Screening the healthy neonate for IEM is discussed in Chapter 17. For the symptomatic patient, an investigation for IEM begins by a careful examination of routine metabolic studies followed by specific studies. For the patient with a developmental disability who is not acutely ill, examine CBC, electrolytes, and liver function test results, since abnormalities in any of these would suggest further studies are indicated. There is not necessarily any physical finding in patients with macrocytic anemia, renal tubular or metabolic acidosis, or liver dysfunction. For the acutely ill patient, inappropriately low ketosis is also an important clue and can be detected by urinalysis. Acidosis out of proportion to clinical status or the presence of alkalosis should increase suspicion of IEM. Be certain to consider IEM as the cause of findings on imaging. For example, patients with mitochondrial disease may have stroke-like episodes, true stroke, or evidence of brain injury in a pattern indistinguishable from hypoxia. They may also have classic presentations that are clearly due to IEM, such as the white matter disease of adrenoleukodystrophy or the basal ganglia injury and extra-axial fluid of classical glutaric acidemia.

Check ammonia level in any patient with acutely altered mental status or acute ataxia, and consider an ammonia level in a neonate with suspected sepsis, but see Table 7-2 for caution regarding collection and handling. In the acutely ill patient or patient with hypotonia, consider also testing lactate levels; be aware lactate is also sensitive to collection and handling but unlike ammonia, lactate levels can change in minutes. Lactate can be normal on a sample collected incorrectly, so it will not be possible to be sure incorrect handling is the cause of elevation. Collecting lactate incorrectly may therefore lead to added testing that could have been avoided if the sample was collected properly. (See Table 7-2.)

Testing for biochemical analytes is guided by clinical presentation. Like testing for toxins, the yield for specific biochemical (analyte) testing for IEM will vary with the presentation. Biochemical studies of the patient with an ammonia level 100 times the upper limit of normal is highly likely to identify a disorder of the urea cycle. Plasma amino acids in a patient with nonspecific developmental disability will have low yield compared with studies such as comparative genome hybridization. However, the total cost of testing the most commonly measured analytes (PAA, UOA, ACP, total and free carnitine, CSF amino acids, and urine MPS) is a very small fraction of the cost of the care of the acutely ill patient or the neurodevelopmentally disabled child, because typically that panel of studies can be done for less than the cost of MRI or of comparative genomic hybridization. In addition, patients identified with chromosomal deletions are at higher risk than the general population to have IEM. For example, boys with certain deletions of the X chromosome have glycerol kinase deficiency, causing recurrent episodes of acidosis and altered mental status, and also have Duchenne muscular dystrophy.

Testing of DNA can assist in the diagnosis of IEM, and is addressed in more detail in Chapters 10 and 11. As with any DNA testing, be sure that the interpretation (including sensitivity) is discussed with genetic experts if experience in interpreting these test results is lacking. Consider, too, whether the purpose of DNA testing is to guide management of the patient or is to determine whether it will be possible to provide carrier testing to other family members or prenatal testing in the future.

Since most IEMs are autosomal recessive, testing of parents (DNA or enzyme assay) can provide critical help in making or excluding a diagnosis. For example, if galactosemia is suspected in a newborn who has been transfused, testing of the mother that demonstrates she is not a carrier will virtually exclude the possibility that galactosemia is the cause of the presentation (paternal uniparental isodisomy from a carrier father could still cause galactosemia, but this is rare). However, DNA testing of family members is not always necessary and can lead to some problems. For example, when a child's father has just been diagnosed with hemochromatosis with homozygosity for the common mutation, testing the child and finding the mutation does not add any new information to guide management. Finding no mutation will suggest misattributed paternity (non-paternity).

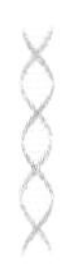

IEM Testing for the Dying Child

A special consideration in testing for IEM is in the acute setting when the child is dying. When a diagnosis that excludes IEM is not conclusively established, studies for IEM could identify living or future relatives at risk and in need of treatment. In addition, studies for IEM could establish cause of death, and prevent inappropriate prosecution of a parent, as happened in the case of a mother who was incarcerated until the diagnosis of methylmalonic acidemia in her second child led to her release. Samples for IEM testing should therefore be sent even if there is no expectation that the patient will respond to efforts at resuscitation. Some samples can be collected after death; however, a full metabolic autopsy requires immediate collection of samples suitable for testing of analytes and enzymes within the first hour after death, and requires collaboration of emergency or intensive care unit (ICU) care providers, pathology, and metabolic geneticists, and in some circumstances will require permission from a medical examiner.

Managing IEM in Pediatric Primary Care, on the Wards, in the Emergency Department, and in the ICU

The first step to management of IEM in the pediatric and pediatric specialty practice is making the diagnosis. The diagnosis can only be made when IEM is appropriately suspected and testing initiated. The stakes can be high for emergency recognition of IEM (eg, in a child with overwhelming acidosis or a child in a coma that proves to be caused by hyperammonemia). The PCP or nongenetics pediatric specialist will typically work with a geneticist in the management of IEM; however, management is often initiated in the acutely ill patient by excluding potentially harmful dietary components, and by providing glucose in amounts sufficient to prevent catabolism. It should be emphasized that patients who have an IEM, once stabilized and in the chronic phase of management, typically are not hospitalized because of the underlying IEM. Rather, a viral illness, fasting, etc, will tip the balance and cause a metabolic crisis unless the child is treated promptly. Primary care physicians, therefore, are at the forefront of management of these children. In addition, the importance of maintaining vaccination schedules as recommended by the American Academy of Pediatrics and obtaining annual influenza (killed) vaccinations in both the affected child and family members are simple, yet critically important, aspects of pediatric care.

Specific management is available for many IEMs, such as the branched chain amino acid restricted diet for MSUD, or provision of cofactor for B_6-responsive seizures. Some conditions that in the recent past were untreatable and fatal (eg, Pompe disease) can now be treated with enzyme infusions that can reverse some symptoms and prevent further injury. Specific therapy for long-recognized conditions continues to evolve. For example, some individuals with PKU are now recognized to respond to therapy with the cofactor biopterin. Phenylketonuria is also an example of an IEM that requires lifelong therapy. Patients with poor compliance in late childhood and teen years are at risk to develop progressive white matter disease of the brain, and since elevated phenylalanine is a teratogen, young women with poorly controlled PKU will have offspring with intellectual disability and malformations. Other examples of the preventable adverse consequences of poor compliance are liver cancer in those with glycogen storage disease or a stroke in those with homocystinuria.

For other IEMs, current treatment consists solely or primarily of supportive, symptomatic management, while research efforts continue to develop specific treatments. Patients and families often wish to participate in experimental therapies, especially for conditions that are fatal and have no current proven effective therapy. Anticipatory guidance is critical for the management of all IEMs, and genetic counseling is important for families and for the patients themselves when they consider future reproductive risks.

Management is a collaborative effort with the geneticist, and any other appropriate medical specialists. For example, management of cystinosis will typically require collaboration with nephrology and ophthalmology specialists, and management of Pompe disease will involve a cardiologist. For most IEMs there is a role for the specifically trained metabolic dietitian, genetics/metabolic nurse, and genetic counselor, working as a team with the geneticist to provide care and support for the PCP and other pediatric specialists. Transition to adult care is an issue for all pediatric patients with chronic disease, and in many cases the genetics team will remain constant after transition to adult care, as the metabolic genetics team typically sees adults as well as children.

Key Points

- Most IEMs are individually rare, but collectively (including mitochondrial disease) affect at least 1/1,000 individuals.
- Inborn errors of metabolism are important causes of neurodevelopmental and health problems in pediatrics.

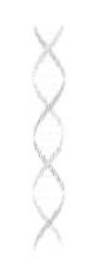

- Many IEMs have specific treatments that can reduce or even prevent disability and death.
- Inborn errors of metabolism are by definition genetic, and recurrence risk within families is therefore significant.
- Inborn errors of metabolism can present at any age and cause virtually any symptom.
- Particularly consider IEM in the newborn, infant, child, or adolescent with
  - Neurodevelopmental abnormalities with
    - Acute altered mental status
    - Recurrent/intermittent symptoms or progression
    - Hypotonia after 1 year of age
    - A movement disorder
  - Acidosis out of proportion to systemic illness
  - Hypoketosis (low ketones for a state of fasting or catabolism), especially if there is hypoglycemia
  - Cardiomyopathy, liver failure, FTT, and renal tubular acidosis individually or in combination with each other or with abnormal neurologic status
- Basic laboratory testing for IEM starts with CBC, electrolytes, liver enzymes, and urinalysis in almost all cases, and proper use of blood amino acids, UOA studies and acylcarnitine profile, and total and free carnitine, and with properly collected ammonia and lactate levels where appropriate.

Resources

Fernandes J, Saudubray J-M, van den Berghe, G, Walter JH, eds. *Inborn Metabolic Diseases: Diagnosis and Treatment*. 4th ed. Springer Medizin Verlag; 2006

Hoffman GF, Zschocke J, Nyhan WL, eds. *Inherited Metabolic Diseases: A Clinical Approach*. Springer Verlag; 2010

Valle D, et al, eds. The Online Metabolic and Molecular Bases of Inherited Disease. http://www.ommbid.com/

Chapter 8

Assessing Dysmorphology in Primary Care

H. Eugene Hoyme, MD

Introduction

Because primary care physicians (PCPs) are the first, and often only, point of contact with the health care system for children, it is crucial that physicians caring for children be able to recognize and diagnose a genetic disease in children whose only presenting symptom may be a dysmorphic feature. The importance of a correct diagnosis for the affected child and his or her family cannot be overstated. The correct diagnosis allows for discussion of the prognosis and natural history of the disorder, accurate treatment planning, and genetic counseling for the parents of the affected child and other family members, particularly concerning the risk of recurrence with future pregnancies. Accurate clinical classification is also important for precise phenotyping (for ongoing molecular genetic research into the causation of malformations) and for the training of pediatric residents in clinical genetics and dysmorphology in order to serve the needs of children with disabilities in the post-genome era.

The diagnostic workup of children with dysmorphic features is conducted in the context of the clinical setting. A higher level of suspicion for genetic disorder is present in a child with a single obvious dysmorphic feature when there is an associated developmental delay. Any child with developmental delay should be assessed for dysmorphic features in a logical, stepwise manner similar to that used in clinical pediatrics in general (Box 8-1). Despite the landmark advances that have taken place in molecular genetic diagnostic methodologies over the past decade, the best tools available to the pediatrician continue to be careful clinical observation and assessment followed by any appropriate genetic laboratory tests.

Box 8-1. Evaluation of a Child With Suspected Dysmorphic Features

- **When to Assess for Dysmorphic Features**
  - Presence of an obvious minor anomaly
  - Presence of developmental delay or intellectual disability
    (Presence of a major anomaly requires referral to geneticist.)
- **History and Interview**
  - Review pregnancy history—pregnancy losses, pregnancy planning, parental occupations, parental health at conception, exposure to illicit drugs, prescription drugs, nonprescription drugs, alcohol, cigarettes, maternal fever, rash, acute or chronic illness, possible teratogenic exposures, natural or assisted conception
  - Birth history—birth weight, length, head circumference, infant growth curves analyzed, Apgar scores, transition difficulties, any neonatal hospitalization
  - Review medical history (see Chapter 5 for history and pedigree tools)—photographs of the older child or adolescent at various ages may be helpful; photographs of family reveal common features
  - Create 3-generation pedigree (see Chapter 5)
  - Assess developmental milestones
- **Assessing for Dysmorphic Features**
  Growth, including head circumference
  - Craniofacial features
    - Head shape—size, shape
    - Forehead—prominence or sloping
    - Eyes—distance between eyes, interpupillary distance, shape, slant, measurement of palpebral fissures, presence of epicanthal folds
    - Nose—shape, appearance of nasal bridge, nares shape and orientation
    - Malar region—presence of hypoplasia, philtrum appearance
    - Ears—size, ear shape, ear position and orientation
    - Mouth—cleft lip/palate, bifid uvula, natal teeth, single central maxillary incisor
    - Jaw—size and appearance
  - Neck—presence of webbing, posterior hairline, size of thyroid gland
  - Trunk—chest shape and symmetry, presence of scoliosis
  - Genitalia—hypoplasia, structure
  - Extremities
    - Proportion of limbs to trunk and head
    - Joints—range of motion
    - Hands—number of digits, finger shape, nail formation, palmar creases
    - Feet—shape, number of digits, arch formation
- **Summarizing the Information**
  - List positive findings
  - Create differential diagnosis
- **Next Steps**
  - Laboratory evaluation
    - Microarray analysis —usually in consultation with geneticist
    - Chromosome analysis—if indicated, usually in consultation with geneticist
    - Molecular diagnostic test—only when clinical diagnosis is questionable
    - Biochemical laboratory test—if storage disease suspected
  - Radiography
    - Skeletal—if bony abnormalities suspected
    - Cranial or visceral imaging—if indicated
  - Refer to a geneticist if diagnosis is unclear.

Dysmorphology: Definition and Relevance

In pediatrics, the term *dysmorphology* was coined by Dr David W. Smith in the 1960s to describe the study of human malformations.[1] Dysmorphology is derived from the Greek *dys* (abnormal or impaired) and morphology (the study of form or structure). A child with *dysmorphic* features displays structural development that is out of the ordinary. What constitutes abnormal structure is to some extent a statistical definition, with findings that occur in more than 5% of the population defined as variants of normal, and those observed in less than 5% of the population termed structural anomalies, either major or minor.[2]

Anomalous structure results from 1 of 3 basic mechanisms during prenatal development: malformation, deformation, or disruption (Figure 8-1). A malformation is defined as a structural defect arising from an intrinsically abnormal developmental process during embryogenesis (eg, cleft lip with or without cleft palate). A deformation is considered to be an abnormal structure resulting from nondisruptive mechanical forces applied to a once normally formed part (eg, club feet in a child who gestated in a malformed uterine cavity). Finally, a disruption follows destruction of a

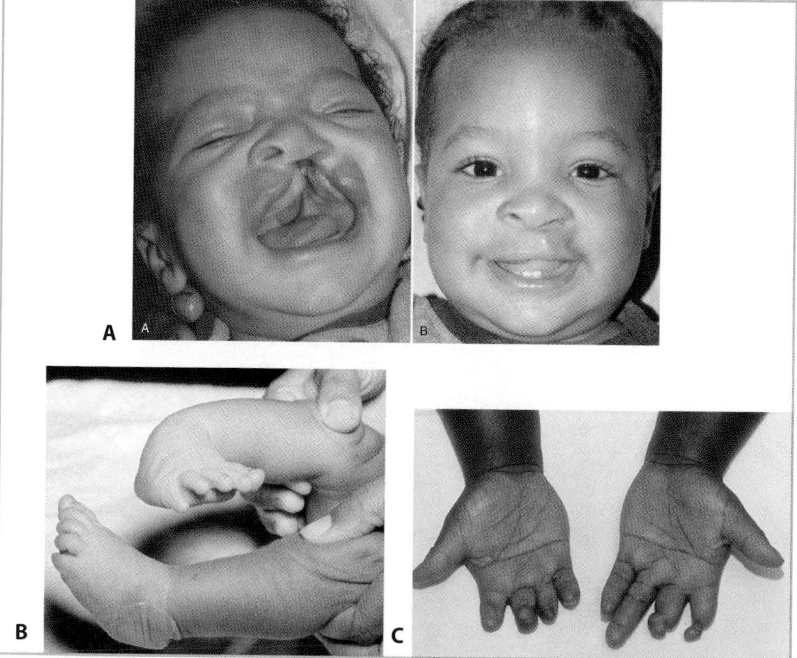

Figure 8-1. Mechanisms by which congenital structural defects occur. **A.** Malformation (cleft lip sequence); **B.** deformation (club feet); **C.** disruption (digital amputations/constriction ring secondary to amniotic bands).

once normally formed part (eg, the amniotic band sequence). The importance of assigning one of these mechanisms to the observed anomaly lies in discussing prognosis with the family: Malformations and disruptions never self-correct, and even with surgical intervention, prognosis can be guarded. On the other hand, deformations often resolve with nonsurgical intervention, either spontaneously or by applying the opposite force postnatally to that applied in utero. For example, in a child with club feet, through serial casting the orthopedic surgeon might correct the underlying deformation by persistently applying the opposite force to the lower extremities from that applied in utero by the constraining forces of the abnormal intrauterine environment.[3]

Anomalies can be further deconstructed into major anomalies and minor anomalies. A minor anomaly is a structural finding observed in less than 5% of the general population, which is of no significant cosmetic or functional significance to the affected child. An example of a minor anomaly is a single transverse palmar crease. Conversely, a major anomaly is a structural variation that is observed in less than 5% of the general population and is

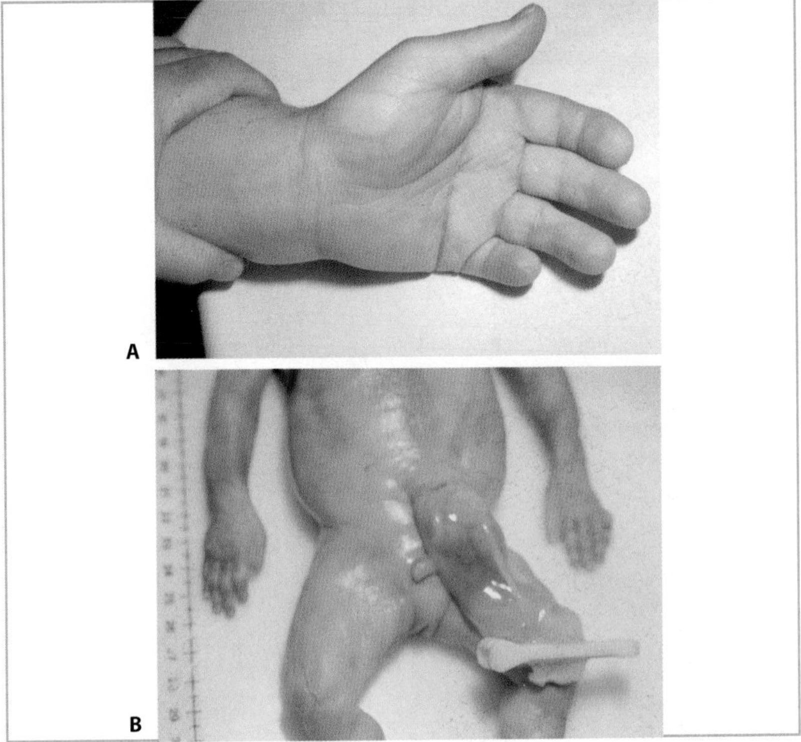

Figure 8-2. Minor vs major anomaly. **A.** Minor anomaly (defect of no significant cosmetic/functional significance): single transverse palmar crease; **B.** major anomaly (defect of significant cosmetic/functional significance): omphalocele.

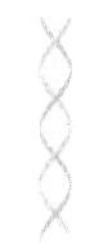

Box 8-2. Partial Listing of Minor Anomalies[5–12]

Craniofacial	Hands and Feet
Brachycephaly	Camptodactyly
Prominent metopic ridge	Digital pad, prominent
Hair whorls, abnormal number	Fingers/toes, long
Widow's peak	Fingers/toes, overlapping
Malar flattening	Finger/toe, tapered
Chin, H-shaped crease	Thumb/hallux, broad
Low nasal bridge	Hand, radial/ulnar deviation of
Neck webbing	Hand, trident
Palpebral fissure, upslanted	Metacarpal/metatarsal, short
Palpebral fissure, short	Sandal gap
Eyes, closely/widely spaced	Fingers/toes, cutaneous syndactyly of
Telecanthus	Palmar crease, single transverse
Ptosis	Nail, hyperconvex
Epicanthus	Nail, small
Ear, low set	**Skin**
Helix, overfolded	Hypopigmented patches
Pit/tag, preauricular	Aplasia cutis congenita
Philtrum, smooth	Pigmented nevi
Vermilion upper lip, thin	Hairy patch on lower spine
Tooth, natal	Café au lait macules
Central incisor, single maxillary	Pigmentary streaks along the lines of Blaschko
Micrognathia	
Uvula, cleft	

associated with significant cosmetic and/or functional impairment.[2,4] An example of a major anomaly is omphalocele (Figure 8-2). A partial listing of minor anomalies is set forth in Box 8-2.

Major anomalies are readily apparent at birth; minor anomalies are often more subtle, and unless the astute clinician is searching for them, they may easily be overlooked. However, recognizing minor anomalies is important, since their presence or absence can alter the overall diagnosis of a child with disabilities. Seventy-one percent of minor anomalies are present in the craniofacies and the hands. Careful examination of these parts is, therefore, most likely to be helpful in diagnosis.[4] Figures 8-2 through 8-56 are images of minor anomalies.

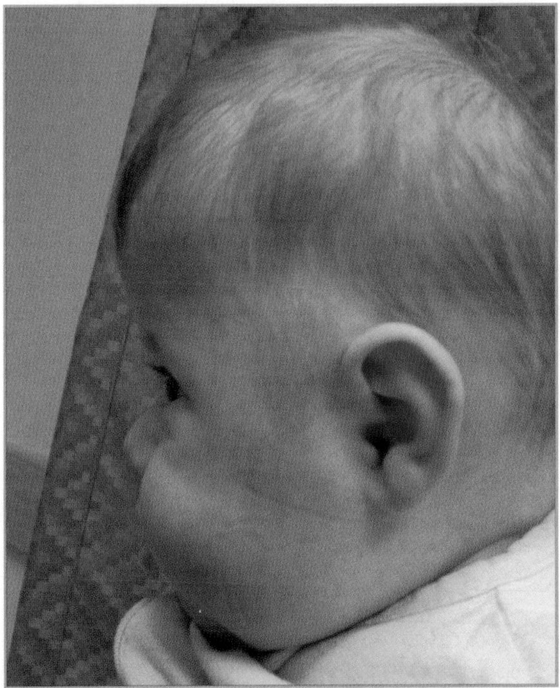

Figure 8-3. Brachycephaly. Courtesy of John Johnson, MD.

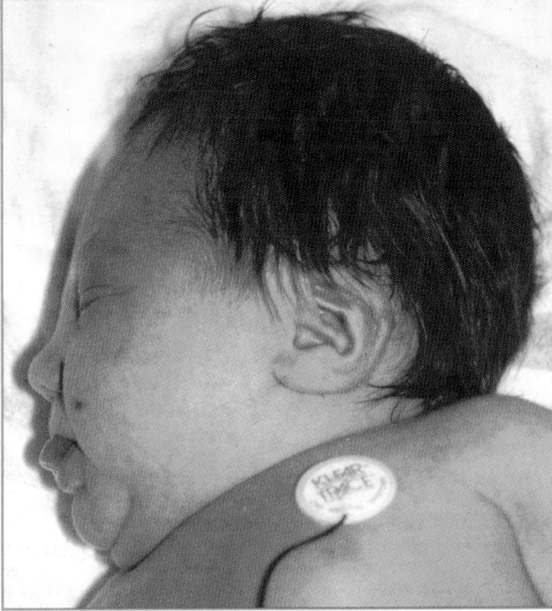

Figure 8-4. Brachycephaly. Courtesy of Lynne Bird, MD.

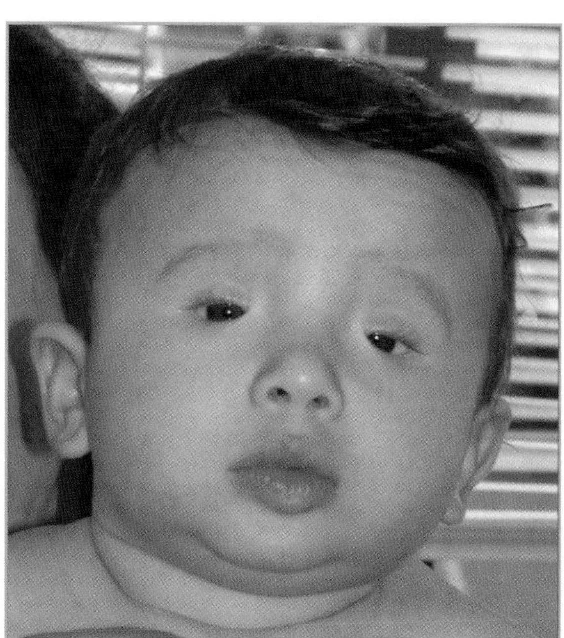

Figure 8-5. Epicanthus-blepharophimosis. Courtesy of Lynne Bird, MD.

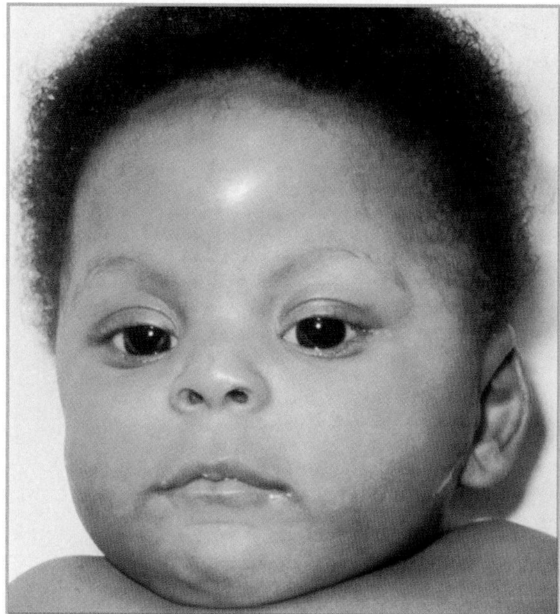

Figure 8-6. Wide-spaced eyes (hypertelorism). Courtesy of Greenwood Genetic Center, Greenwood, SC.

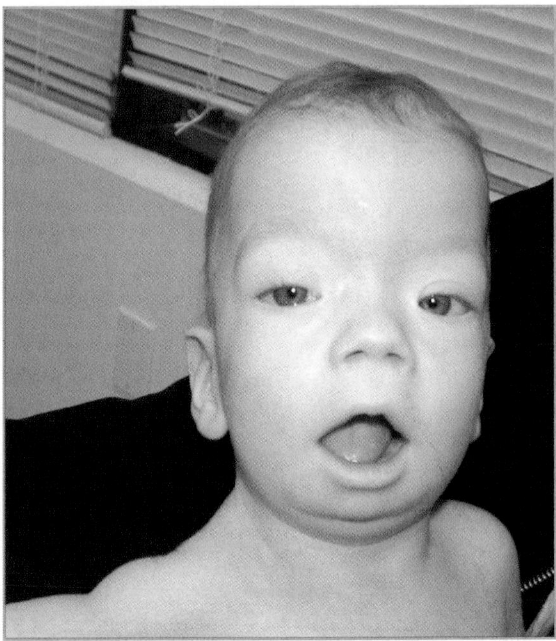

Figure 8-7. Telecanthus. Courtesy of Lynne Bird, MD.

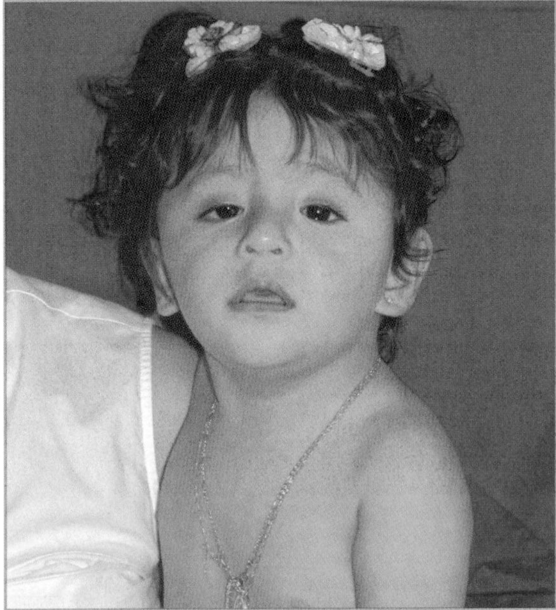

Figure 8-8. Ptosis. Courtesy of Lynne Bird, MD.

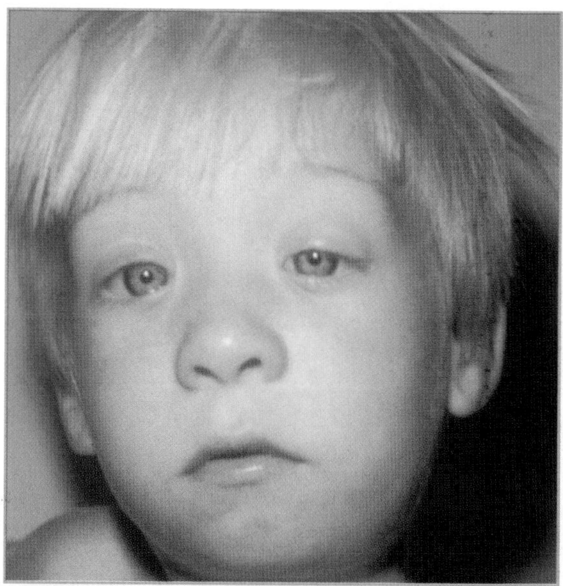

Figure 8-9. Ptosis. Courtesy of Greenwood Genetic Center, Greenwood, SC.

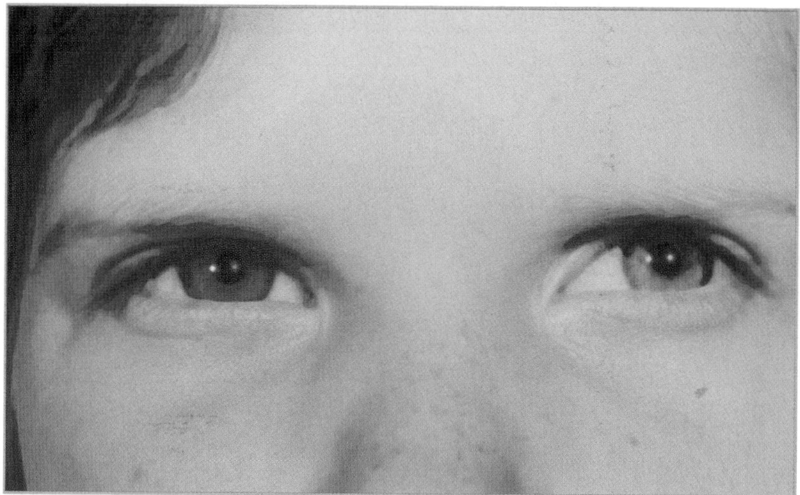

Figure 8-10. Heterochromia. Courtesy of Greenwood Genetic Center, Greenwood, SC.

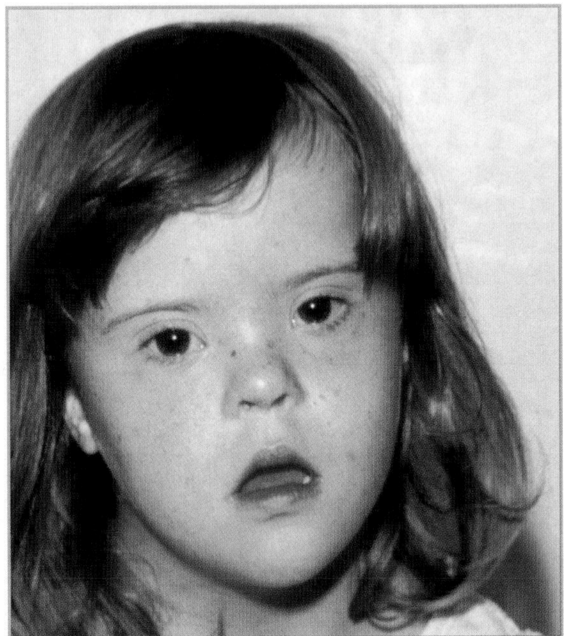

Figure 8-11. Palpebral fissures, upslanted. Courtesy of Greenwood Genetic Center, Greenwood, SC.

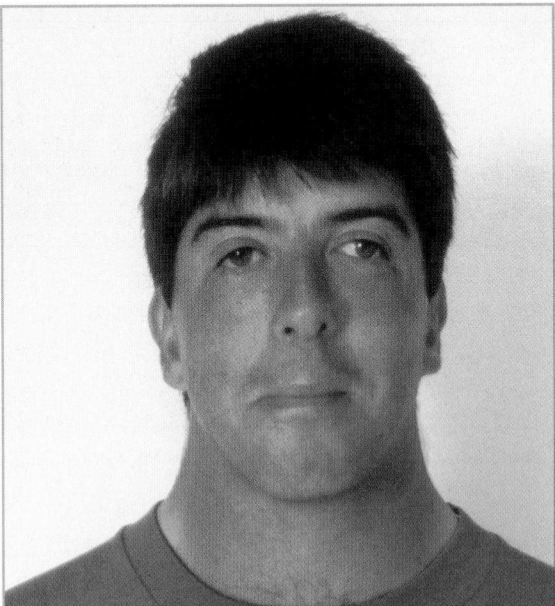

Figure 8-12. Palpebral fissures, downslanted. Courtesy of Greenwood Genetic Center, Greenwood, SC.

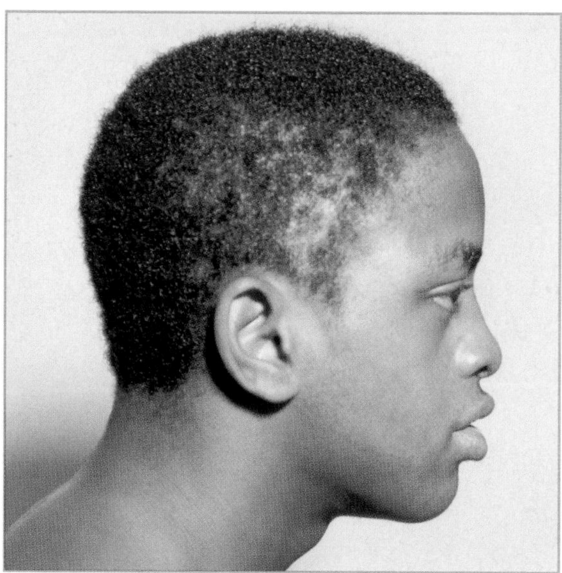

Figure 8-13. Midface hypoplasia/malar flattening. Courtesy of Greenwood Genetic Center, Greenwood, SC.

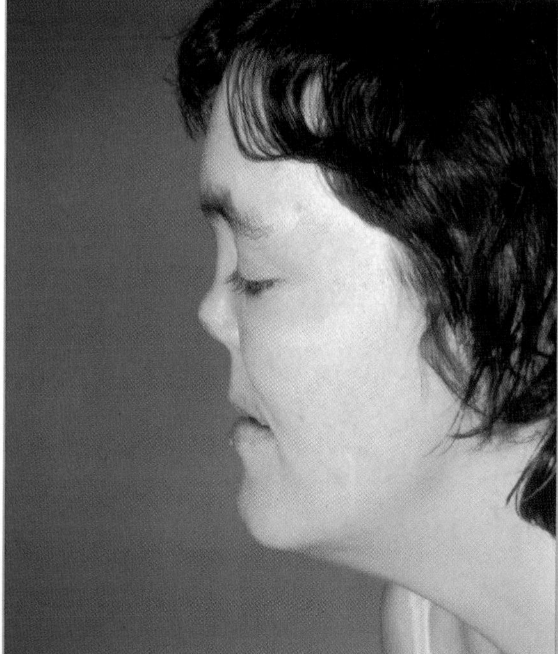

Figure 8-14. Facial flattening. Courtesy of Greenwood Genetic Center, Greenwood, SC.

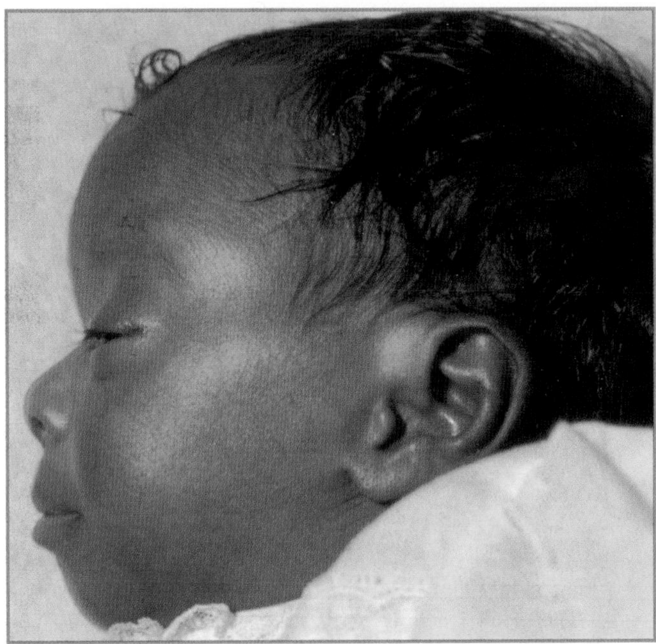

Figure 8-15. Low-set ears. Courtesy of Greenwood Genetic Center, Greenwood, SC.

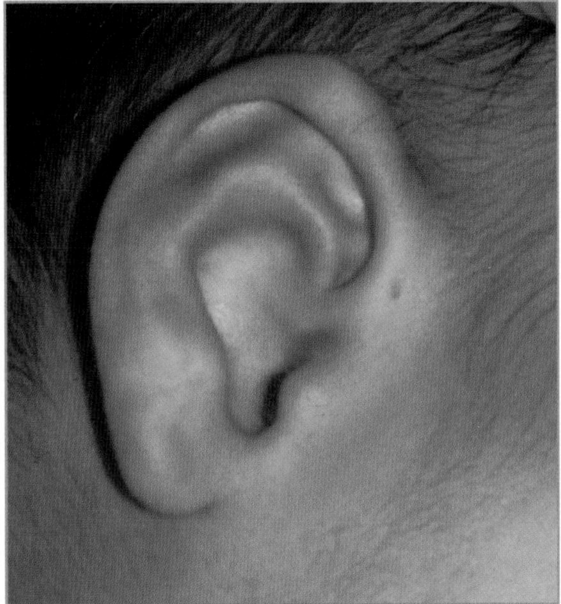

Figure 8-16. Preauricular pit. Courtesy of Lynne Bird, MD.

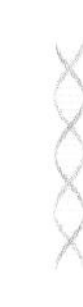

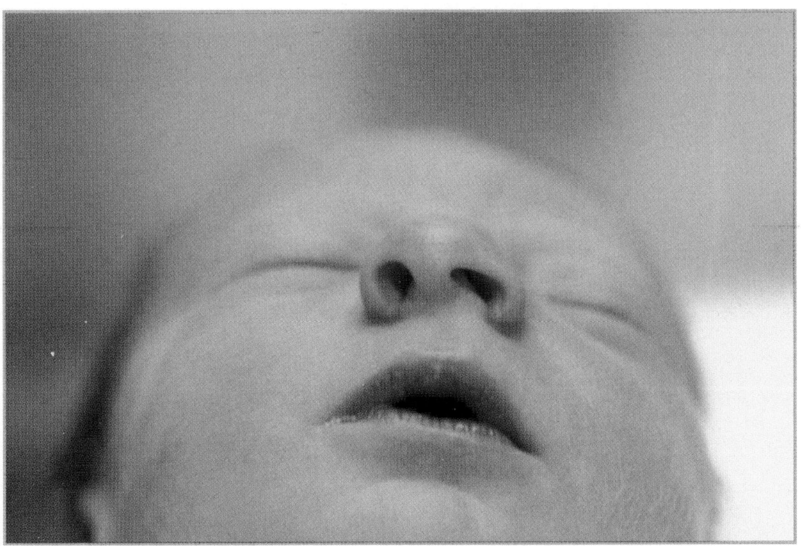

Figure 8-17. Dislocated nose. Courtesy of Greenwood Genetic Center, Greenwood, SC.

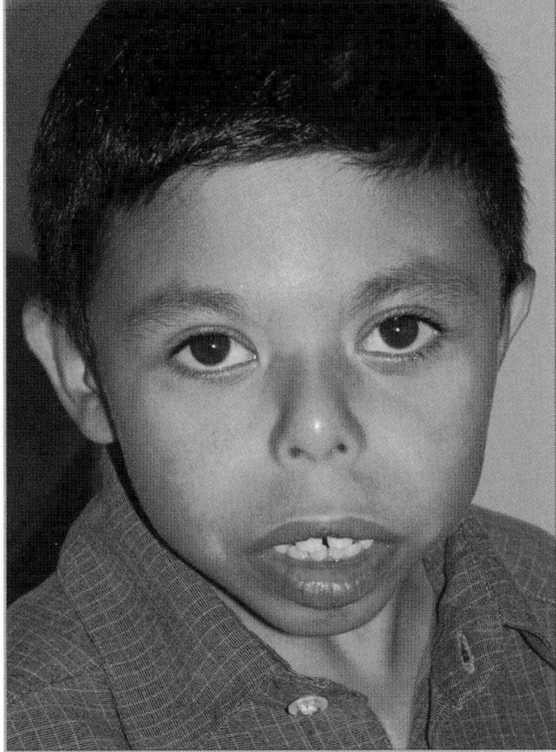

Figure 8-18. Smooth philtrum. Courtesy of Lynne Bird, MD.

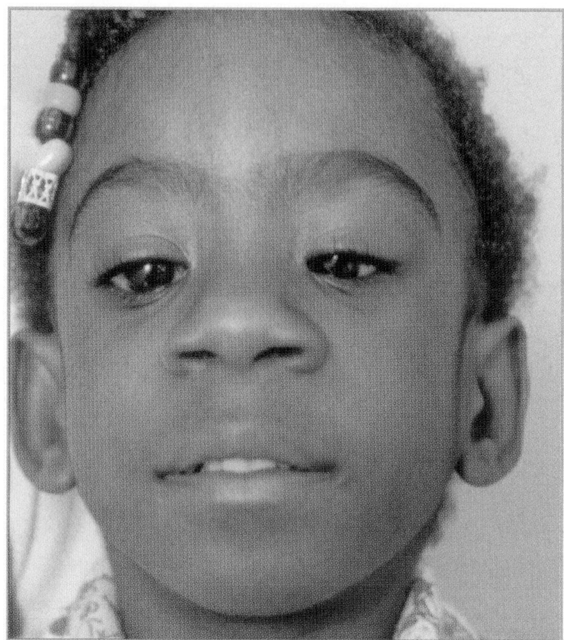

Figure 8-19. Smooth philtrum. Courtesy of Greenwood Genetic Center, Greenwood, SC.

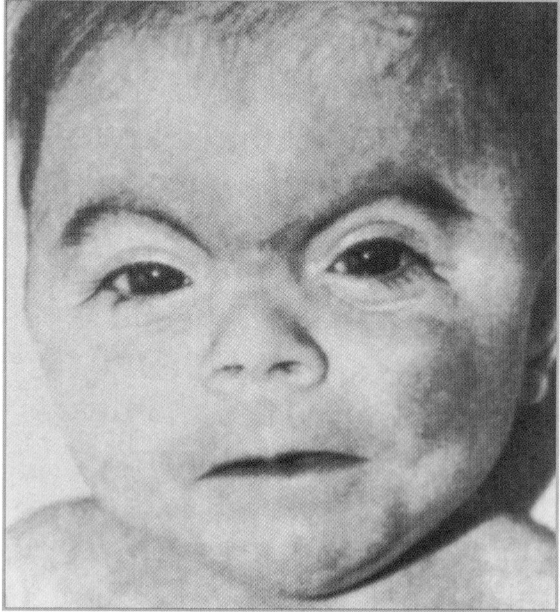

Figure 8-20. Thin upper lip. Courtesy of Greenwood Genetic Center, Greenwood, SC.

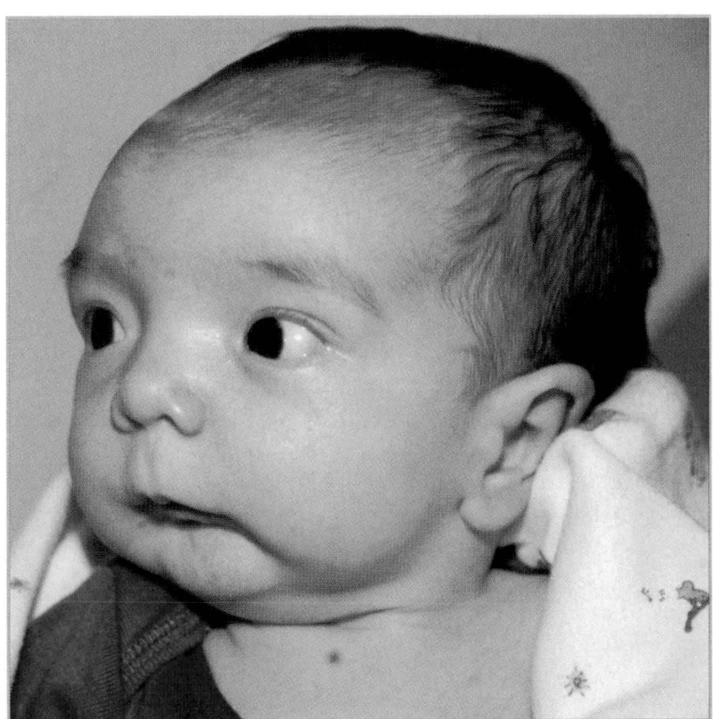

Figure 8-21. Micrognathia. Courtesy of Lynne Bird, MD.

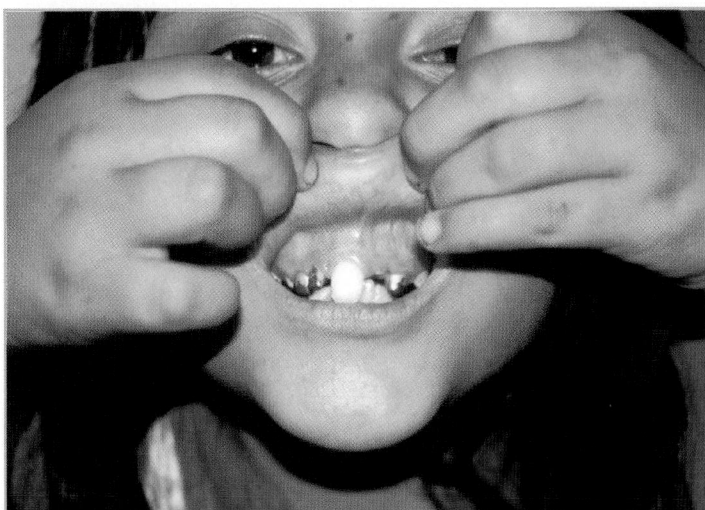

Figure 8-22. Single central incisor. Courtesy of Lynne Bird, MD.

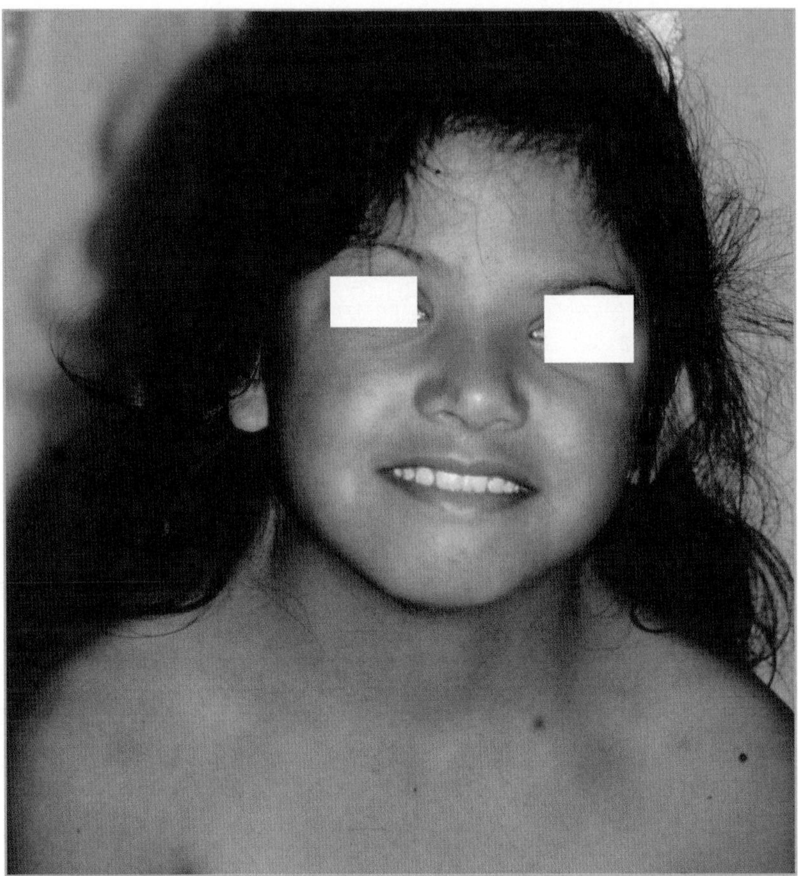

Figure 8-23. Webbed neck, frontal. Courtesy of Lynne Bird, MD.

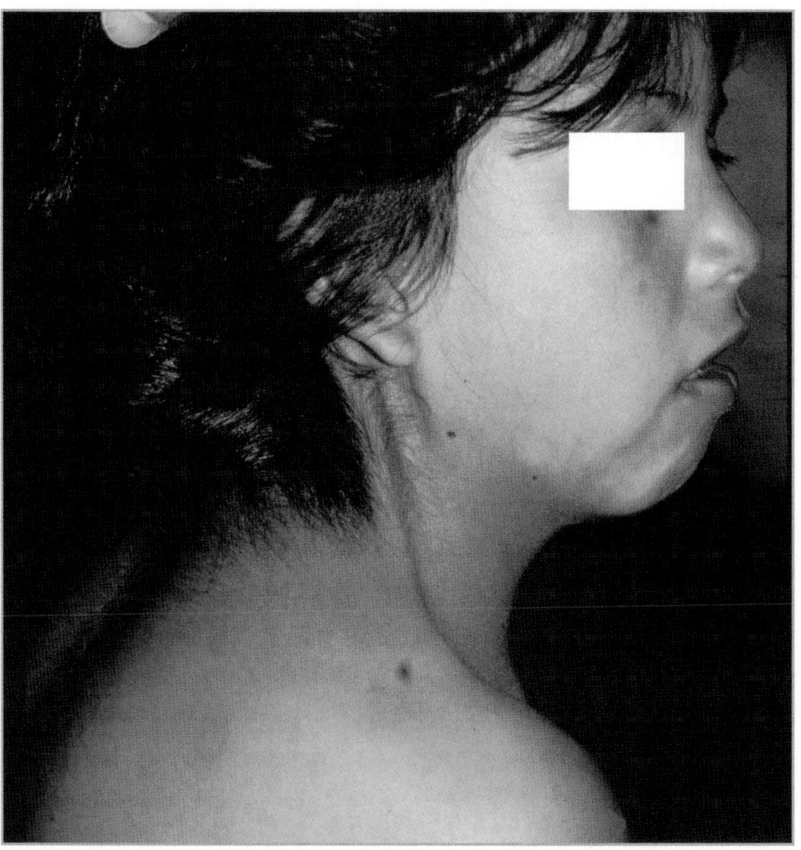

Figure 8-24. Webbed neck, profile. Courtesy of Lynne Bird, MD.

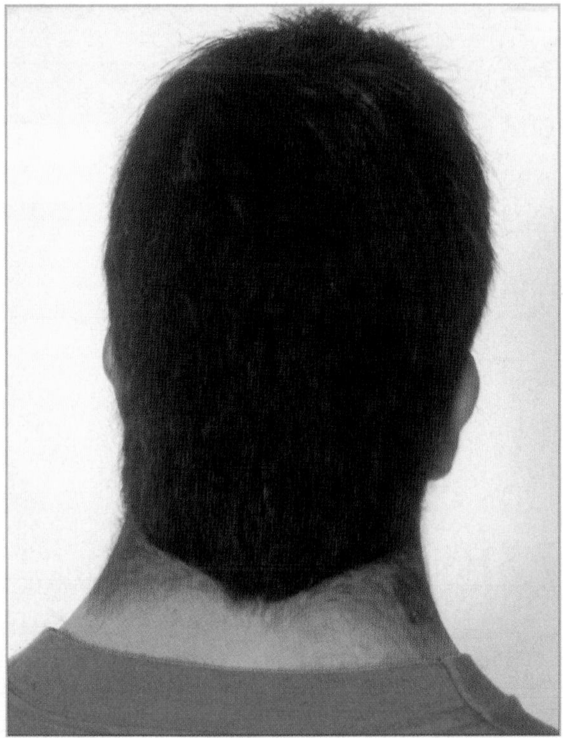

Figure 8-25. Webbed neck, posterior. Courtesy of Greenwood Genetic Center, Greenwood, SC.

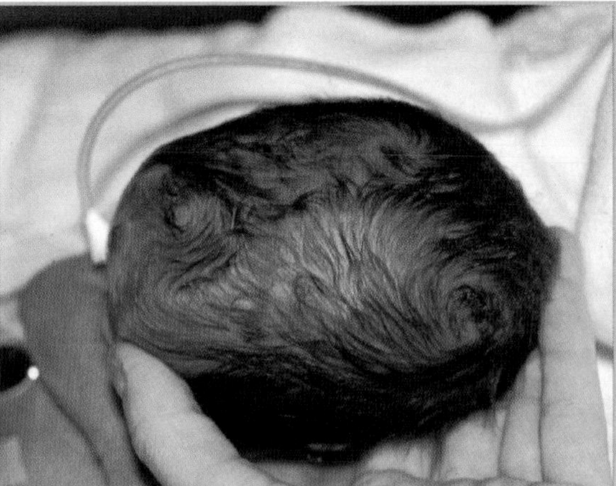

Figure 8-26. Three hair whorls. Courtesy of Lynne Bird, MD.

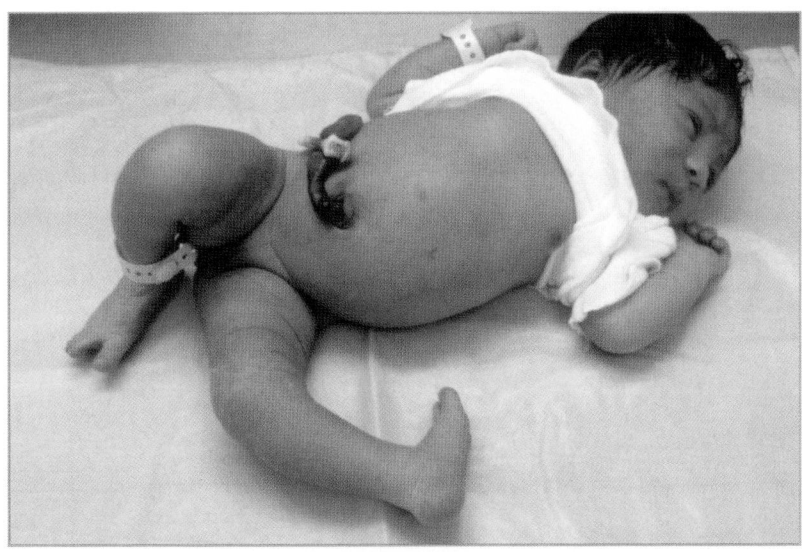

Figure 8-27. Genu recurvatum. Courtesy of Greenwood Genetic Center, Greenwood, SC.

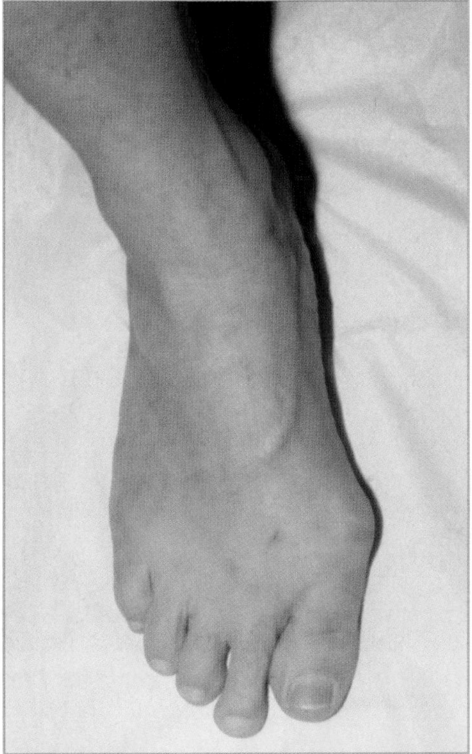

Figure 8-28. Hallux valgus. Courtesy of Greenwood Genetic Center, Greenwood, SC.

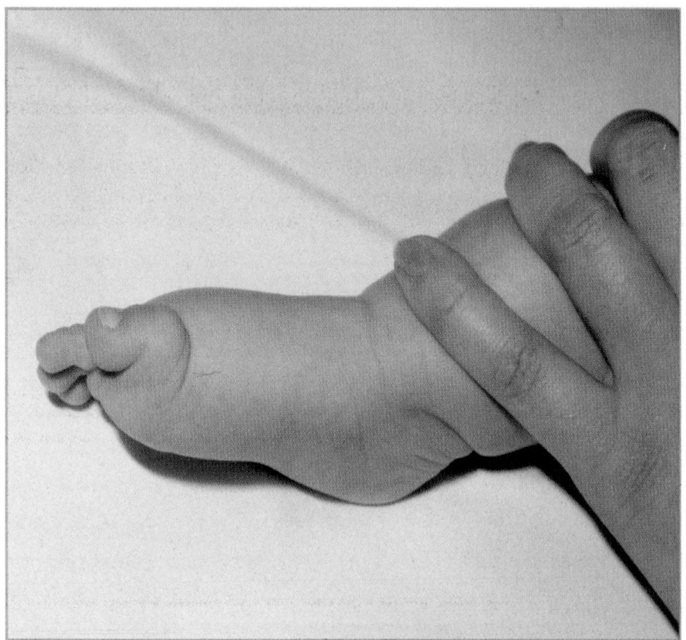

Figure 8-29. Hammer toe. Courtesy of Greenwood Genetic Center, Greenwood, SC.

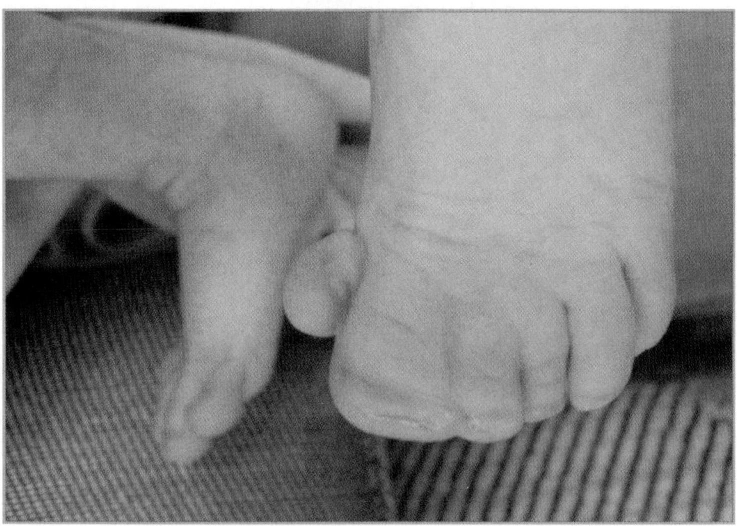

Figure 8-30. 1-2 syndactyly of the toes (pre-axial polydactyly is also present). Courtesy of John Johnson, MD.

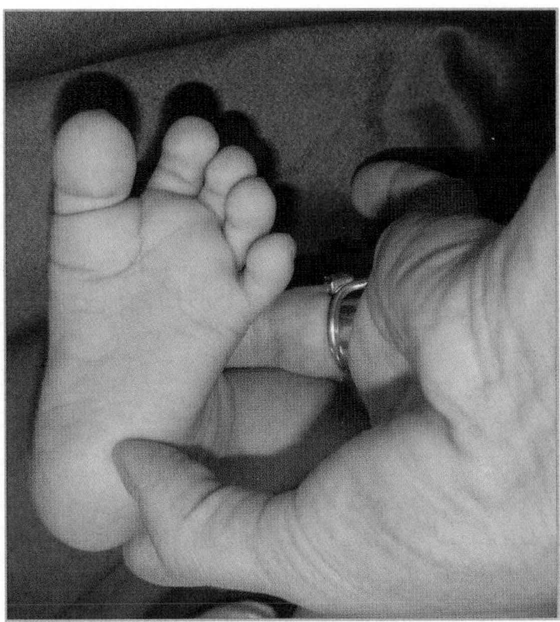

Figure 8-31. Sandal gap. Courtesy of Lynne Bird, MD.

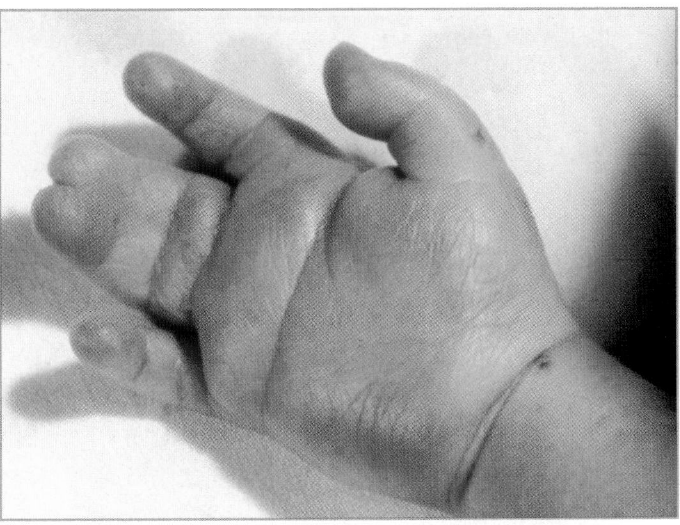

Figure 8-32. 3-4 syndactyly of the hand. Courtesy of Greenwood Genetic Center, Greenwood, SC.

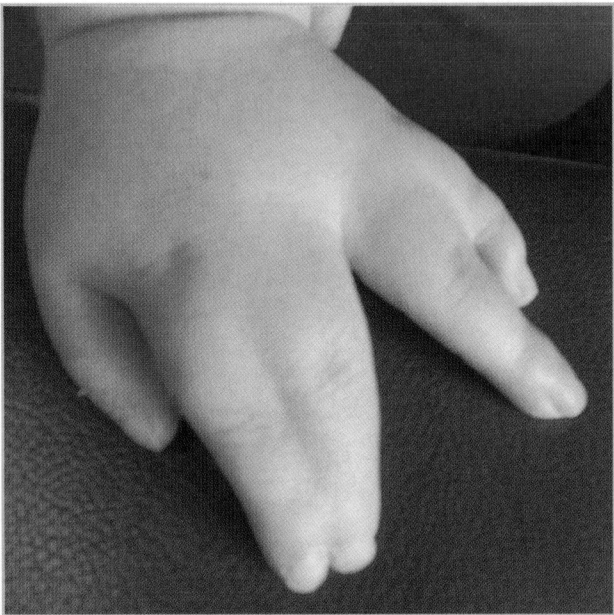

Figure 8-33. 2-3 syndactyly of the hand. Courtesy of John Johnson, MD.

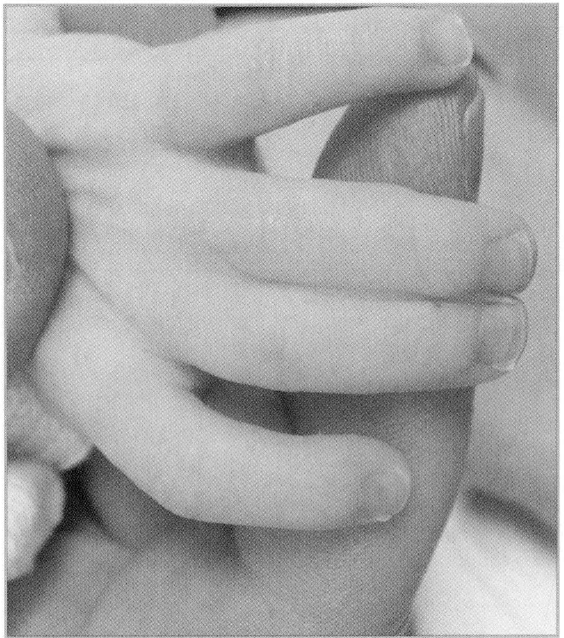

Figure 8-34. 3-4 syndactyly of the hand. Courtesy of John Johnson, MD.

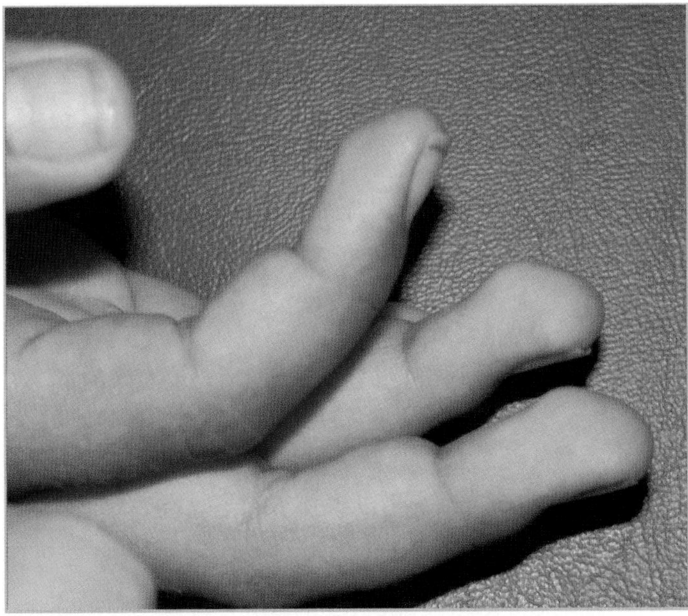

Figure 8-35. Digital pads. Courtesy of Lynne Bird, MD.

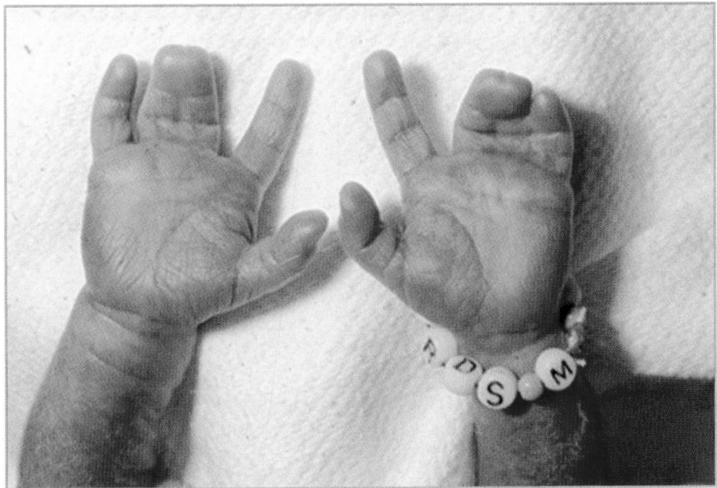

Figure 8-36. Cutaneous syndactyly. Courtesy of Greenwood Genetic Center, Greenwood, SC.

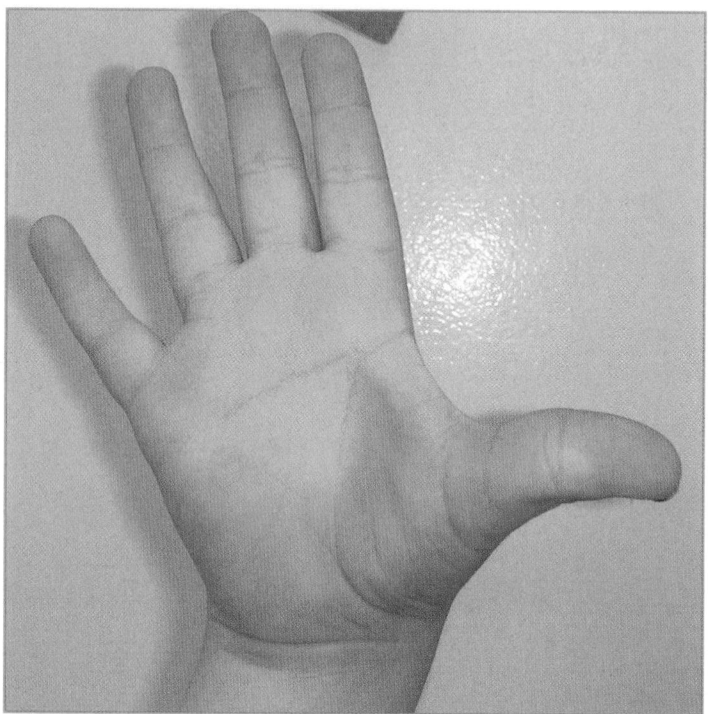

Figure 8-37. Single palmar crease. Courtesy of Lynne Bird, MD.

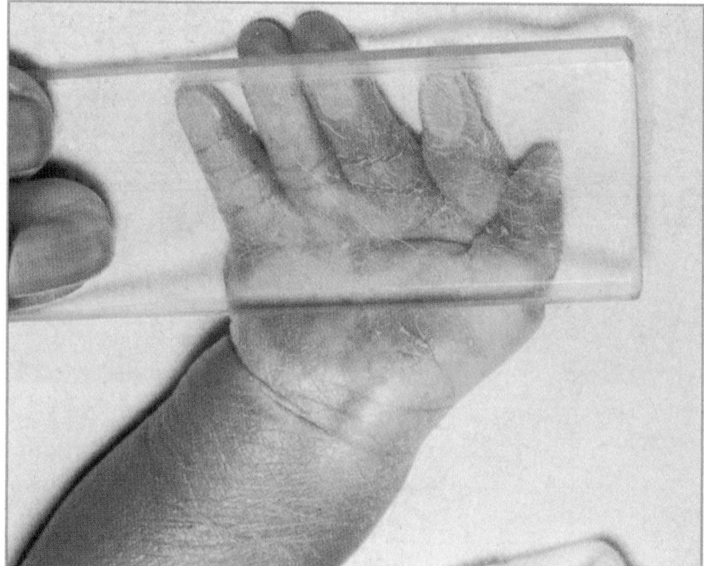

Figure 8-38. Palmar crease, single transverse. Courtesy of Greenwood Genetic Center, Greenwood, SC.

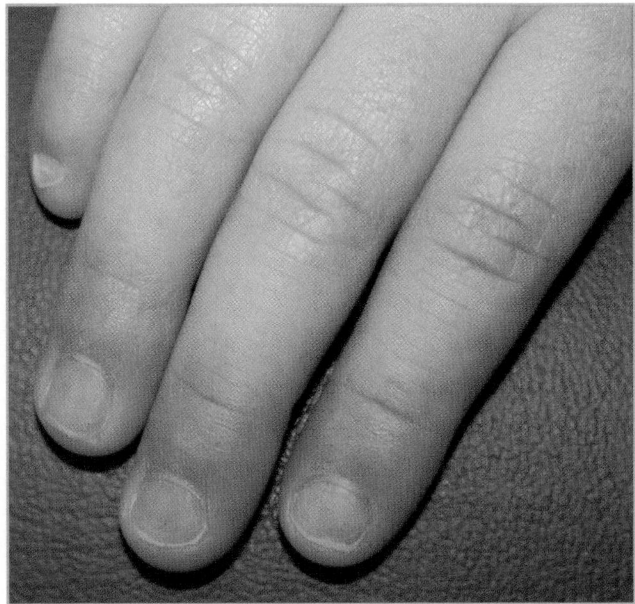

Figure 8-39. Small fifth fingernail. Courtesy of Lynne Bird, MD.

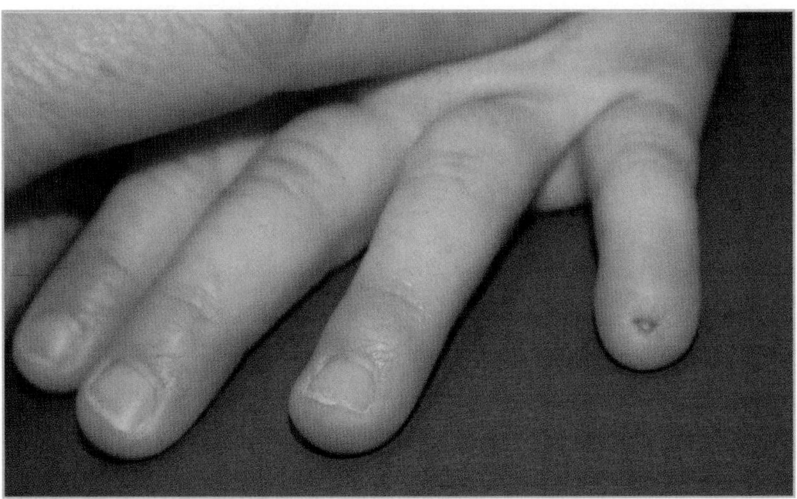

Figure 8-40. Small fifth fingernail. Courtesy of Lynne Bird, MD.

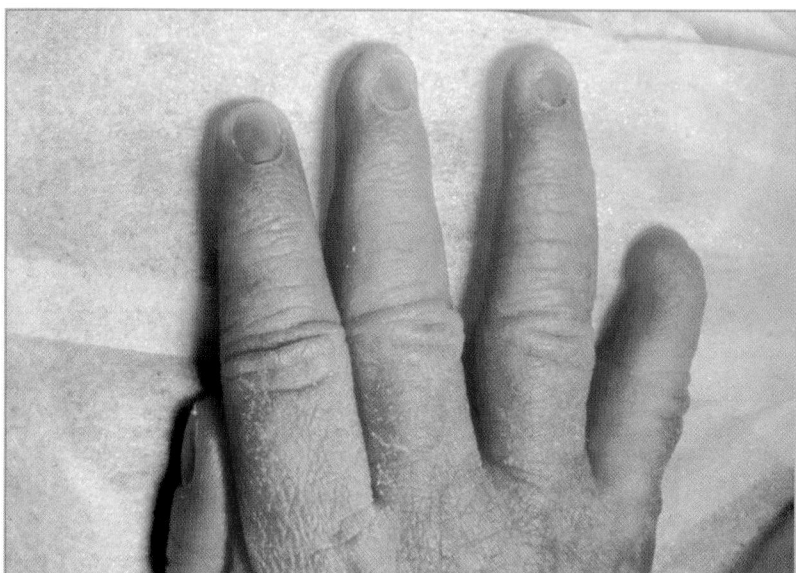

Figure 8-41. Tapered fingers, distal phalanx amputation, digit 5. Courtesy of Greenwood Genetic Center, Greenwood, SC.

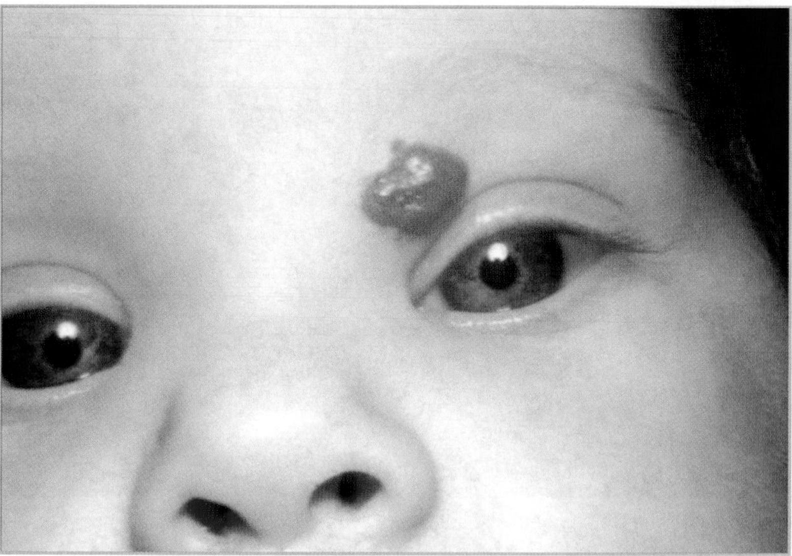

Figure 8-42. Hemangioma. Courtesy of Greenwood Genetic Center, Greenwood, SC.

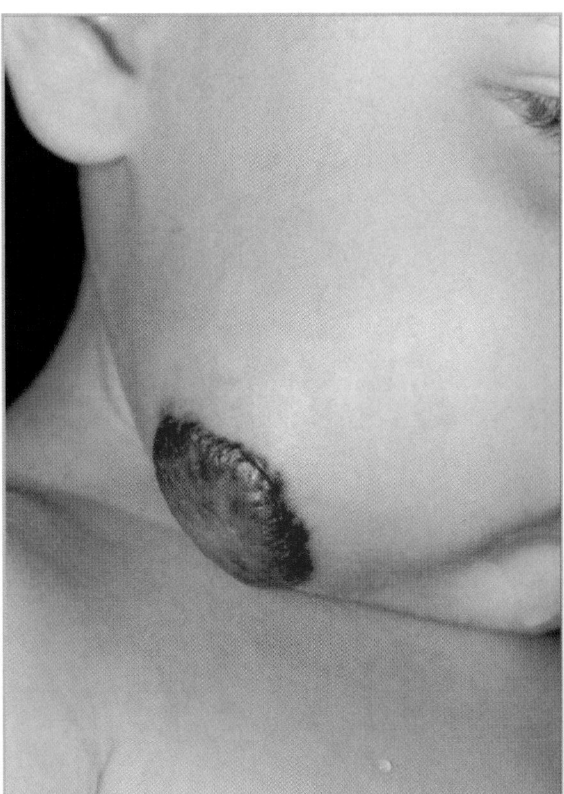

Figure 8-43. Hemangioma. Courtesy of Greenwood Genetic Center, Greenwood, SC.

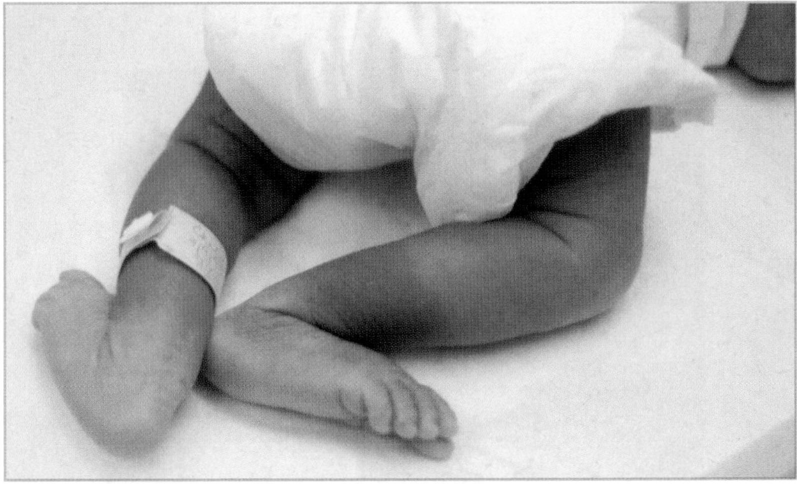

Figure 8-44. Mongolian spot. Courtesy of Greenwood Genetic Center, Greenwood, SC.

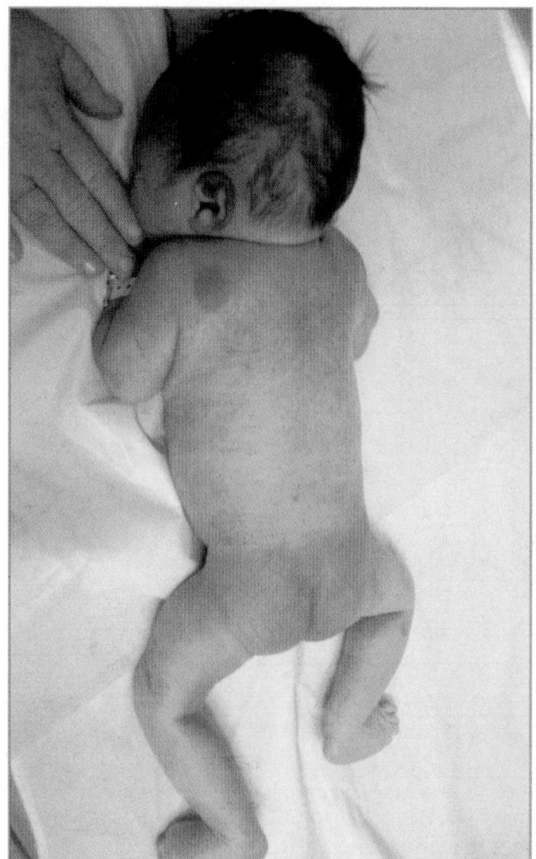

Figure 8-45. Mongolian spot. Courtesy of Greenwood Genetic Center, Greenwood, SC.

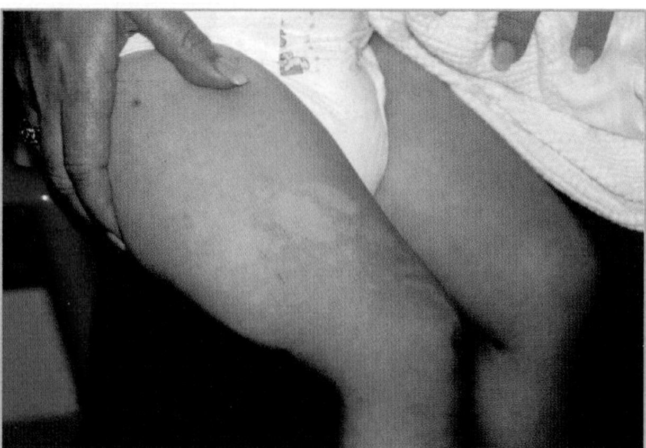

Figure 8-46. Hypopigmented patches. Courtesy of Lynne Bird, MD.

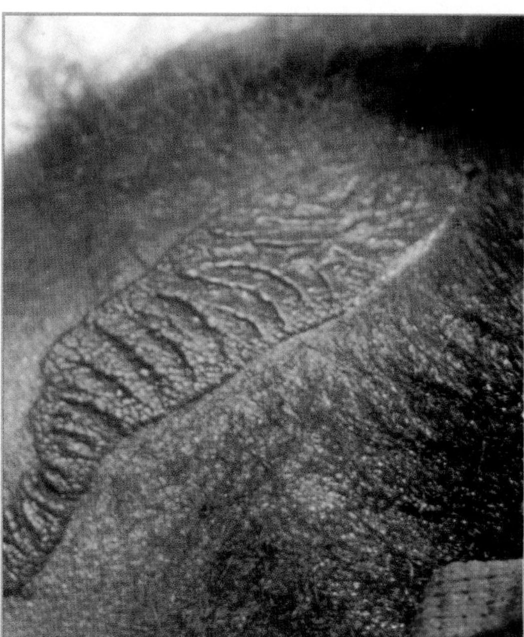

Figure 8-47. Nevus sebaceous of Jadassohn. Courtesy of Greenwood Genetic Center, Greenwood, SC.

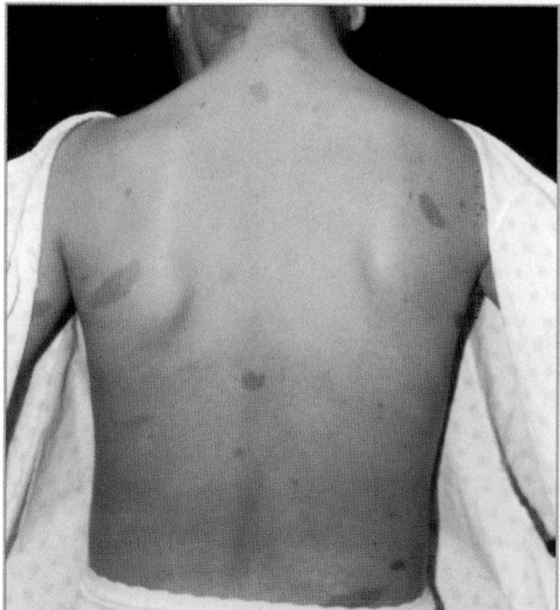

Figure 8-48. Café au lait macules. Courtesy of Greenwood Genetic Center, Greenwood, SC.

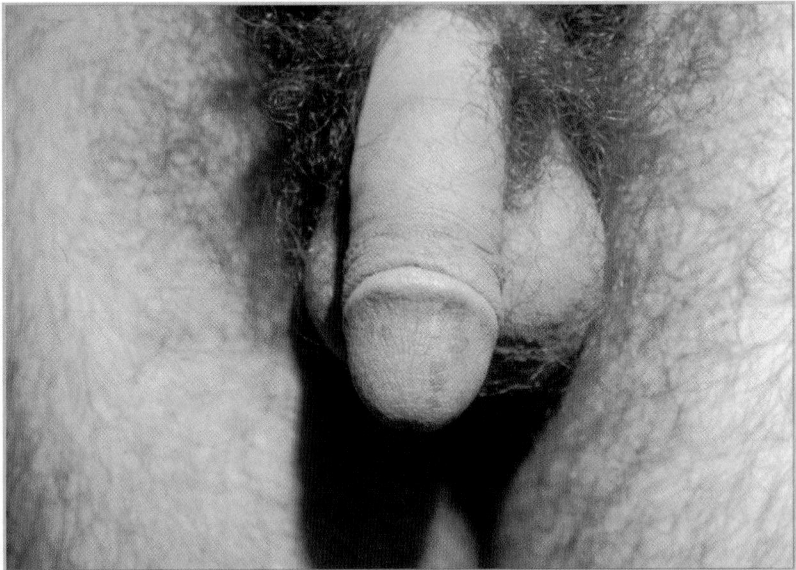

Figure 8-49. Café au lait macules on glans penis. Courtesy of Greenwood Genetic Center, Greenwood, SC.

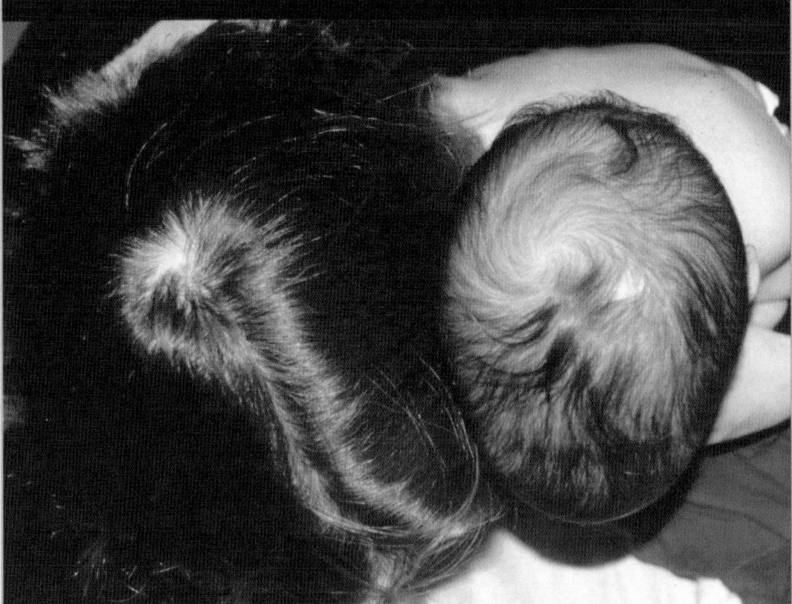

Figure 8-50. Aplasia cutis in mother and son. Courtesy of Lynne Bird, MD.

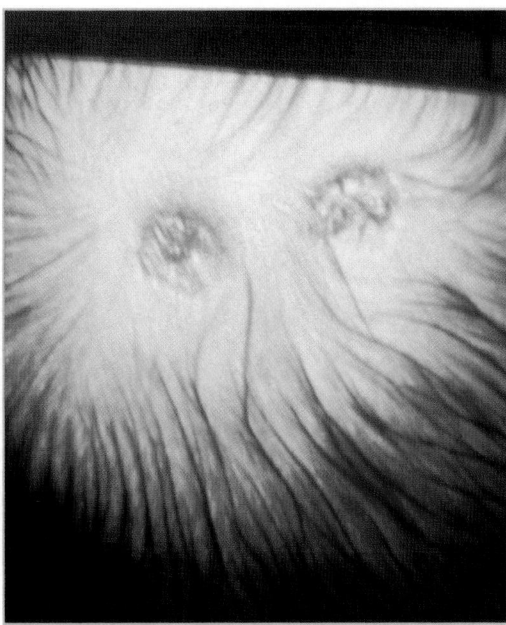

Figure 8-51. Cutis aplasia, scalp. Courtesy of Greenwood Genetic Center, Greenwood, SC.

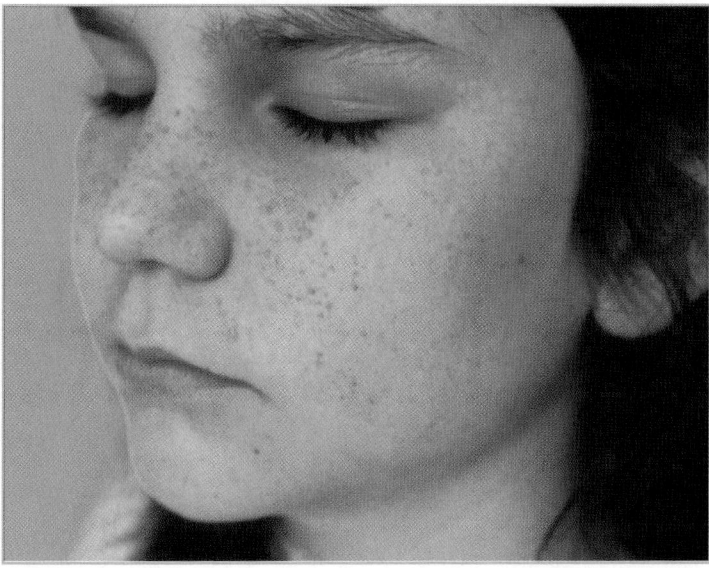

Figure 8-52. Facial angiofibromas. Courtesy of Greenwood Genetic Center, Greenwood, SC.

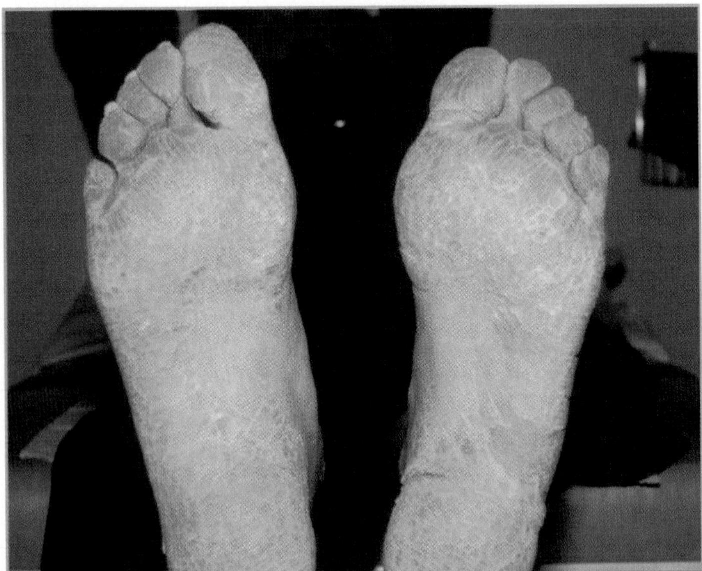

Figure 8-53. Hyperkeratosis of the feet. Courtesy of Greenwood Genetic Center, Greenwood, SC.

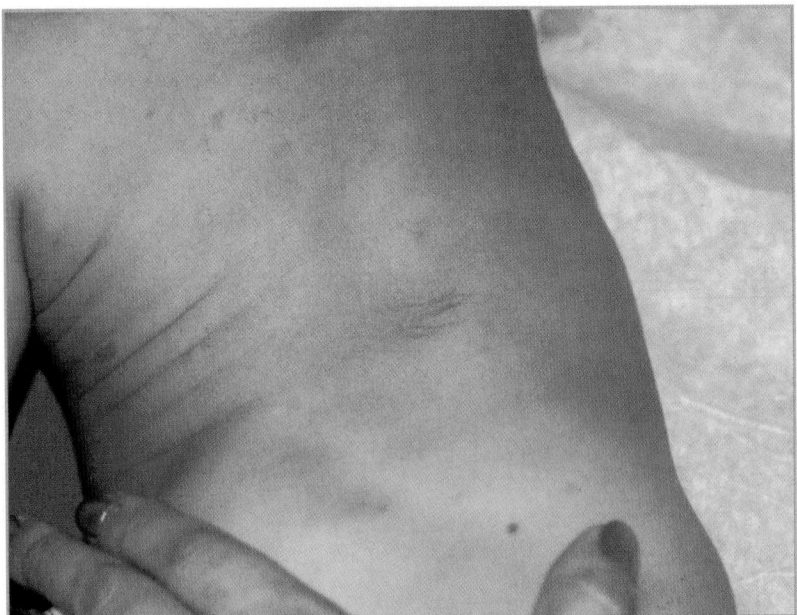

Figure 8-54. Hair tuft over lower spine. Courtesy of Lynne Bird, MD.

Minor anomalies are useful diagnostic features in 1 of 3 ways: Single minor anomalies may be the external "red flags" indicating the presence of specific occult major anomalies (Table 8-1), patterns of minor anomalies constitute most features by which multiple malformation syndromes are defined (Table 8-2), and 3 or more minor anomalies may be a nonspecific indicator of an occult major anomaly (~20%–25% risk). With respect to the latter, 1 or 2 minor anomalies are not associated with an increased frequency of associated major anomalies and warrant no further clinical investigation. Additional clinical investigation into the child with 3 or more minor anomalies depends on the overall diagnosis of the child and the presence or absence of additional symptoms and signs.[2]

Table 8-1. Minor Anomalies as Markers of Occult Major Anomalies[2,4]

Minor Anomaly	Associated Occult Major Anomaly or Syndrome
Pit/tag, preauricular	Malformed structures of the middle ear; congenital hearing loss
Central incisor, single maxillary	Holoprosencephaly
Oligodontia/hypodontia	Ectodermal dysplasias, various
Café au lait macules	Neurofibromatosis, type 1 or type 2
Hypopigmented patches	Tuberous sclerosis complex
Pigmentary streaks along the lines of Blaschko	Mosaicism for a chromosome anomaly or single gene abnormality
Hairy patch in lumbosacral area	Tethered spinal cord
Neck webbing	Jugular lymphatic obstruction sequence (Turner syndrome, Noonan syndrome, others)

Table 8-2. Patterns of Minor Anomalies in Representative Multiple Malformation Syndromes[3]

Syndrome	Pattern of Minor Anomalies
Trisomy 21 (Down syndrome)	3rd fontanelle, brachycephaly, low nasal bridge, epicanthus, upslanting palpebral fissures, Brushfield spots, short hands, clinodactyly of 5th fingers, single transverse palmar crease, sandal gap
Williams syndrome	Stellate irises, medial eyebrow flare, periorbital fullness, low nasal bridge, large mouth, large tongue, widely spaced teeth, hallux valgus, small nails, clinodactyly of 5th fingers
Noonan syndrome	Curly hair, downslanting palpebral fissures, ptosis, epicanthus, low nasal bridge, low-set ears, posteriorly angulated ears, short neck, webbed neck, pectus excavatum/carinatum
Fetal alcohol syndrome	Railroad track ears, short palpebral fissures, thin vermilion border of upper lip, smooth philtrum, hockey stick palmar creases, small nails, camptodactyly, limited pronation/supination at elbows
Waardenburg syndrome, type 1	White forelock, premature graying of hair, iris heterochromia, telecanthus, wide nasal bridge, hypopigmented patches
Neurofibromatosis, type 1	Café au lait macules, axillary/inguinal freckling, iris Lisch nodules, subcutaneous nodules (neurofibromas)
Tuberous sclerosis complex	Hypopigmented patches, facial angiofibromas (adenoma sebaceum), fibrous facial plaques, Shagreen patches, split nails, periungual fibromas

The Medical History of a Dysmorphic Child

Developmental disabilities often begin during prenatal life. The pregnancy history should include details of previous pregnancy losses, pregnancy planning, parental occupation and health at the time of conception, exposure to drugs (prescription, nonprescription, and illicit), alcohol, cigarettes, maternal fever, rash, acute or chronic illness, or other potential teratogenic exposures. Children with malformation syndromes associated with central nervous system malformations frequently exhibit altered gestational timing, late-onset or decreased fetal activity, polyhydramnios (accompanying deficient fetal swallowing), or an increased prevalence of non-vertex presentation at delivery. Congenital renal anomalies may be associated with oligohydramnios. Finally, the results of any prenatal genetic screening, fetal ultrasound or other imaging studies, genetic amniocentesis, chorionic villus sampling, or other genetic testing should be reviewed.

With respect to the neonatal period and infancy, prenatal onset growth deficiency or excess that persists postnatally is a frequent accompaniment

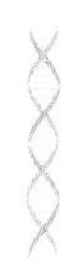

of many malformation syndromes. Thus birth weight, length, and head circumference should be recorded, and infant growth curves should be analyzed. Since children with anomalous brain development may exhibit difficulties with neonatal transition, assigned Apgar scores and any history of neonatal resuscitation should be obtained. The length of the neonatal hospitalization and any associated medical problems, consultations, and/or diagnostic studies should be ascertained. A careful developmental history with an emphasis on gross and fine motor milestones and formal assessments of behavior and development should also be sought. If available, medical records should be reviewed to validate any diagnosis or treatment of an isolated major malformation or malformation syndrome.[5]

Regarding childhood and adolescence, a comprehensive history should include hospitalizations, surgical procedures, medication use, major illnesses, growth, pubertal transition, behavioral problems, school performance, required educational or therapeutic interventions, and diagnostic imaging or laboratory procedures.

Finally, assessment of photographs of the child at various ages may be helpful, especially if assessing an older child or adult. Review of family photographs may also serve to identify other family members with similar features.

The Family History in Evaluating a Dysmorphic Child

A comprehensive family history should be obtained in the form of a 3-generation pedigree (a family history diagram). (See Chapter 5 for information on how to construct a pedigree.) The PCP, often in consultation with a dysmorphologist, uses information from the pedigree to determine if the disorder in question appears to have a genetic predisposition and, if so, what pattern of inheritance is most likely. In acquiring data for the pedigree, the following information is important to obtain in family members: known genetic conditions, malformation syndromes, intellectual disability, structural birth defects, pregnancy losses, stillbirths, and cause(s)/age(s) of death.[5]

The Essential Parts of a Dysmorphology Physical Examination

A detailed description of complete anatomy, landmarks, variations of normal, and minor anomalies is beyond the scope of this chapter; however, this information is available in many of the references listed at the end of the discussion.

It is axiomatic that careful observation and attention to detail are essential in examining a child with disabilities since, as stated earlier, recognition of patterns of minor anomalies constitutes the method by which most malformation syndromes are recognized.[2] It is important to approach the physical examination in an objective manner, avoiding subjective or pejorative descriptions (eg, "elfin facies" or "FLK"). Children with dysmorphic features always have discrete minor anomalies, which taken as a whole result in a phenotype that varies from normal. These findings should be described with standard terminology. (An international group of dysmorphologists has recently formulated universally accepted standardized terms for describing human morphology.)[6–12]

The examiner should begin with an accurate assessment of height, weight, and head circumference, the latter being an essential component of any examination of a child with disabilities, regardless of age (eg, a child with growth deficiency in the presence of accompanying microcephaly should prompt a completely different diagnostic assessment from that pursued in a growth-deficient child with a normal head circumference). A systematic examination of structure should then follow, using observation, palpation, auscultation, and simple morphometric techniques when clinically indicated (eg, measuring palpebral fissure length, inner canthal distance, middle finger and hand length; or assessing arm span or upper to lower segment ratio). Depending on the chief complaint of the child, a variety of morphometric norms are readily available for such measurements.[13,14] A standardized dysmorphology assessment form may be helpful in recording findings.

Formulating a Differential Diagnosis

Once historical and physical assessments are complete, it is useful to compose a short list of the most striking features of the child. For example, in a child with Williams syndrome, the list might include hypercalcemia, supravalvar aortic stenosis, and stellate iris pattern. Common findings, not likely to help differentiate the child from a diagnostic standpoint, would not be included (eg, short stature, microcephaly, or intellectual disability). A search for the observed pattern of malformations among electronic databases or print textbooks of malformation syndromes then follow.[3,15–19] Once a list of possible diagnoses is compiled, further laboratory assessments, imaging studies, and other diagnostic studies can be planned.

If a diagnosis is not forthcoming, the general pediatrician should consider referral of the child and his or her family to a dysmorphologist for further evaluation and counseling. In the United States, most dysmorphologists are pediatric clinical geneticists, certified by the American Board of Pediatrics and the American Board of Medical Genetics and Genomics, and are members of the American College of Medical Genetics and Genomics. An online directory of genetics professionals is available.[20] When and whether to make a referral will depend on the pediatrician's own background, training, and comfort in assessing children with disabilities. Occasionally the dysmorphologist will also be unable to assign a diagnosis to a child with birth defects or developmental disabilities. However, even in the absence of a formal diagnosis, the dysmorphologist may be able to reassure the family, suggest treatment or interventional strategies, and explore prenatal diagnostic planning for potential future pregnancies.

Laboratory Investigation in Assessing Dysmorphology

In general, genetic laboratory diagnostic tests are more likely to be helpful in diagnosing children with multiple minor anomalies or intellectual disability than in diagnosing those who appear to be structurally normal. The mainstay of laboratory diagnosis in dysmorphic children remains a high-resolution G-banded karyotype (>550 bands). However, chromosome analysis depends on visual inspection of microscopic chromosome structure and is thus limited. In general, visual chromosome inspection cannot routinely detect rearrangements smaller than 5 to 8 megabases, and much larger abnormalities escape notice if they occur in regions where the banding pattern is not distinctive. New molecular cytogenetic techniques (array comparative genomic hybridization or virtual karyotyping) can detect copy number changes in DNA at the level of 10 to 20 kilobases, about the size of a gene. This is approximately 1,000-fold greater resolution than high-resolution karyotypes obtained from conventional cytogenetics. As this technology becomes more widespread and more affordable, it may eventually supplant most conventional chromosome analysis. However, virtual karyotypes cannot detect balanced translocations and inversions. Therefore, for the time being PCPs in association with clinical geneticists will continue to order conventional chromosome analysis if such structural chromosome changes are sought.[21]

The sequences of many genes associated with malformation syndromes are known, and mutation analyses are now commercially available and can be ordered by pediatricians. However, availability alone is not a good reason to order mutation analysis. An unambiguous clinical diagnosis does not require molecular laboratory confirmation. Molecular diagnosis is indicated only in those single gene disorders in which a clinical diagnosis is questionable, where parents desire additional children and would take advantage of prenatal diagnosis if the particular mutation were known, or where presymptomatic testing for at-risk family members would be useful. In all cases, the practitioner must be aware of the limitations of the testing, such as etiologic heterogeneity of a syndrome or the frequent inability to find all of the mutations in a gene or genes.[5] A continuously updated directory of laboratories offering mutational analysis for many single gene disorders is available online.[15]

Biochemical genetic laboratory testing may be helpful in many cases, particularly in children in whom storage diseases are suspected (eg, mucopolysaccharidoses), or when clinical features suggest specific biochemical pathways. Examples include peroxisomal disorders (eg, Zellweger syndrome or chondrodysplasia punctata), mitochondrial disorders, and disorders of cholesterol metabolism (eg, Smith-Lemli-Opitz syndrome).[5]

Management and Counseling

Accurate diagnosis in a child with multiple malformations is important for families in order to counsel them appropriately about the prognosis and natural history of the disorder, discuss treatment and prenatal diagnostic options, provide genetic counseling about risks of recurrence with future pregnancies, alleviate guilt and blame, and make appropriate recommendations for diagnosis-specific support organizations.[19] Options for the management of genetic diseases are varied and expanding rapidly. Although a significant number of genetic diseases still have no effective treatment, for others many treatment options exist. Current treatment modalities include dietary management (eg, the restriction of phenylalanine in phenylketonuria), protein or enzyme replacement (eg, in Gaucher syndrome and some of the mucopolysaccharidoses), and tissue replacement (eg, blood transfusions or bone marrow transplantation in sickle cell anemia and β-thalassemia). Multidisciplinary teams (such as craniofacial or myelodysplasia clinics) can fulfill a vital function in the care of children with multiple congenital anomalies. Pediatric surgical and dental specialists provide additional services as needed. Other treatments are strictly symptomatic, such as the use of β-blockers to slow the rate of aortic dilation in Marfan syndrome, administration of antibiotics in early cystic fibrosis, or female hormone replacement in Turner syndrome. Many textbooks and online resources discuss management of specific genetic disorders.[15–19,22]

Key Points

- An organized clinical approach to diagnosis in children with multiple anomalies remains the mainstay of pediatric assessment for children with dysmorphic features.
- Approximately 70% of minor anomalies are present in the craniofacies and hands.
- Anomalous structures result from prenatal malformation, deformation, or disruption.
- Single minor anomalies may be red flags indicating the presence of specific occult major anomalies. Patterns of minor anomalies constitute most features by which multiple malformation syndromes are defined. Three or more minor anomalies may be a nonspecific indicator of an occult major anomaly.
- One or 2 minor anomalies are not associated with an increased frequency of associated major anomalies and warrant no further clinical investigation.
- Evaluating a child with a dysmorphism should include creating a 3-generation pedigree.

References

1. Smith DW. Dysmorphology (teratology). *J Pediatr.* 1966;69(6):1150–1169
2. Aase JM. *Diagnostic Dysmorphology.* New York, NY: Plenum Medical Book Co.; 1990
3. Jones KL. *Smith's Recognizable Patterns of Human Malformation.* 6th ed. Philadelphia, PA: Elsevier Saunders; 2006
4. Hoyme HE. Minor anomalies: diagnostic clues to aberrant human morphogenesis. *Genetica.* 1993;89:307–315
5. Hunter AGW. Medical genetics 2: the diagnostic approach to the child with dysmorphic signs. *CMAJ.* 2002;167(4):367–372
6. Allanson JE, Biesecker LG, Carey JC, Hennekam RC. Elements of morphology: introduction. *Am J Med Genet Part A.* 2009;149A:2–5
7. Allanson JE, Cunniff C, Hoyme HE, McGaughran J, Muenke M, Neri G. Elements of morphology: standard terminology for the head and face. *Am J Med Genet Part A.* 2009;149A:6–28
8. Hall BD, Graham JM Jr, Cassidy SB, Opitz JM. Elements of morphology: standard terminology for the periorbital region. *Am J Med Genet Part A.* 2009;149A:29–39
9. Hunter A, Frias J, Gillessen-Kaesbach G, Hughes H, Jones K, Wilson L. Elements of morphology: standard terminology for the ear. *Am J Med Genet Part A.* 2009;149A: 40–60
10. Hennekam RC, Cormier-Daire V, Hall J, Mehes K, Patton M, Stevenson R. Elements of morphology: standard terminology for the nose and philtrum. *Am J Med Genet Part A.* 2009;149A:61–76
11. Carey JC, Cohen MM Jr, Curry C, Devriendt K, Holmes L, Verloes A. Elements of morphology: standard terminology for the lips, mouth, and oral region. *Am J Med Genet Part A.* 2009;149A:77–92

12. Biesecker LG, Aase JM, Clericuzio C, Gurrieri F, Temple K, Toriello H. Elements of morphology: standard terminology for the hands and feet. *Am J Med Genet Part A.* 2009;149A:93–127
13. Hall JG, Allanson JE, Gripp KW, Slavotinek AM. *Handbook of Physical Measurements.* 2nd ed. New York, NY: Oxford University Press; 2007
14. Farkas LG. *Anthropometry of the Head and Face in Medicine.* New York, NY: Elsevier; 1981
15. Gene Tests/Gene Reviews. http://www.ncbi.nlm.nih.gov/sites/GeneTests/?db=GeneTests. Accessed March 5, 2010
16. Winter RM, Baraitser M. London Dysmorphology Database. London Medical Databases; 2003
17. Online Mendelian Inheritance in Man. http://www.ncbi.nlm.nih.gov/omim/. Accessed March 5, 2010
18. POSSUM (Pictures of Standard Syndromes and Undiagnosed Malformations). http://www.possum.net.au/. Accessed March 5, 2010
19. Clinical Genetics Computer Resources. http://www.kumc.edu/gec/prof/genecomp.html. Accessed March 5, 2010
20. American College of Medical Genetics. http://www.acmg.net/. Accessed March 5, 2010
21. Li MM, Andersson HC. Clinical application of microarray-based molecular cytogenetics: an emerging new era of genomic medicine. *J Pediatrics.* 2009;155(3):311–317
22. Cassidy SB, Allanson JE, ed. *Management of Genetic Syndromes.* 2nd ed. Hoboken, NJ: John Wiley & Sons, Inc; 2005

Chapter 9

Specific Genetic Conditions

Michael J. Lyons, MD

Introduction

Genetic syndromes are generally considered rare conditions. However, most pediatricians and primary care physicians will take care of individuals with known genetic syndromes. Select, common heritable conditions, grouped by the primary system of involvement are listed in Table 9-1. Mode of inheritance, prevalence, and characteristic findings demonstrate the factors that primary care physicians (PCPs) should consider as they manage patients with these disorders.

In addition, included here are 15 genetic conditions with recognizable features that reflect relatively common disorders likely to be encountered in primary care practice. The underlying cause of each condition is known, and testing is clinically available. Management issues are important for all of the syndromes included in the chapter. Case presentations highlight clinical features, laboratory testing, counseling issues, and management recommendations. The cases refer to a specific presentation and may not be generalizable to all such affected patients. Pictures and tables are provided to emphasize certain clinical features. Specific references are included with each case and general resources are provided at the end of the chapter.

Table 9-1. Select Common Heritable Pediatric Conditions[a]

Primary System	Condition	Inheritance	Prevalence	Characteristic Clinical Findings
Audiologic				
	Sensorineural hearing loss	AD, AR, XL (majority AR)	1:500 newborns	Bilateral permanent hearing loss ≥40 dB
	Waardenburg syndrome, type I	AD	1:20,000–40,000	Sensorineural hearing loss Heterochromia White forelock
Cardiovascular				
	Arrhythmogenic right ventricular cardiomyopathy	AD	1:1,000–1:2,500	Ventricular tachycardia Sudden death
	Dilated cardiomyopathy	AD, AR, XL	1:2,700	Congestive heart failure Arrhythmias Thromboembolic disease
	Familial hypercholesterolemia	AD	1:500	Elevated LDL cholesterol (from birth) Early-onset cardiovascular disease
	Familial hypertrophic cardiomyopathy	AD	1:500–1,000	Heart failure Shortness of breath Syncope
	Long Q-T syndrome	AD	1:3,000–1:7,000	Prolonged QT interval, T-wave abnormalities on ECG Syncope
	Wolff-Parkinson-White syndrome	AD	1-3:1,000	Supraventricular tachycardia Short PR interval, wide QRS complex on ECG

Primary System	Condition	Inheritance	Prevalence	Characteristic Clinical Findings
Dermatologic				
	Hereditary hemorrhagic telangiectasia	AD	1:10,000	Telangiectasias Nosebleeds Multiple arteriovenous malformations
	Neurofibromatosis, type I	AD	1:3,000	Café au lait macules Neurofibromas Lisch nodules
	Tuberous sclerosis	AD	1:5,800	Hypomelanotic macules Facial angiofibromas Cortical tubers Seizures Intellectual disability
Genitourinary				
	Polycystic kidney disease, autosomal dominant	AD	1–2:1,000	Renal cysts (bilateral) Intracranial aneurysms
	Polycystic kidney disease, autosomal recessive	AR	1:10,000–40,000	Large, echogenic kidneys in infants
	Renal adysplasia	AD	1:4,000	Bilateral or unilateral renal agenesis

Table 9-1. Select Common Heritable Pediatric Conditions[a] *(continued)*

Primary System	Condition	Inheritance	Prevalence	Characteristic Clinical Findings
Growth				
	Beckwith-Wiedemann syndrome	AD, UPD, imprinting disorder	1:13,700	Overgrowth Macroglossia Hemihyperplasia Abdominal wall defect
	Turner syndrome	Chromosomal	1:2,500–3,000 live-born females	Short stature Webbed neck Coarctation of the aorta
Hematologic				
	Hemophilia A	XL	1:4,000–5,000 males	Prolonged bleeding Excessive bruising Hemarthrosis
	Sickle cell disease	AR	1:300–500 African Americans	Chronic hemolytic anemia Intermittent pain crises Dactylitis
	Von Willebrand disease	AD, AR	1:100–1,000	Bruising Prolonged bleeding
Musculoskeletal				
	Achondroplasia	AD	1:26,000–28,000	Disproportionate short stature Macrocephaly Midface hypoplasia
	Ehlers-Danlos syndrome, classic type	AD	1:20,000	Joint hypermobility Skin hyperextensibility Abnormal wound healing

Primary System	Condition	Inheritance	Prevalence	Characteristic Clinical Findings
	Marfan syndrome	AD	1:5,000–1:10,000	Aortic root dilatation Ectopia lentis Disproportionately long extremities
	Osteogenesis imperfecta, type I	AD	1:30,000	Multiple fractures Wormian bones Blue sclerae
Neurodevelopment				
	Angelman syndrome	Chromosome deletion, paternal UPD, imprinting, *UBE3A* mutation	1:12,000–20,000	Intellectual disability Ataxia Seizures Acquired microcephaly
	Down syndrome	Chromosomal	1:650–800	Intellectual disability Congenital heart defect Brushfield spots Upslanting palpebral fissures Transverse palmar creases
	Fragile X syndrome	XL	1:2,500–3,700 males 1:7,000 females	Intellectual disability Long face Large ears Macroorchidism
	Klinefelter syndrome	Chromosomal	1:500–1,000	Develomental delay Gynecomastia Delayed puberty Infertility

Table 9-1. Select Common Heritable Pediatric Conditions[a] *(continued)*

Primary System	Condition	Inheritance	Prevalence	Characteristic Clinical Findings
Neurodevelopment *(continued)*				
	Noonan syndrome	AD	1:1,000–2,500	Short stature Develomental delay Pulmonic stenosis Broad/webbed neck Ptosis
	Prader-Willi syndrome	Chromosome deletion, maternal UPD, imprinting	1:10,000–30,000	Intellectual disability Hypotonia Hyperphagia Obesity Short stature
	Rett syndrome	XL	1:8,500 females	Developmental regression Stereotypic hand movements Acquired microcephaly Seizures
	Smith-Lemli-Opitz syndrome	AR	1:20,000–40,000	Intellectual disability Microcephaly Growth delay Underdeveloped genitalia Cleft palate 2- to 3-toe syndactyly
	Smith-Magenis syndrome	Chromosome deletion, *RAI1* mutation	1:15,000–25,000	Intellectual disability Sleep disorder Behavior problems

Primary System	Condition	Inheritance	Prevalence	Characteristic Clinical Findings
Neurodevelopment *(continued)*				
	Sotos syndrome	AD	1:14,000	Intellectual disability Overgrowth
	Velocardiofacial syndrome	AD	1:4,000	Developmental delay Cleft palate Immune deficiency Congenital heart defect Hypocalcemia
	Williams syndrome	AD	1:7,500–10,000	Intellectual disability Overly friendly Supravalvular aortic stenosis Hypercalcemia Full cheeks Periorbital fullness
Neuromuscular				
	Charcot-Marie-Tooth syndrome	AD, AR, XL	1:3,300	Distal muscle weakness and atrophy Sensory loss Depressed tendon reflexes High-arched feet
	Duchenne muscular dystrophy	XL	1:4,700 male live births	Delayed milestones Progressive proximal muscle weakness Calf hypertrophy
	Huntington disease	AD	1–2:25,000	Progressive motor, cognitive, psychiatric disturbances
	Spinal muscular atrophy	AR	1:10,000	Muscle weakness Tongue fasciculations Absent tendon reflexes

Table 9-1. Select Common Heritable Pediatric Conditions[a] *(continued)*

Primary System	Condition	Inheritance	Prevalence	Characteristic Clinical Findings
Pulmonary				
	Cystic fibrosis	AR	1:3,200 Caucasians 1:15,000 African Americans 1:31,000 Asian Americans	Pulmonary disease (lower airway inflammation and chronic infections) Meconium ileus at birth (15%–20%) Pancreatic insufficiency

Abbreviations: AD, autosomal dominant; AR, autosomal recessive; ECG, electrocardiogram; LDL, low-density lipoprotein; UPD, uniparental disomy; XL, X-linked.

[a]Not all of the listed conditions are exclusively genetic. Phenocopies (nongenetic presentations of the disorder) may exist.

Achondroplasia

Clinical Features

A 2-year-old male has disproportionate short stature, relative macrocephaly, prominent forehead, low nasal bridge, and trident configuration of the hands (Figure 9-1). Skeletal x-rays reveal short long bones with metaphyseal flare; small, square iliac wings; and narrow sciatic notch. Vertebral films are not adequate to assess for cuboid vertebral bodies, short pedicles, and narrow lumbar interpedicular distance. His features are consistent with achondroplasia (Table 9-2).

Laboratory Diagnosis

Achondroplasia testing of the fibroblast growth factor receptor 3 (*FGFR3*) gene is consistent with achondroplasia. *FGFR3* is the only gene known to be associated with achondroplasia. Most cases (~98%) are due to a guanine-to-adenine mutation at nucleotide 1138 resulting in a substitution of arginine for glycine at amino acid 380 (G380R). Another 1% of cases are due to a guanine-to-cytosine mutation at nucleotide 1138, which also leads to a G380R change.

Genetic Counseling

The family is counseled that the *FGFR3* gene test results confirm the diagnosis of achondroplasia, which is the most common cause of disproportionate short stature, with a birth prevalence of 1:26,000 to 1:28,000. Achondroplasia is an autosomal dominant disorder. The parents both have normal stature, indicating this is likely a new mutation, which is true for most cases (>80%) of achondroplasia. Because the achondroplasia is likely caused by a new mutation, the recurrence risk is low but is higher than the risk in the general population due to possible germline mosaicism for an *FGFR3* mutation in one of the parents. New mutations are seen more commonly in fathers with advanced paternal age. In 20% of cases, one or both parents have achondroplasia. The recurrence risk if one parent is affected is 50%. If both parents are affected, there is a 25% chance of having a child with normal stature, a 50% chance of having a child with achondroplasia, and a 25% chance of having a child who has a mutation in both copies of *FGFR3*, resulting in homozygous achondroplasia, which is typically lethal.

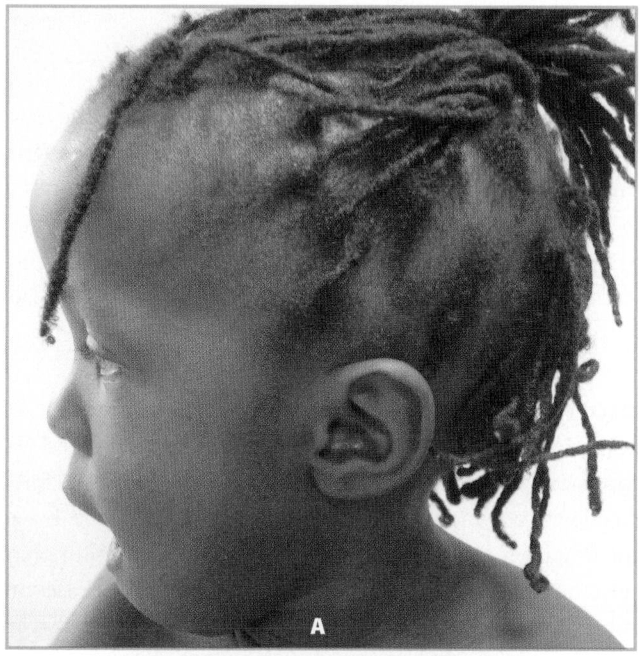

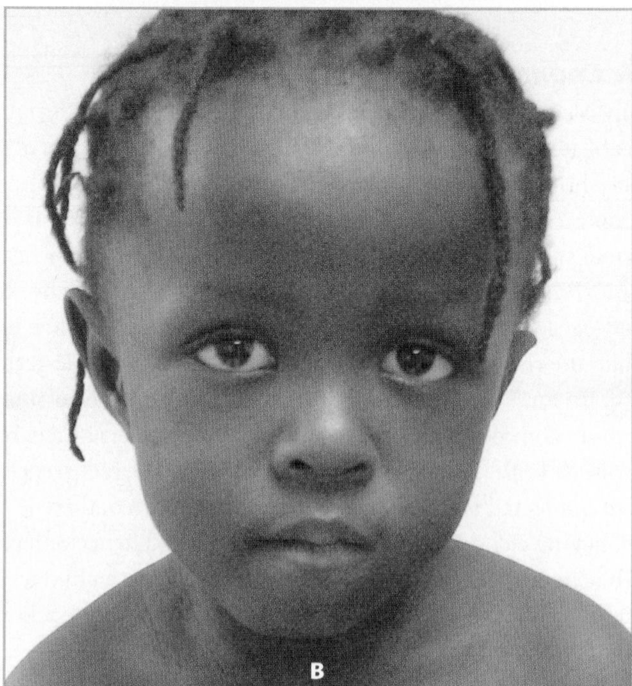

Figure 9-1A–D. Disproportionate short stature, lordosis, prominent forehead, and low nasal bridge in a male with achondroplasia.

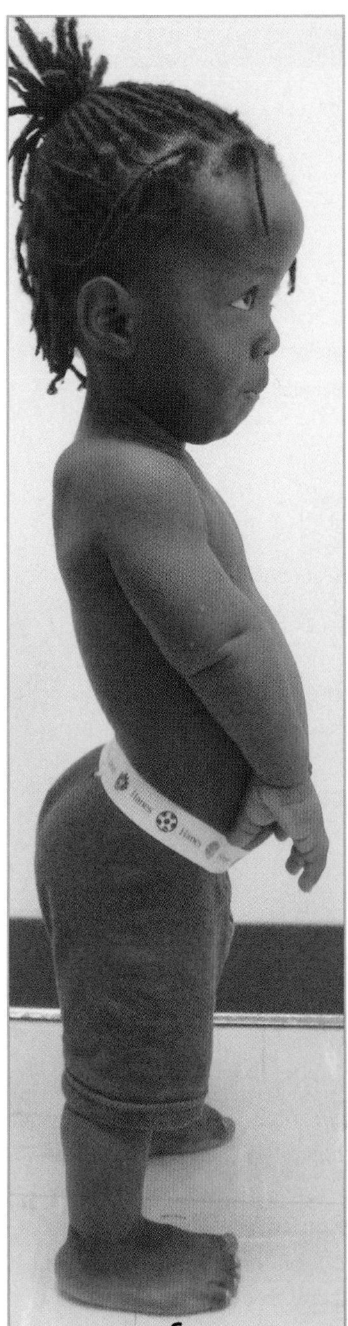
C

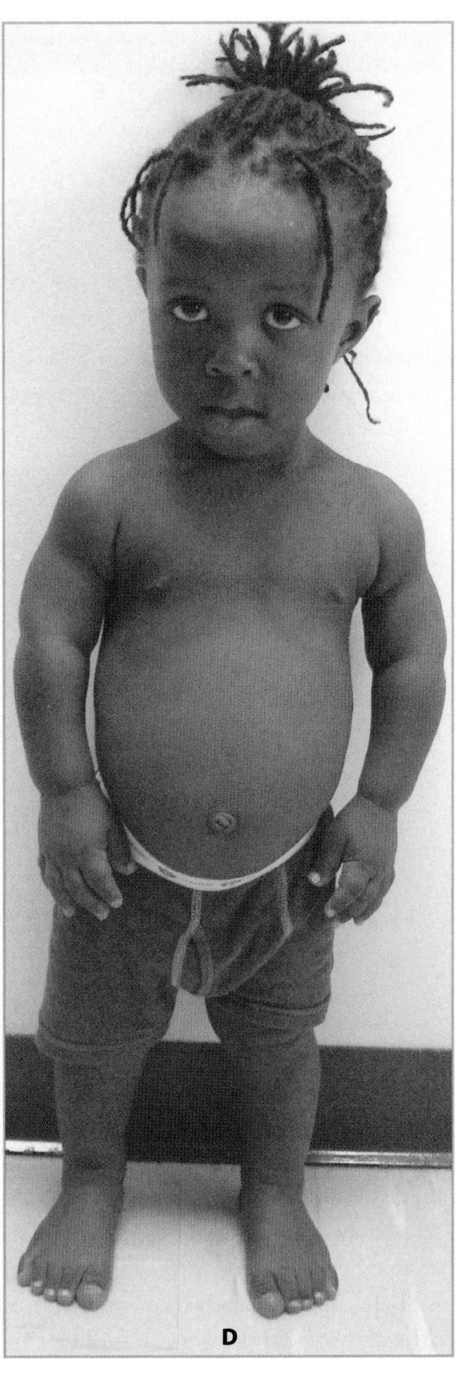
D

Table 9-2. Achondroplasia Characteristic Features

Area	Feature
Craniofacial	Macrocephaly Prominent forehead Midface hypoplasia Low, broad nasal bridge Narrow nasal passages Recurrent ear infections Dental malocclusion
Growth	Short stature (mean adult height: male 130 cm; female 125 cm)
Musculoskeletal	Rhizomelia (short proximal limbs) Short, trident hand Lumbar lordosis, kyphosis Small, cuboid vertebral bodies Short vertebral pedicles Narrow lumbar interpediculate distance Square pelvis with small sacrosciatic notch Bowed legs Incomplete elbow extension
Neurodevelopment	Normal intelligence with motor delays Hydrocephalus Cervicomedullary junction compression related to small foramen magnum Spinal stenosis
Otolaryngologic	Obstructive sleep apnea

Management

Regular monitoring of growth on growth charts specific for achondroplasia is recommended. Although cognitive function is typically normal, development should be closely monitored because motor delays are common. Annual hearing evaluations should be performed. Magnetic resonance imaging or computed tomography is used to look for evidence of hydrocephalus and spinal cord compression. Referral to pediatric neurology or pediatric neurosurgery should be considered if there are significant neurologic changes, such as hyperreflexia or clonus. Individuals should be monitored for signs of obstructive sleep apnea.

Angelman Syndrome

Clinical Features

A 19-month-old male has global developmental delays, frequent laughter, hand-flapping, and a fascination with water. A physical examination reveals microcephaly, a flat occiput, upslanted palpebral fissures, a high-arched palate, and hypotonia (Figure 9-2). His features are consistent with Angelman syndrome (Table 9-3).

Laboratory Diagnosis

High-resolution chromosome analysis is normal. Fluorescent in situ hybridization (FISH) analysis of the Angelman syndrome critical region on chromosome 15q11-q13 reveals a deletion consistent with Angelman syndrome. Chromosome analysis and FISH testing of the Angelman syndrome critical region is performed on the patient's mother and is normal. Angelman syndrome is due to a maternal deletion in 68% to 70% of cases. An additional 10% of cases are due to paternal uniparental disomy (UPD) or imprinting defects. Angelman syndrome cases due to deletions, UPD, or imprinting defects can be detected by methylation analysis. Sequence analysis of the *UBE3A* gene detects an additional 10% to 11% of cases. Methylation analysis and *UBE3A* testing identifies approximately 90% of Angelman syndrome cases. Chromosome analysis detects less than 1% of cases of Angelman syndrome. An underlying genetic etiology is not identified in the remaining 10% with clinical features of Angelman syndrome.

Genetic Counseling

The family is counseled that the FISH test results confirm the clinical diagnosis of Angelman syndrome. The prevalence of Angelman syndrome is 1:12,000 to 1:20,000. Individuals with Angelman syndrome have an alteration of the area on chromosome 15q11-q13 that is maternally derived. The recurrence risk depends on how the area is altered. The patient's deletion occurred for the first time in the family, which confers a low recurrence risk of less than 1% in future offspring. Uniparental disomy is typically a sporadic event with a low recurrence risk of less than 1%. An imprinting defect or *UBE3A* mutation that occurred for the first time in an individual would confer a low recurrence risk of less than 1%. The presence of a maternally inherited imprinting defect or *UBE3A* mutation can result in a recurrence risk as high as 50%. If a parent carries a chromosome rearrangement, the recurrence risk may be relatively high depending on the type of rearrangement.

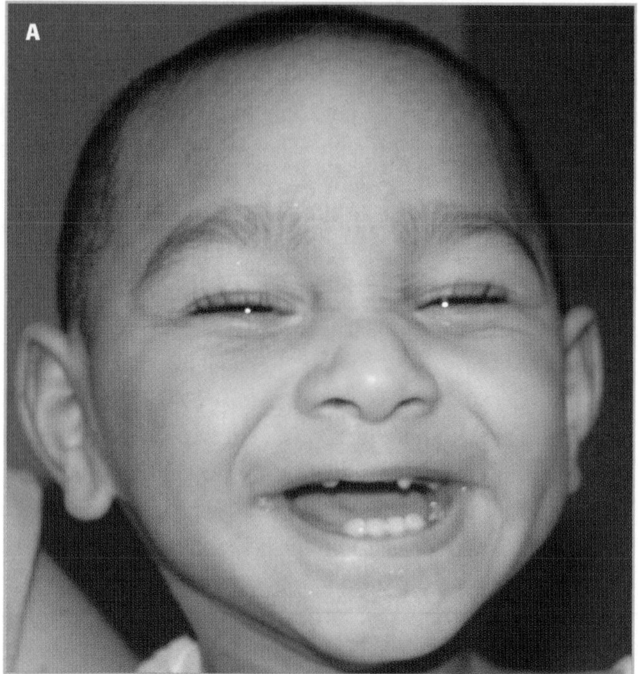

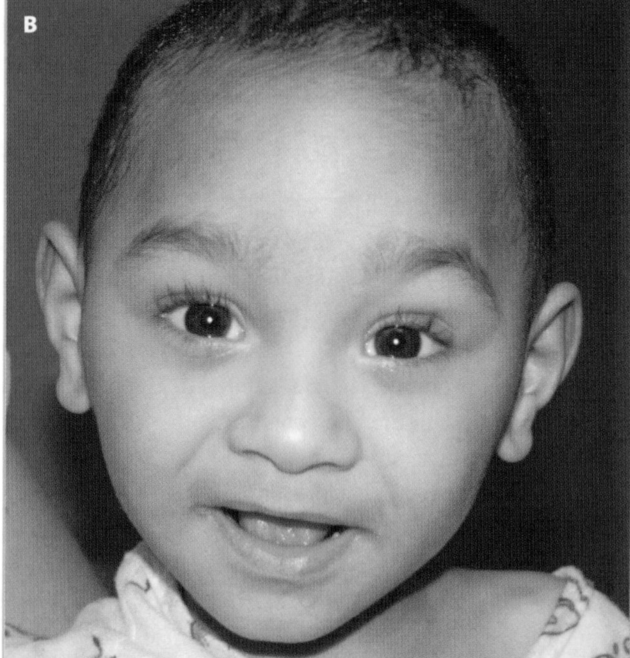

Figure 9-2A–E. Microcephaly and wide mouth with frequent laughter in a male with Angelman syndrome.

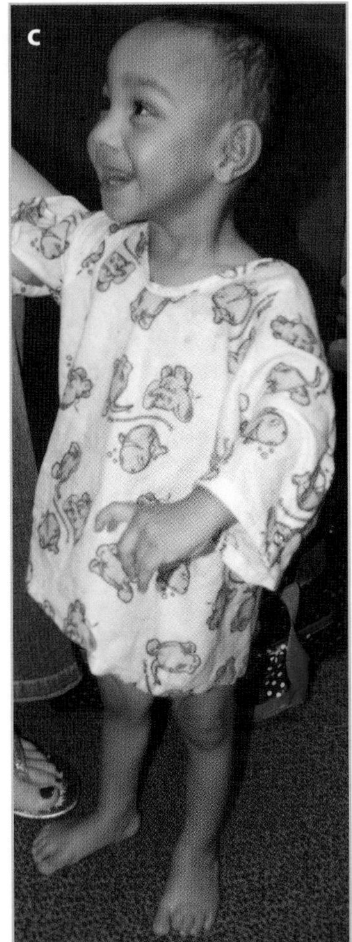
C

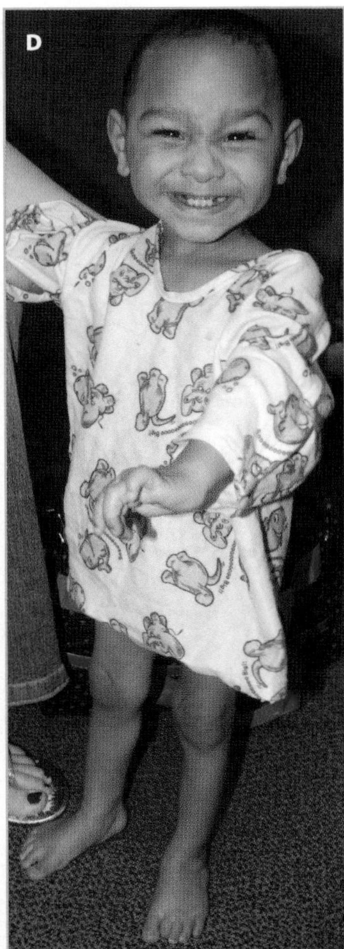
D

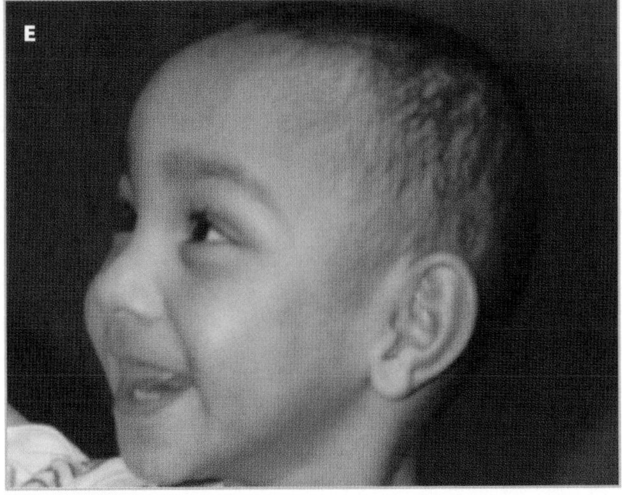
E

Table 9-3. Angelman Syndrome Characteristic Features

Area	Feature
Craniofacial	Microcephaly (acquired)
	Brachycephaly
	Maxillary hypoplasia
	Wide mouth
	Wide-spaced teeth
	Prominent mandible
Dermatologic	Hypopigmented skin and eyes
Gastrointestinal	Feeding difficulties
Musculoskeletal	Scoliosis
Neurodevelopment	Intellectual disability with severe speech impairment
	Gait ataxia with uplifted and flexed arms during walking
	Tremulousness of the limbs
	Unique behavior with frequent laughter and excitability
	Seizures
	Increased sensitivity to heat
	Sleep disturbance
	Fascination with water
Ophthalmologic	Strabismus

Management

The patient has been evaluated for seizures but has not had any definitive seizure activity. His development is monitored regularly. He receives early education planning and therapies focusing on nonverbal means of communication. He continues to be monitored for behavior problems, feeding issues, sleep disturbance, scoliosis, constipation, and gastroesophageal reflux disease.

Beckwith-Wiedemann Syndrome

Clinical Features

A 3-month-old male has an enlarged tongue and an umbilical hernia. A physical examination reveals height at the 90th percentile, weight greater than the 97th percentile, and head circumference at the 95th percentile. He has subtle creases on his earlobes, macroglossia, umbilical hernia, and nevus flammeus over the glabella (Figure 9-3). His clinical features are consistent with Beckwith-Wiedemann syndrome (Table 9-4).

Laboratory Diagnosis

A chromosome analysis is normal with a 46,XY karyotype. Chromosome abnormalities are an uncommon cause of Beckwith-Wiedemann syndrome. Molecular genetic testing has been discussed with the family but not yet initiated. Methylation analysis of 2 differentially methylated regions (DMRs) on chromosome 11p15.5 detects abnormalities in 2% to 7% of cases for DMR1 and 50% to 60% of cases for DMR2. Paternal UPD accounts for 10% to 20% of cases. As most of these UPD cases appear to be mosaic, testing other tissues may be indicated. Sequence analysis of the *CDKN1C* gene can detect mutations in sporadic or familial cases.

Genetic Counseling

The incidence of Beckwith-Wiedemann syndrome is approximately 1:13,700. Because the expression is variable, the incidence may be higher due to lack of recognition of milder cases. Most cases of Beckwith-Wiedemann syndrome are sporadic with a low recurrence risk. Autosomal dominant inheritance is identified in 15% of cases. Parents of an individual with Beckwith-Wiedemann syndrome caused by a chromosome abnormality may have a balanced chromosome rearrangement with a recurrence risk as high as 50%. Paternal duplications of 11p15.5 are associated with developmental delay. There have been reports indicating a possible increased risk for Beckwith-Wiedemann syndrome associated with assistive reproductive technology.

Management

The patient should have his growth followed regularly. Developmental evaluations should be performed to detect early signs of developmental delay. In the neonatal period, individuals with Beckwith-Wiedemann syndrome should be screened for hypoglycemia. Feeding difficulties related to macroglossia should

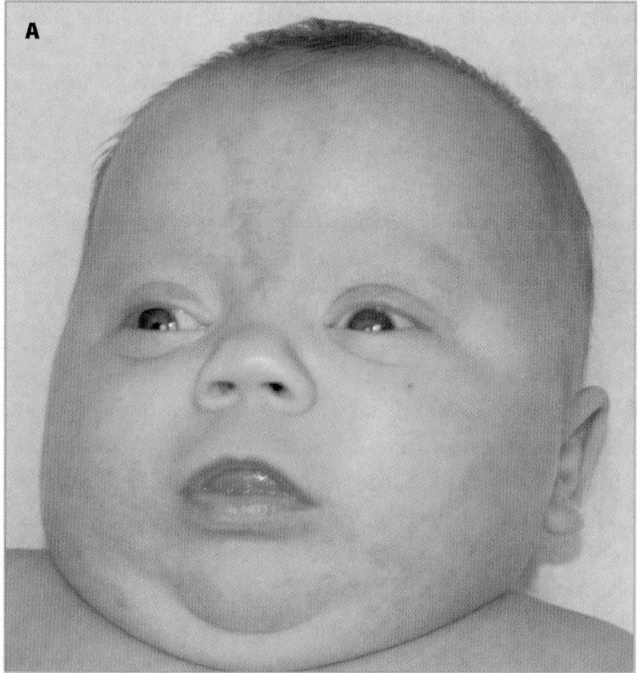

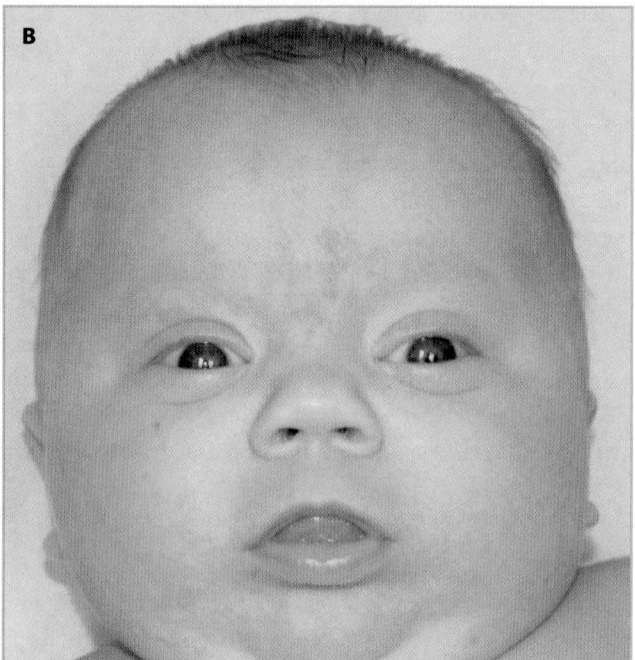

Figure 9-3A–D. Macroglossia, subtle earlobe crease, and umbilical hernia in a male with a clinical diagnosis of Beckwith-Wiedemann syndrome.

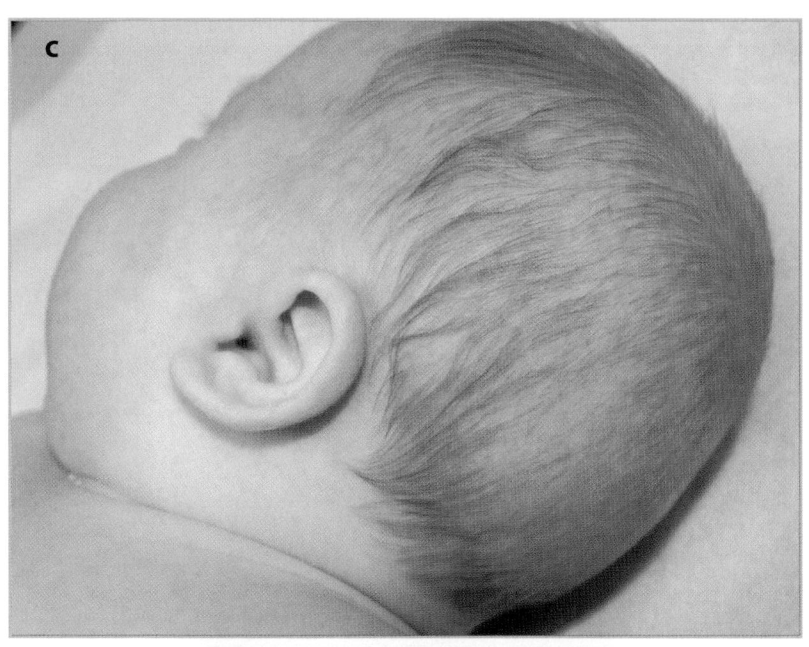
C

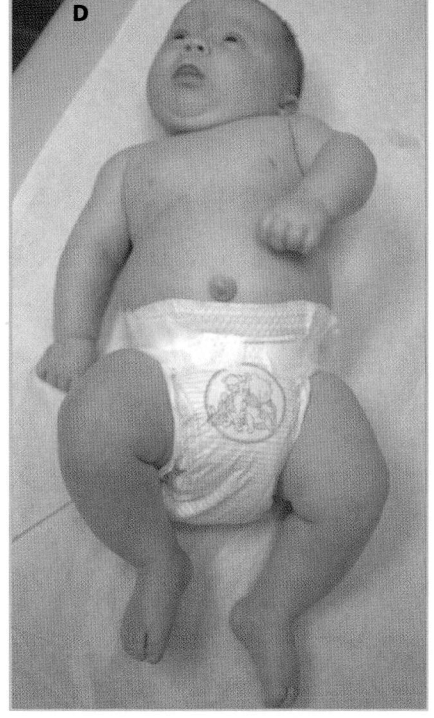
D

Table 9-4. Beckwith-Wiedemann Syndrome Characteristic Features

Area	Feature
Cardiovascular	Cardiomegaly Cardiac malformation
Craniofacial	Macroglossia Earlobe creases and helical pits Midface hypoplasia Cleft palate
Dermatologic	Facial nevus flammeus
Endocrine	Neonatal hypoglycemia
Gastrointestinal	Abdominal wall defect: omphalocele, umbilical hernia, diastasis recti Visceromegaly Adrenocortical cytomegaly
Genitourinary	Renal anomalies
Growth	Macrosomia
Musculoskeletal	Hemihyperplasia
Neurodevelopment	Normal development in most cases
Oncology	Increased risk for embryonal tumors: Wilms, hepatoblastoma
Ophthalmologic	Prominent eyes with infraorbital creases
Perinatal	Polyhydramnios Prematurity Enlarged placenta

be addressed. Significant complications related to macroglossia may require surgical intervention. If leg length discrepancy related to hemihyperplasia develops, orthopedic intervention may be necessary. Due to an increased risk for cardiac malformations, a cardiology evaluation should be considered. Renal ultrasounds and urinary calcium-to-creatinine ratio are used to screen for renal anomalies. Abdominal wall defects may require surgical correction. Due to an increased risk for embryonal tumors, regular screening with abdominal ultrasounds and α-fetoprotein is recommended.

Down Syndrome

Clinical Features

A 13-month-old female born at 37 weeks' gestation to a 25-year-old mother has upslanting palpebral fissures, Brushfield spots, hypoplastic midface, small ears, small nose, and protruding tongue (Figure 9-4). Her features are consistent with Down syndrome (Table 9-5).

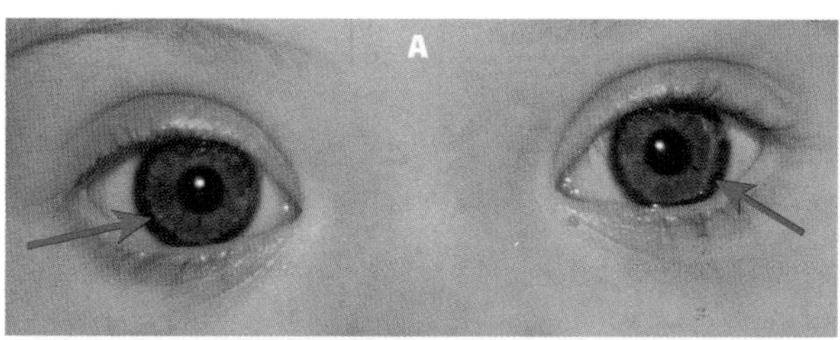

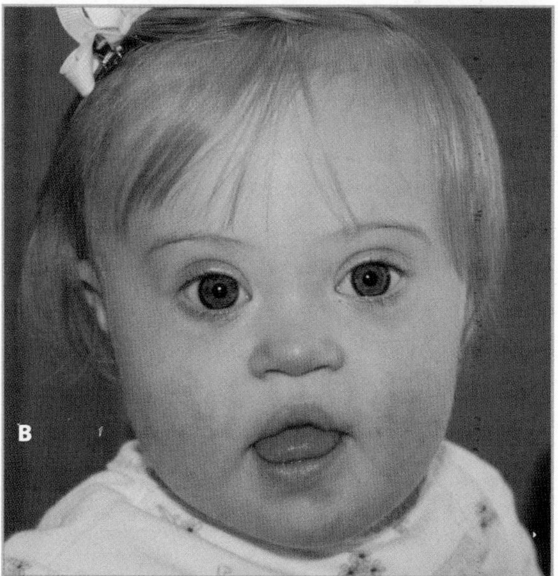

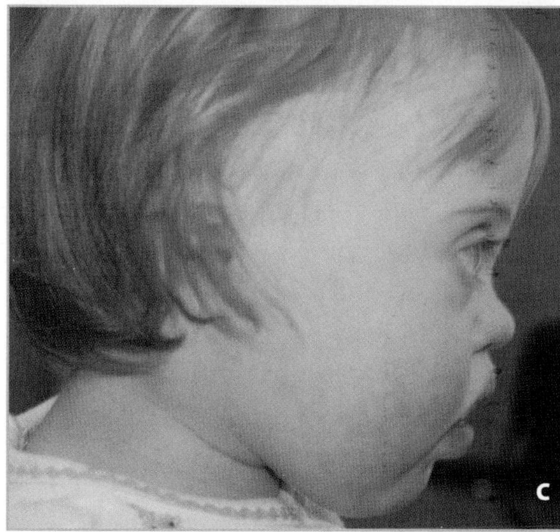

Figure 9-4A–C. Brushfield spots (arrows) and characteristic facial features in a female with Down syndrome.

Table 9-5. Down Syndrome Characteristic Features

Area	Feature
Cardiovascular	Congenital heart defect (endocardial cushion defect)
Craniofacial	Brachycephaly
	Midface hypoplasia
	Upslanting palpebral fissures
	Epicanthal folds
	Flat nasal bridge
	Small ears
	Small mouth with a protruding tongue
	Obstructive sleep apnea
	Excess nuchal skin
Endocrine	Hypothyroidism
Gastrointestinal	Duodenal atresia
	Hirschsprung disease
Growth	Short stature
Hematology	Increased risk for leukemia
Musculoskeletal	Increased risk for atlantoaxial instability
	Short and incurved fifth finger
	Transverse palmar crease
	Gap between first and second toes
Neurodevelopment	Intellectual disability
	Hypotonia
	Increased risk for Alzheimer disease
Ophthalmologic	Brushfield spots
	Cataracts
Otolaryngologic	Hearing loss with frequent ear infection

Laboratory Diagnosis

Chromosome analysis reveals a 46,XX,+21,der(21;21)(q10;10) karyotype. This is an unbalanced Robertsonian translocation consistent with Down syndrome. Robertsonian translocations account for 3% to 4% of Down syndrome cases and result from the fusion of an extra copy of chromosome 21 with another acrocentric chromosome (usually 14 or 21). In 95% of cases, Down syndrome is due to trisomy 21 in which there are 3 copies of chromosome 21. The clinical features are the same in individuals with

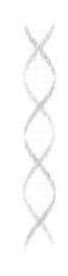

Down syndrome due to a Robertsonian translocation or trisomy 21. Mosaicism is identified in 1% to 2% of Down syndrome cases. Individuals who are mosaic for trisomy 21 have 1 cell line with 2 copies of chromosome 21 and 1 cell line with 3 copies of chromosome 21. Clinical features may be milder in individuals with mosaicism.

Genetic Counseling

The family is counseled that the chromosome results are consistent with Down syndrome, which is the most common genetic cause of intellectual disability (incidence 1:650 to 1:800 live births). Although there is an increased risk for Down syndrome with advanced maternal age, most children with Down syndrome are born to younger mothers. The recurrence risk for trisomy 21 is 1% or the maternal age risk if greater than 1%. The recurrence risk if a parent is a balanced translocation carrier is 10% to 15% if maternal, 2% to 5% if paternal, and 100% if a parent carries a 21;21 translocation. Because the patient has a Robertsonian translocation, chromosome analysis is performed on both parents. The results are normal, indicating that the translocation occurred for the first time. There is therefore a low recurrence risk (~1%).

Management

Growth is monitored on a regular basis. Development and behavior should be followed closely. She receives early education planning and therapies. Normal newborn screening for thyroid disease is confirmed. Hearing and vision are evaluated and found to be normal. Annual evaluations of hearing, vision, and thyroid function are recommended. She will be monitored for feeding problems, sleep disturbances, skin issues, and constipation. An echocardiogram is performed due to a 50% risk of a congenital heart defect. The echocardiogram is normal.

Fragile X Syndrome

Clinical Features

A 3-year-old male has unexplained developmental delay and autism. A physical examination reveals prominent forehead, large ears, and blue irides (Figure 9-5). The clinical features of fragile X syndrome can be difficult to detect prior to puberty, but the history and examination findings in this child are felt to be consistent with fragile X syndrome (Table 9-6).

Laboratory Diagnosis

A clinical diagnosis of fragile X syndrome is confirmed by detection of a CGG trinucleotide repeat expansion of greater than 200 repeats with abnormal methylation in the *FMR1* gene. The patient's mother is

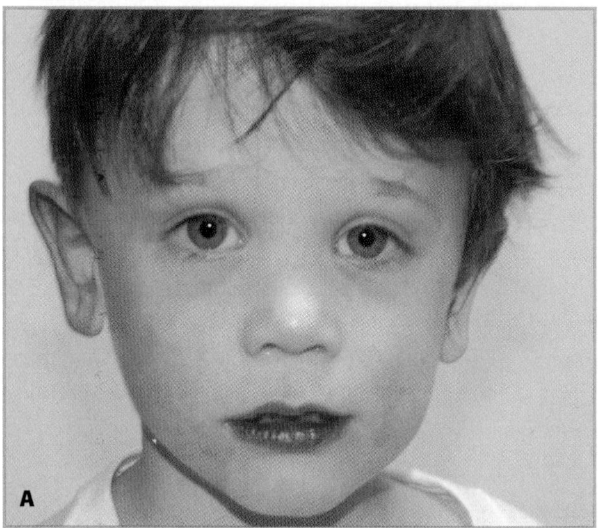

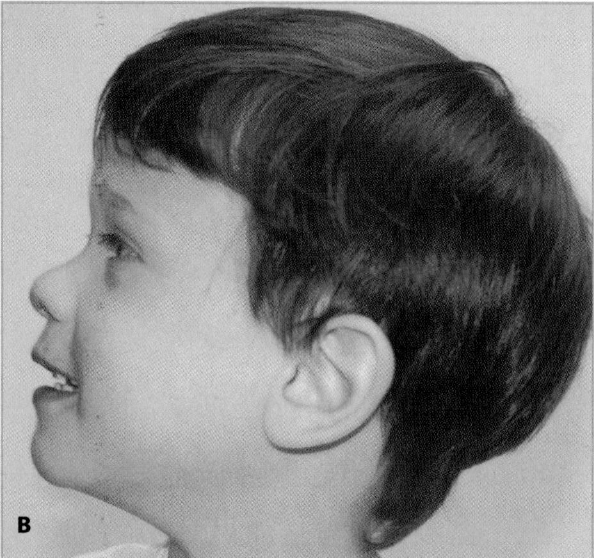

Figure 9-5A–C. Prominent forehead and large ears in a male with fragile X syndrome.

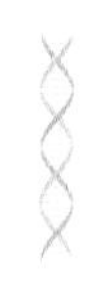

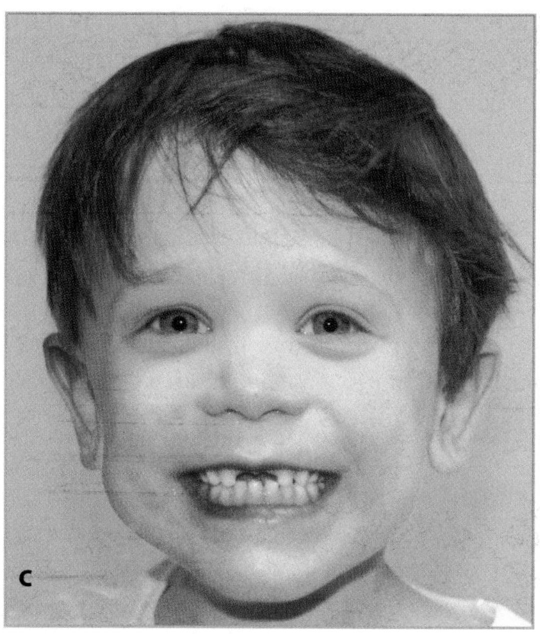

Table 9-6. Fragile X Syndrome Characteristic Features

Area	Feature
Cardiovascular	Mitral valve prolapse
Craniofacial	Long face Prominent forehead Large ears Prominent jaw Craniofacial features become more prominent with age
Dermatologic	Soft, smooth skin
Genitourinary	Macroorchidism (postpubertal)
Musculoskeletal	Joint hyperextensibility Large fleshy hands Pes planus
Neurodevelopment	Intellectual disability Hypotonia Seizures Autism in 20%–25% Behavior issues (hyperactivity, temper tantrums, anxiety, shyness)
Ophthalmologic	Strabismus

found to be a full mutation carrier. She had learning difficulties in school but no evidence of intellectual disability. Although females with a full mutation in *FMR1* may have physical and behavior features of fragile X syndrome, they are typically less severely affected. Individuals with mosaicism for CGG repeat size or methylation status often have milder involvement. Rarely, fragile X syndrome can be due to *FMR1* deletions or missense mutations. Individuals with premutations have approximately 55 to 200 repeats. Males with premutations have an increased risk for fragile X tremor ataxia syndrome, which is associated with ataxia and an intention tremor in later adulthood. Females with premutations have an approximately 20% risk for primary ovarian insufficiency in which menses cease before age 40.

Genetic Counseling

The family is counseled that fragile X syndrome is the most common inherited cause of intellectual disability, affecting 1:2,500 to 1:3,700 males and 1:7,000 females. Fragile X syndrome is an X-linked disorder. The family history is significant for developmental delay in a maternally related male cousin and premature ovarian insufficiency in the patient's maternal grandmother and maternal great aunt. The offspring of other family members are at an increased risk of having fragile X syndrome. The risk depends on the gender of the offspring, the gender of the carrier parent, and the size of the CGG repeat expansion in the carrier parent. Premutations in males do not expand to full mutations in the next generation. Female premutation carriers with larger CGG repeat expansions are at an increased risk to have a child with a full mutation.

Management

Regular monitoring of development and behavior is recommended. The patient should receive early education planning and therapies. Behavior problems can often be managed with a multidisciplinary approach, including medications. Feeding issues in infants should be addressed. Regular evaluations should look for evidence of vision problems, recurrent ear infections, hypertension, mitral valve prolapse, scoliosis, and pes planus. Individuals with seizures should receive close neurologic follow-up with appropriate anticonvulsant medications.

Klinefelter Syndrome

Clinical Features

A 17-year-old male has a history of developmental delay and pervasive developmental disorder. A physical examination reveals normal growth parameters, upslanting palpebral fissures, minimal gynecomastia, small-joint hypermobility, and pes planus (Figure 9-6). The patient's history of developmental delay without significant dysmorphic features is consistent with Klinefelter syndrome (Table 9-7). Physical examination findings are typically more obvious in individuals who have additional sex chromosomes, such as 48,XXXY and 49,XXXXY. Cognitive development is also more severely affected. Each extra X chromosome is associated with a decrease in IQ of approximately 15.

Laboratory Diagnosis

A definite diagnosis of Klinefelter syndrome requires chromosome analysis demonstrating at least 1 Y chromosome and 2 X chromosomes. The patient's chromosome analysis reveals a 47,XXY karyotype consistent with Klinefelter syndrome. FISH testing can also be used to confirm the presence of additional sex chromosomes.

Genetic Counseling

The family is counseled that the patient's chromosome analysis is consistent with a diagnosis of Klinefelter syndrome. Klinefelter syndrome is a common chromosome disorder with a prevalence of approximately 1:500 to 1:1,000. There appears to be a maternal age effect, as the risk for Klinefelter syndrome is higher with increased maternal age. The additional X chromosome in individuals with Klinefelter syndrome is of paternal origin in 50% to 60% of cases and of maternal origin in 40% to 50% of cases. The recurrence risk is low. Individuals with Klinefelter syndrome are typically infertile. Klinefelter syndrome is the cause of 5% to 15% of male infertility cases.

Management

Growth and development should be monitored regularly. Early education planning and therapies are indicated for individuals with learning difficulties. Individuals with Klinefelter syndrome should be evaluated for signs of scoliosis. Delayed puberty and gynecomastia should be assessed during

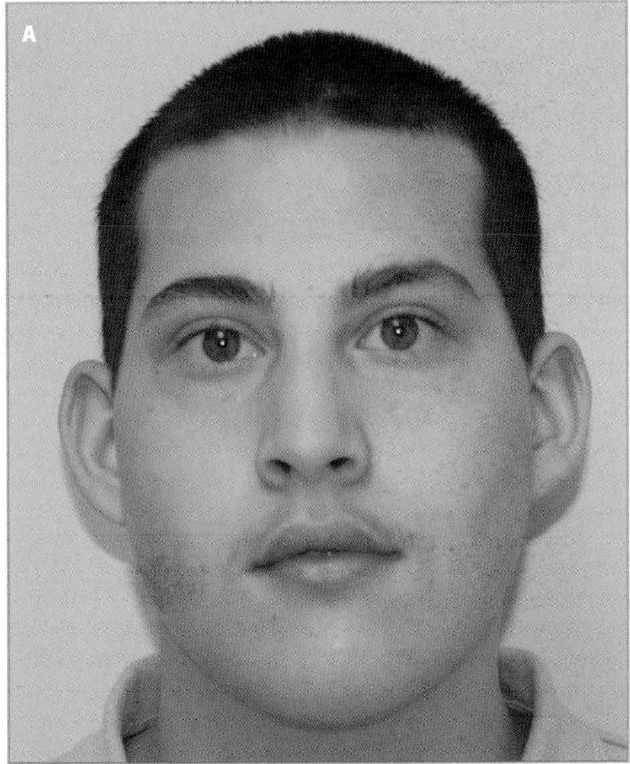

Figure 9-6A, B. Nonspecific facial features in a male with Klinefelter syndrome.

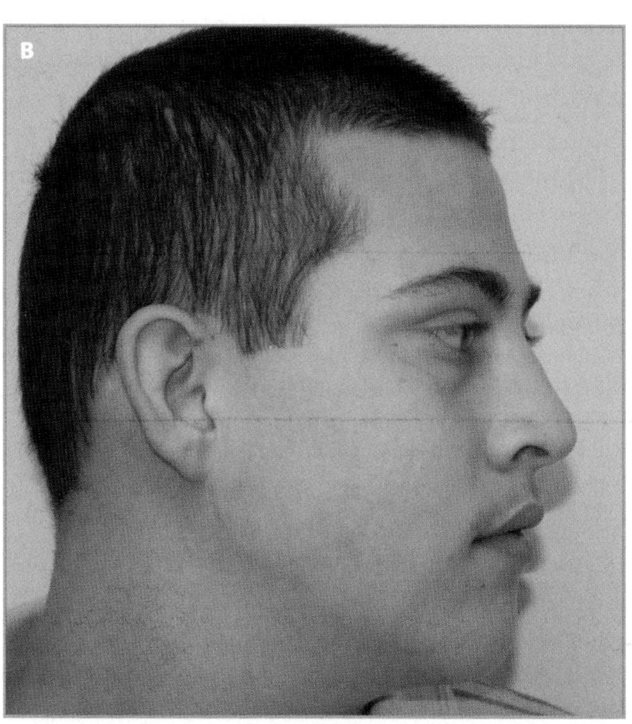

Table 9-7. Klinefelter Syndrome Characteristic Features

Area	Feature
Endocrine	Gynecomastia Hypergonadotropic hypogonadism Delayed puberty Infertility Sparse body hair
Genitourinary	Small testes
Growth	Relative tall stature
Immunologic	Increased risk for autoimmune diseases
Musculoskeletal	Long legs and arms
Neurodevelopment	Developmental delay Speech delay Learning disability Behavior problems Psychosocial issues Hypotonia
Oncology	Increased risk of breast cancer in adults

adolescence. Although prepubertal individuals with Klinefelter syndrome typically have normal gonadotropin and testosterone levels, adolescents often have elevated gonadotropins and low testosterone. Levels of testosterone, luteinizing hormone, and follicle-stimulating hormone are followed annually. Testosterone deficiency is treated with androgen replacement therapy. Thyroid function is followed annually with standard treatment if hypothyroidism is identified.

Marfan Syndrome

Clinical Features

A 9-year-old male has tall stature, recurrent inguinal hernias, and bilateral retinal detachment. A physical examination reveals height at the 97th percentile, long and slender hands and feet, long fingers and toes, positive wrist and thumb signs, pes planus, and joint hypermobility (Figure 9-7). Because of concerns about a possible connective tissue disorder, an echocardiogram is performed, which reveals significant aortic root dilatation. His findings meet the clinical criteria for a diagnosis of Marfan syndrome as he has 2 major criteria (dilatation of the aorta and 4 musculoskeletal features) and

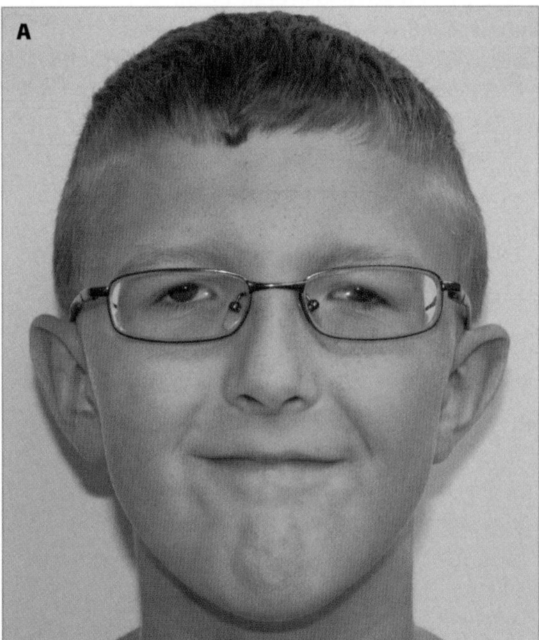

Figure 9-7A–C. Facial features and wrist sign in a male with Marfan syndrome.

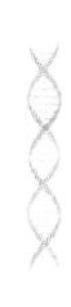

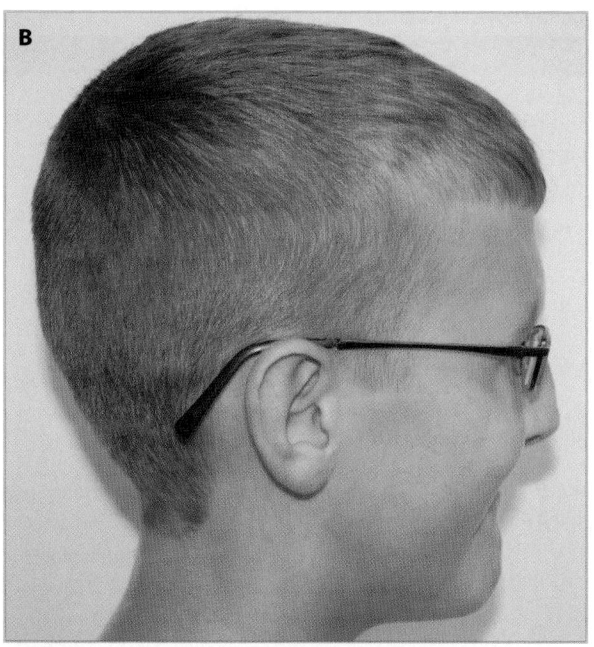
B

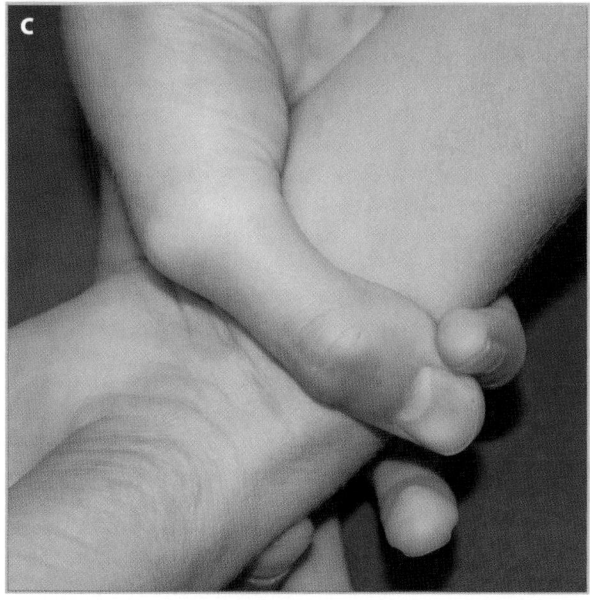
C

Table 9-8. Marfan Syndrome Diagnostic Criteria

Area		Criteria
Cardiovascular Major criterion: ≥1 major finding Minor criterion: ≥1 minor finding	⇒	Aortic root dilatation
	⇒	Ascending aorta dissection
	→	Abdominal aortic dilatation or dissection (<50 years old)
	→	Mitral valve prolapse
	→	Pulmonary artery dilatation (<40 years old)
	→	Mitral annulus calcification (<40 years old)
Dermatologic Minor criterion: ≥1 minor findings	→	Striae
	→	Recurrent hernias
Musculoskeletal Major criterion: ≥4 major findings Minor criterion: 2 major findings or 1 major and ≥2 minor findings	⇒	Pectus excavatum needing surgery or pectus carinatum
	⇒	Upper to lower segment ratio <0.85 or arm span to height ratio >1.05
	⇒	Wrist and thumb signs
	⇒	Scoliosis (>20 degrees) or spondylolisthesis
	⇒	Reduced elbow extension (<170 degrees)
	⇒	Protrusio acetabulae
	⇒	Pes planus due to medial rotation of medial malleolus
	→	Pectus excavatum (moderate)
	→	Joint hypermobility
	→	High-arched palate with crowded teeth
	→	Facial features: dolichocephaly, malar hypoplasia, retrognathia, downslanting palpebral fissures, enophthalmos
Neurodevelopment	⇒	Dural ectasia
Ophthalmologic Minor criterion: ≥2 minor findings	⇒	Ectopia lentis
	→	Elongated globe
	→	Flat cornea
	→	Hypoplastic iris or ciliary muscle
Pulmonary Minor criterion: ≥1 minor findings	→	Spontaneous pneumothorax
	→	Apical blebs

Key: ⇒, major finding; →, minor finding.

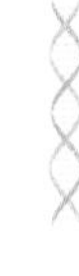

one minor criterion (recurrent hernias) (Table 9-8). Individuals with a family history of Marfan syndrome in a first-degree relative require one major criterion and one minor criterion.

Laboratory Diagnosis

Marfan syndrome testing of the fibrillin 1 (*FBN1*) gene on chromosome 15q21.1 reveals a missense mutation that is thought to be consistent with Marfan syndrome. *FBN1* is the only gene known to be associated with Marfan syndrome. The identification of a pathogenic mutation in the *FBN1* gene is a major diagnostic criterion for Marfan syndrome. However, *FBN1* mutations have also been identified in individuals with distinct disorders that have overlapping features with Marfan syndrome.

Genetic Counseling

Marfan syndrome is an autosomal dominant disorder with a prevalence of 1:5,000 to 1:10,000. The patient's parents are clinically unaffected, indicating that he has a new mutation in the *FBN1* gene. A new mutation is identified in 25% of individuals with Marfan syndrome. The recurrence risk for the family is low but is greater than the population risk; there have been rare cases of germline mosaicism. An affected parent is identified in 75% of Marfan syndrome cases. An individual with Marfan syndrome has a 50% risk of having a child with Marfan syndrome with each pregnancy. There is variable clinical expression within and between families with Marfan syndrome.

Management

Growth should be monitored regularly. Growth charts specific for Marfan syndrome are available. Due to his aortic root dilatation, the patient has been placed on a β-blocker and losartan and is being closely monitored by pediatric cardiology to determine if surgical repair will be necessary. His blood pressure is checked on a regular basis. Individuals with Marfan syndrome should be followed for evidence of skeletal problems. Regular ophthalmologic examinations are recommended. He is advised to avoid contact sports and other activities that may increase the risk of cardiac, pulmonary, or ophthalmologic complications.

Neurofibromatosis Type 1 (NF1)

Clinical Features

A 6-year-old female has multiple café au lait macules. A physical examination reveals more than 5 large café au lait macules and axillary freckling (Figure 9-8). Other clinical features seen in individuals with NF1

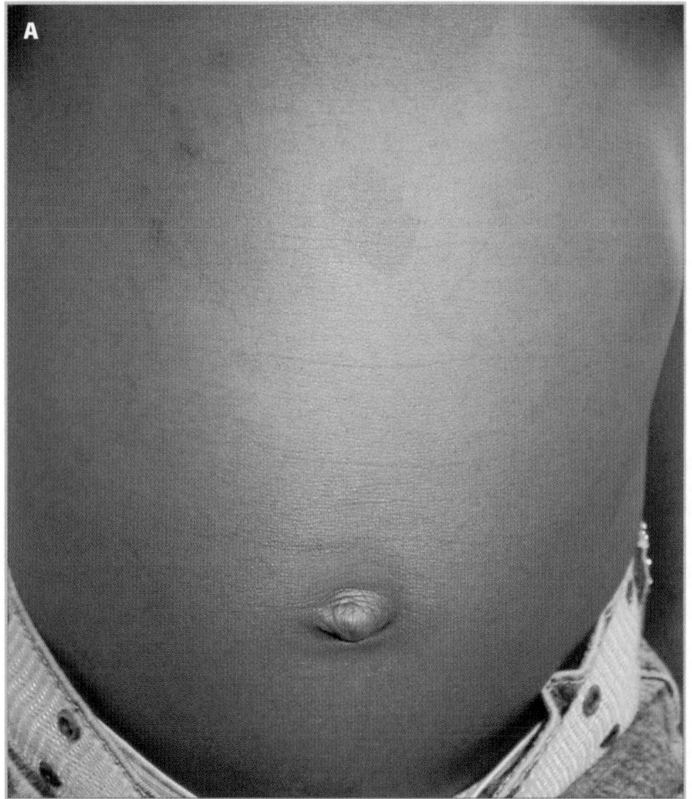

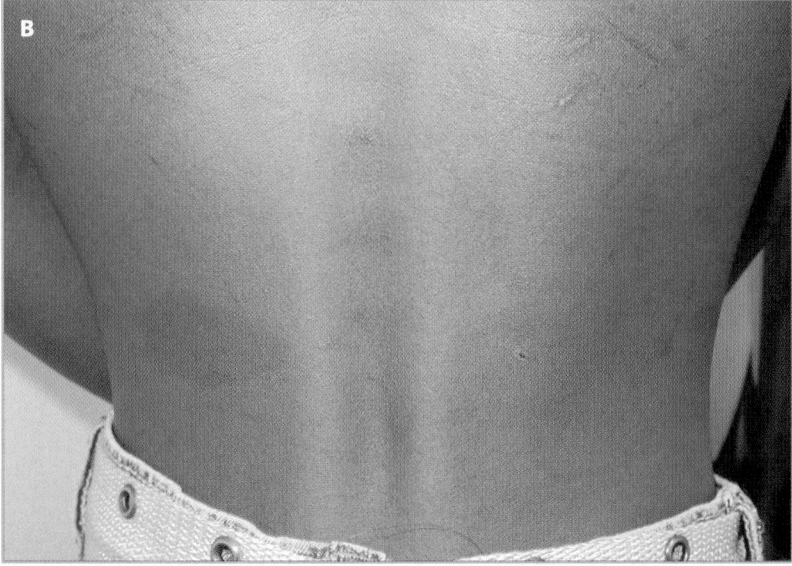

Figure 9-8A, B. Multiple café au lait macules in a female with neurofibromatosis type 1.

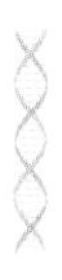

include neurofibromas, Lisch nodules, optic gliomas, and skeletal findings. Because the patient has multiple large café au lait macules and axillary freckling, she is given a clinical diagnosis of NF1. The patient's mother, maternal grandmother, and 2 maternal aunts are suspected to have NF1 because of the presence of multiple café au lait macules and neurofibromas.

Laboratory Diagnosis

A diagnosis of NF1 is made clinically based on the presence of 2 out of 7 clinical criteria (Table 9-9). Molecular testing of the *NF1* gene on chromosome 17q11.2 is available. However, molecular testing is typically not performed as the clinical criteria are generally reliable. Some individuals may be mosaic for an *NF1* mutation with localized or segmental expression.

Genetic Counseling

Neurofibromatosis type 1 is a relatively common autosomal dominant disorder with a prevalence of 1:3,000. The family is counseled that half of individuals with NF1 have an affected parent. Because the family has multiple members who have clinical features consistent with autosomal dominant inheritance of NF1, the recurrence risk is 50%. If the parents of an individual with NF1 are clinically unaffected, the recurrence risk is low. Although penetrance is typically complete, the clinical presentation can be variable within and between families. A clinical diagnosis can be difficult in young children without a family history because the presence of many of the clinical features depends on the age of the individual. In particular, Legius syndrome is a dominant condition that is associated with multiple café au lait macules and axillary freckling, but other clinical features of NF1, such as neurofibromas and Lisch nodules, are not typically seen.

Management

Growth should be monitored on a regular basis. Individuals with NF1 are typically shorter than average with relatively large head sizes. There are specific growth charts for children with NF1. Development should be closely monitored because there is an increased risk for learning disabilities. An ophthalmologic evaluation is recommended to look for evidence of Lisch nodules and optic gliomas. She should have annual ophthalmology evaluations. Annual monitoring of blood pressure is recommended. She should have regular physical examinations with special attention paid to dermatologic and neurologic complaints or findings. Brain magnetic resonance

Table 9-9. Neurofibromatosis Type 1 (NF-1) Diagnostic Criteria (≥ 2 of the Following)

Area		Criteria
Dermatologic	⇒	6 or more café au lait macules (>5 mm prepubertal, >15 mm postpubertal)
	⇒	Axillary and/or inguinal freckling
	⇒	≥2 neurofibromas or 1 plexiform neurofibroma
Family history	⇒	First-degree relative with NF-1
Musculoskeletal	⇒	Distinctive osseous lesions: sphenoid dysplasia or thinning of long-bone cortex
Ophthalmologic	⇒	Optic glioma
	⇒	≥2 Lisch nodules (iris hamartomas)

Key: ⇒, major finding.

imaging may be indicated if there are neurologic complaints or visual changes, or if there is an increase in head size. Early orthopedic referral is indicated if tibial dysplasia is identified. Regular monitoring for scoliosis is recommended.

Noonan Syndrome

Clinical Features

A 20-month-old female has mild developmental delay, pulmonic stenosis, and dysmorphic facial features. A physical examination reveals normal growth parameters, low-set and posteriorly rotated ears, epicanthal folds, broad neck, low posterior hairline, pectus carinatum superiorly and pectus excavatum inferiorly, and widely spaced nipples (Figure 9-9). Her clinical features are consistent with Noonan syndrome (Table 9-10).

Laboratory Diagnosis

Because the clinical features suggest Noonan syndrome, molecular testing of the *PTPN11* gene is ordered. *PTPN11* testing reveals a missense mutation consistent with Noonan syndrome. *PTPN11* testing of the patient's parents is normal. *PTPN11* mutations account for 50% of Noonan syndrome cases. Individuals with Noonan syndrome have also been found to have mutations in the *SOS1* (~13%), *RAF1* (~3%–17%), and *KRAS* (<5%) genes. Pulmonic stenosis has been associated with *PTPN11* mutations, while hypertrophic cardiomyopathy has been associated with *RAF1* mutations.

Genetic Counseling

The family is counseled that the *PTPN11* gene test results confirm the diagnosis of Noonan syndrome, which is a relatively common autosomal dominant disorder with a prevalence of 1:1,000 to 1:2,500. An affected parent is identified in 30% to 75% of Noonan syndrome cases. Noonan syndrome is often the result of a new mutation, which would confer a low recurrence risk. Parents of a newly diagnosed case should be evaluated for signs of Noonan syndrome by performing a physical examination and cardiac evaluation or molecular testing if the proband's mutation is known. Because the parental testing was normal, the recurrence risk for future offspring is low.

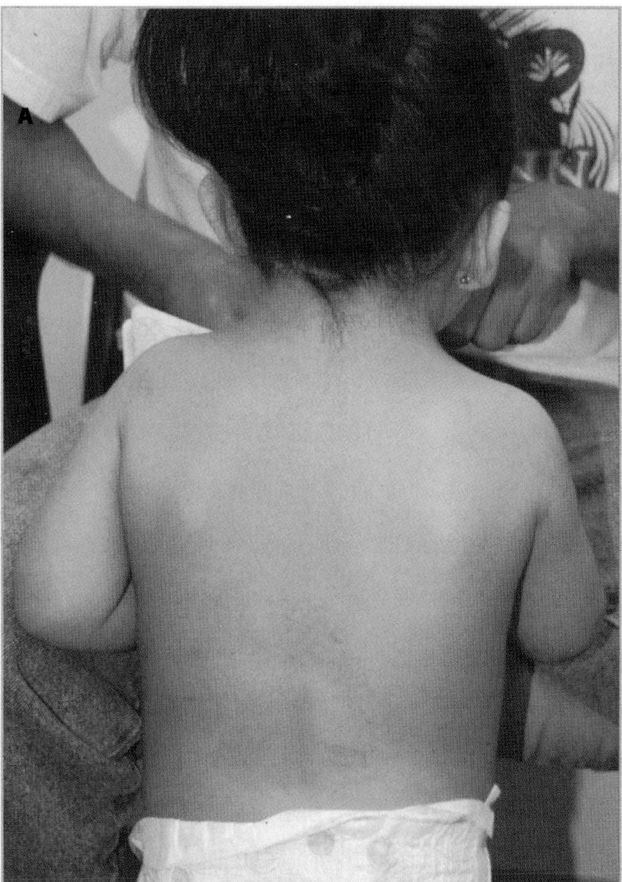

Figure 9-9A–D. Broad neck, wide-spaced nipples, and facial features in a female with Noonan syndrome.

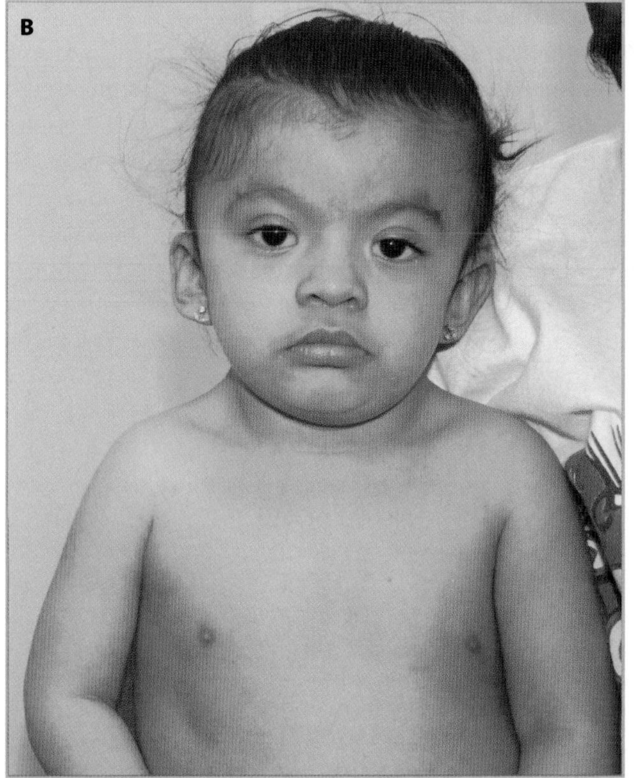
B

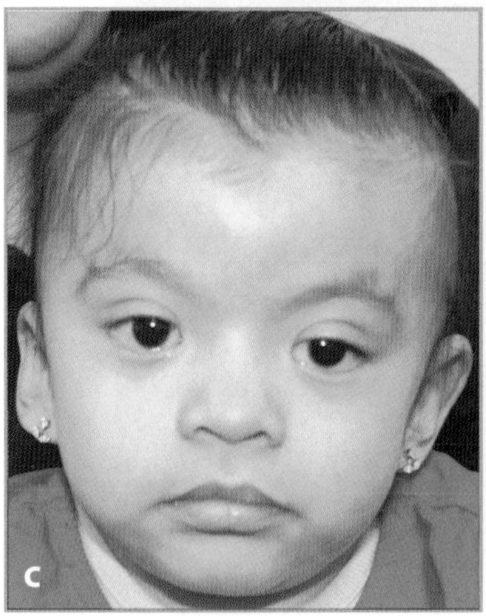
C

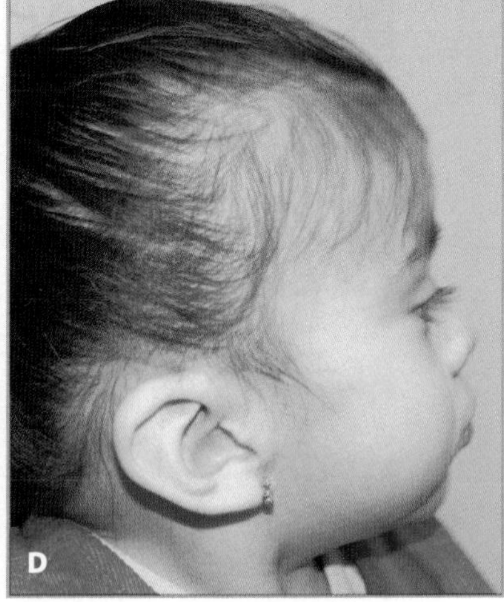
D

Table 9-10. Noonan Syndrome Characteristic Features

Area	Feature
Cardiovascular	Pulmonic stenosis Hypertrophic cardiomyopathy Lymphatic abnormalities
Craniofacial	Low-set ears Posteriorly rotated ears Fleshy helices Hypertelorism Downslanting palpebral fissures Epicanthal folds Ptosis Thick eyelids Broad/webbed neck
Genitourinary	Cryptorchidism in males Renal abnormalities
Growth	Short stature
Hematology	Coagulation defects
Musculoskeletal	Superior pectus carinatum with inferior pectus excavatum Low-set nipples
Neurodevelopment	Developmental delay Mild intellectual disability (may be present in one-third of cases)
Ophthalmologic	Strabismus Refractive errors
Otolaryngologic	Hearing loss

Management

Growth should be monitored regularly. Growth charts specific for Noonan syndrome are available. The use of growth hormone therapy in individuals with Noonan syndrome varies among different countries and institutions. Regular monitoring of development, vision, and hearing is recommended. Following the diagnosis of Noonan syndrome, an echocardiogram and electrocardiogram should be ordered because there is a significant risk for congenital heart disease. Regular echocardiograms are advised to detect cardiac hypertrophy. Due to an increased risk for bleeding or bruising in individuals with Noonan syndrome, a coagulation screen should be ordered. A renal ultrasound and x-rays of the spine and rib cage are also recommended.

Osteogenesis Imperfecta (OI) Type I

Clinical Features

A 7-year-old female has blue sclerae and recurrent fractures. She was found to have bilateral femur fractures on prenatal ultrasound. She did not have any subsequent fractures until 2 weeks ago when she broke her right ankle while kicking a basketball. She does not have any hearing or dental problems. A physical examination reveals normal growth parameters with strikingly blue sclerae (Figure 9-10). Her history and examination findings are thought to be consistent with OI type I (Table 9-11).

Laboratory Diagnosis

A skin biopsy is performed in order to send fibroblasts for collagen screening. The biochemical findings from the collagen screening are consistent with OI type I. Biochemical testing looks at the structure and quantity of

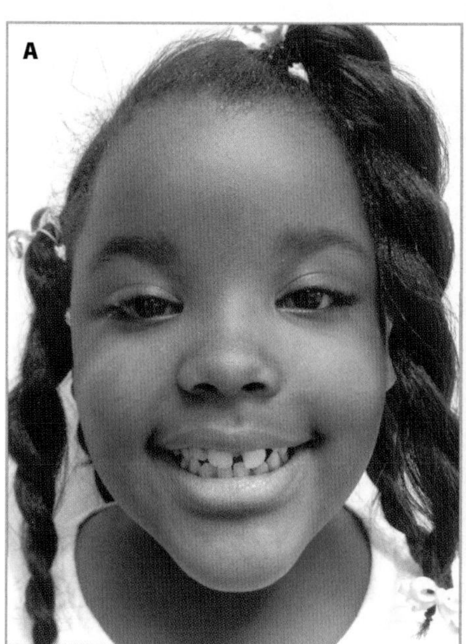

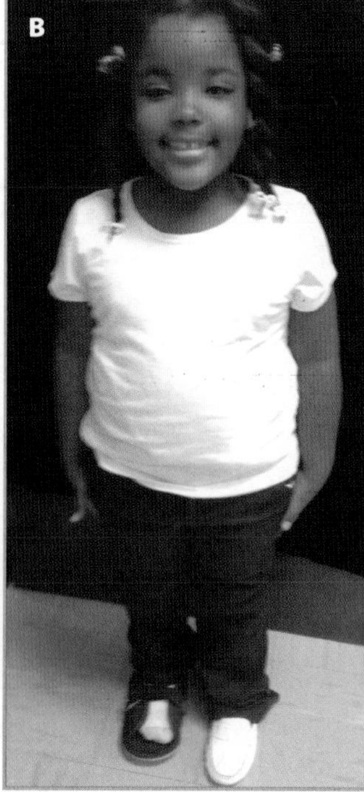

Figure 9-10A, B. Blue sclerae and broken foot in a female with osteogenesis imperfecta type I.

Table 9-11. Osteogenesis Imperfecta Type I Characteristic Features

Area	Feature
Craniofacial	Dentinogenesis imperfecta (type IB)
Growth	Normal height or mild short stature for family
Hematologic	Easy bruising
Musculoskeletal	Fractures with minimal trauma (a few to a hundred) Bone deformity uncommon Joint hypermobility Wormian bones on skull x-rays Codfish vertebrae on spine x-rays Osteopenia and thin cortices on skeletal x-rays
Neurodevelopment	Normal intellect
Ophthalmologic	Blue sclerae
Otolaryngologic	Hearing loss (progressive)

type I collagen. Abnormalities on biochemical testing are identified in 90% of individuals with OI type I. Mutation analysis of the *COL1A1* and *COL1A2* genes is also clinically available. A mutation in the *COL1A1* or *COL1A2* genes is detected in approimately 90% of those with OI.

Genetic Counseling

Osteogenesis imperfecta consists of a number of overlapping types. There is variable expression within and between families, but type I OI is generally the mildest form. Individuals with OI type I have a decreased amount of type I collagen that is structurally normal, while more severe types of OI typically have structurally abnormal type I collagen. Osteogenesis imperfecta type I is an autosomal dominant disorder with a prevalence of approximately 1:30,000. A new mutation is identified in 60% of individuals with OI type I. The patient has an extensive family history of individuals with recurrent fractures and blue sclerae consistent with autosomal dominant inheritance. The patient and other affected family members have a 50% risk of having a child with OI type I.

Management

Osteogenesis imperfecta type I needs to be differentiated from non-accidental trauma in an individual with multiple fractures in the absence of significant trauma. The patient is counseled to be cautious in terms of participation in contact sports but is encouraged to be physically active. Regular hearing and dental evaluations are recommended. Growth should be monitored. Some individuals with OI type I have responded to growth hormone treatment. Bisphosphonates decrease bone resorption and are used in some individuals with OI. However, given the patient's mild presentation, treatment with bisphosphonates has not been initiated.

Prader-Willi Syndrome

Clinical Features

A 17 year-old male has mild intellectual disability and obesity. He has a history of congenital hypotonia, skin-picking, and hyperphagia. A physical examination reveals a narrow bifrontal diameter, upslanted palpebral fissures, obesity, hypogonadism, and small hands (Figure 9-11). His clinical features meet the diagnostic criteria for Prader-Willi syndrome (Table 9-12).

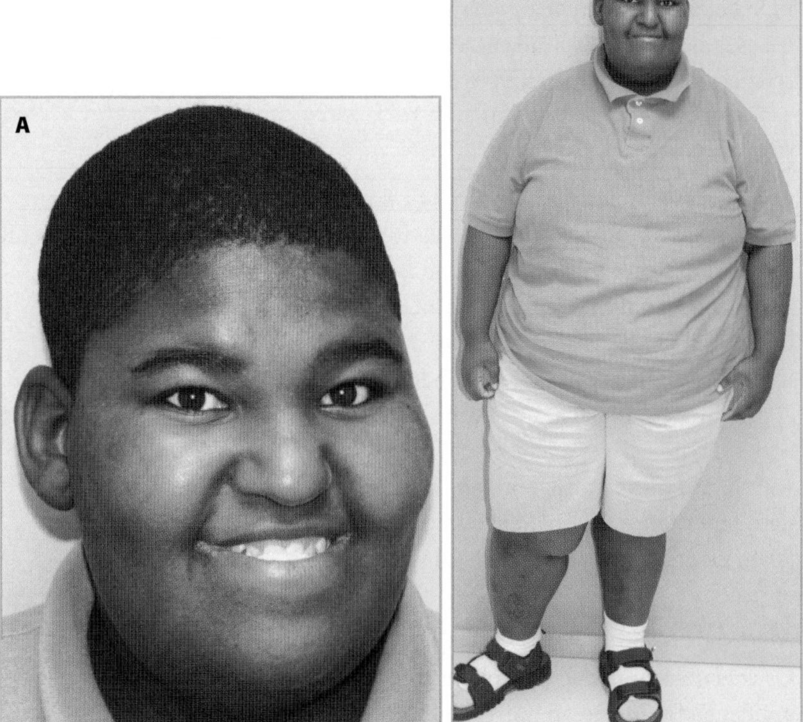

Figure 9-11A, B. Facial features and obesity in a male with Prader-Willi syndrome.

Table 9-12. Prader-Willi Syndrome Diagnostic Criteria[a]

Area		Criteria
Craniofacial	⇒	Characteristic facial features: narrow bifrontal diameter, almond-shaped palpebral fissures, down-turned corners of mouth
	→	Saliva that is thick and viscous
Dermatologic	→	Hypopigmentation
	→	Skin-picking
Genitourinary	⇒	Hypogonadism: genital hypoplasia, delayed puberty, infertility
Growth	→	Short stature for the family (by age 15 years)
Musculoskeletal	→	Small hands and feet
	→	Narrow hands with straight ulnar borders
Neurodevelopment	⇒	Neonatal/infantile hypotonia with poor suck improving with age
	⇒	Feeding problems in infancy needing special feeding
	⇒	Rapid weight gain 1–6 years old leading to central obesity
	⇒	Hyperphagia
	⇒	Developmental delay/intellectual disability
	→	Articulation defects
	→	Decreased fetal movements
	→	Behavior problems: temper tantrums, compulsive, stubborn
	→	Sleep disturbance
Ophthalmologic	→	Strabismus, myopia

Key: ⇒, major finding; →, minor finding.
[a]<3 years: 5 points with 4 major criteria; ≥3 years: 8 points with 5 major criteria.

Laboratory Diagnosis

Certain clinical features should lead to testing for Prader-Willi syndrome at specific ages (Table 9-12). Because of the patient's history of neonatal hypotonia, intellectual disability, and hyperphagia, FISH analysis is performed to look for a deletion involving the Prader-Willi syndrome critical region on chromosome 15q11-q13. The FISH analysis is normal. Methylation analysis is then performed and is abnormal. Methylation analysis identifies 99% of individuals with Prader-Willi syndrome. Deletions, UPD, and imprinting defects can all be detected by methylation

Table 9-13. Prader-Willi Testing Based on Age-Dependent Features

Age (y)	Criteria
0–2	Hypotonia with poor suck as a neonate
2–6	Hypotonia with history of poor suck PLUS developmental delay
6–12	History of hypotonia with poor suck PLUS developmental delay PLUS hyperphagia with central obesity
13+	Cognitive impairment PLUS hyperphagia with central obesity PLUS hypothalamic hypogonadism and/or behavior problems

analysis. **P**ra**d**er-Willi syndrome is due to a **p**aternal **d**eletion in 70% of cases. Maternal UPD is responsible for 20% to 30% of Prader-Willi syndrome cases and is the most likely cause in this case.

Genetic Counseling

The prevalence of Prader-Willi syndrome is 1:10,000 to 1:30,000. Individuals with Prader-Willi syndrome have an alteration of the paternally derived Prader-Willi syndrome critical region on chromosome 15q11-q13. The recurrence risk depends on how the region is altered. If the paternally derived region is missing due to a deletion or UPD, the recurrence risk is less than 1%. As the patient likely has Prader-Willi syndrome as a result of UPD, the recurrence risk is very low. If a parent carries a mutation affecting the imprinting control center, the recurrence risk can be as high as 50%. A de novo imprinting defect would confer a low recurrence risk. If a parent carries a chromosome rearrangement, the recurrence risk may be relatively high depending on the type of rearrangement.

Management

Due to feeding problems in infancy, the patient has a history of needing gavage feeding followed by the use of special nipples. His food intake now needs to be closely monitored because of the development of hyperphagia. Growth should be followed closely. Growth charts specific for Prader-Willi syndrome are available. Growth hormone therapy has shown benefits in increasing lean body mass and decreasing fat mass. Regular monitoring of development, vision, sleep, and behavior is recommended. Serotonin reuptake inhibitors have shown benefit in treating behavior problems. Hormone replacement can aid secondary sexual development. Males should be evaluated for evidence of cryptorchidism and managed with hormone treatment or surgery as needed.

Smith-Magenis Syndrome

Clinical Features

A 17-year-old male has intellectual disability and behavior problems. He pulls his nails, rocks back and forth, and hits himself when frustrated. He has a high pain tolerance, has been diagnosed with obsessive-compulsive disorder, and has poor sleep. The family history is noncontributory. A physical examination reveals broad and square face, upslanting palpebral fissures, strabismus, everted upper lip, and open mouth expression (Figure 9-12). Although he has relatively tall stature, his features are consistent with Smith-Magenis syndrome (Table 9-14).

Laboratory Diagnosis

To look for evidence of Smith-Magenis syndrome, chromosome analysis and FISH for Smith-Magenis syndrome are sent and are normal. Individuals with Smith-Magenis syndrome typically have a deletion on chromosome 17p11.2 that can be detected by FISH analysis in 90% of cases. A recurrent 3.5 Mb deletion is present in 70% of cases and can often be

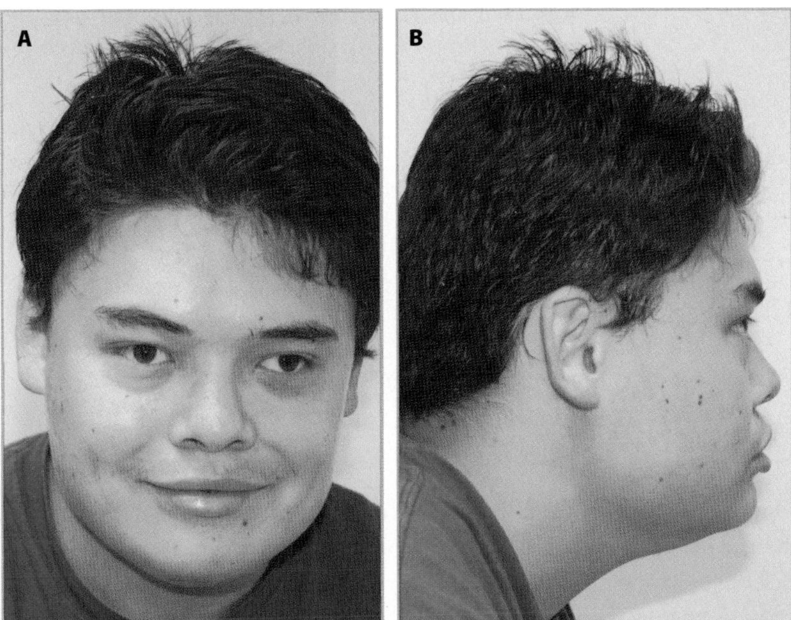

Figure 9-12A, B. Broad and square face, upslanting palpebral fissures, and strabismus in a male with Smith-Magenis syndrome.

Table 9-14. Smith-Magenis Syndrome Characteristic Features

Area	Feature
Cardiovascular	Cardiac defects
Craniofacial	Brachycephaly Midface hypoplasia Broad, square face Upslanting palpebral fissures Deep-set eyes Prognathism Everted upper lip
Gastrointestinal	Constipation Hypercholesterolemia/hypertriglyceridemia
Genitourinary	Renal anomalies
Growth	Failure to thrive Short stature
Musculoskeletal	Brachydactyly Scoliosis
Neurodevelopment	Intellectual disability Scoliosis Behavior problems: self-injurious behaviors, attention-seeking behaviors, temper tantrums, stereotypic behaviors (upper-body squeeze) Sleep disorder Hypotonia Peripheral neuropathy Seizures
Ophthalmologic	Strabismus Microcornea Refractive errors
Otolaryngologic	Hearing loss Hoarse voice Velopharyngeal incompetence

identified by chromosome analysis. The *RAI1* gene is responsible for most clinical features associated with Smith-Magenis syndrome. Small, atypical deletions may be missed if the FISH probe does not contain the *RAI1* gene. In order to look for a small deletion, chromosome microarray analysis is sent on the patient and detects a 0.55 Mb deletion, which includes the *RAI1* gene. The result is confirmed by a FISH probe, which includes the *RAI1* gene. The deletion is consistent with Smith-Magenis syndrome, but small deletions are less commonly associated with short stature and structural anomalies.

Genetic Counseling

Smith-Magenis syndrome has a prevalence of 1:15,000 to 1:25,000. This disorder is typically caused by an interstitial 17p11.2 deletion that involves multiple contiguous genes including *RAI1*. An intragenic mutation involving only the *RAI1* gene accounts for 5% to 10% of cases. Smith-Magenis syndrome is almost always due to a new deletion or mutation that occurred for the first time in an affected individual. There have been rare familial reports of chromosome rearrangements involving chromosome 17p11.2. As a result, chromosome analysis and FISH of the patient's parents is performed. The results are normal, indicating that there is a low recurrence risk.

Management

After a diagnosis of Smith-Magenis syndrome is confirmed, a renal ultrasound, echocardiogram, and spine x-rays are ordered. In addition, a sample is sent for qualitative immunoglobulins. Thyroid function studies, lipid profile, and urinalysis are routinely monitored. Growth, development, behavior, and sleep are closely followed. Individuals with Smith-Magenis syndrome should receive early education planning and therapies. The use of medications such as melatonin may be helpful for sleep disturbance. Regular monitoring for hearing problems, vision issues, and scoliosis is recommended.

Turner Syndrome

Clinical Features

A newborn female has a history of increased nuchal translucency and fluid around the heart, lungs, and neck on prenatal ultrasound. A physical examination reveals wide-spaced nipples, puffy feet, and normal growth parameters (Figure 9-13). Her clinical features are consistent with Turner syndrome (Table 9-15). The presentation of Turner syndrome is extremely variable. The diagnosis is typically suspected in girls with lymphedema at birth, short stature in childhood, or delayed puberty in adolescence.

Laboratory Diagnosis

A clinical diagnosis of Turner syndrome is confirmed by chromosome analysis, which reveals a 45,X karyotype. Turner syndrome is due to the absence of all or part of the second sex chromosome. A complete absence of the second sex chromosome resulting in a 45,X karyotype accounts for half of Turner syndrome cases. Mosaic Turner syndrome, in which at least one other cell line is present in addition to cells with a 45,X karyotype, is responsible for approximately 20% of cases. Individuals with Turner syndrome can also have a partial deletion of an X chromosome, an isochromosome in which the short arm (Xp) is missing and the long arm (Xq) is duplicated, or a ring X chromosome.

Genetic Counseling

Turner syndrome is a chromosome disorder that affects 1:2,500 to 1:3,000 live-born females. The diagnosis is much more common among pregnancy losses. Turner syndrome is typically sporadic with a low recurrence risk. Mosaic cases of Turner syndrome with a 45,X/46,XX karyotype may have milder features. Mosaicism for a 45,X/46,XY karyotype accounts for approximately 5% to 6% of Turner syndrome and is associated with an increased risk for gonadoblastoma. Screening for Y chromosome material may be indicated in certain cases. Individuals with Turner syndrome who have a ring X or marker chromosome may have more severe clinical features. Deletion of genes on the short arm of the X chromosome seems to account for many clinical features of Turner syndrome, including the association of short stature with loss of the *SHOX* gene on Xp22.33.

Management

Growth should be followed regularly. Growth charts specific for Turner syndrome are available. Although intelligence is typically normal, development should be monitored with particular attention to the increased risk for nonverbal learning difficulties. A cardiology evaluation is recommended. Regular monitoring of the aortic arch in individuals with Turner syndrome has been suggested. A renal ultrasound is ordered to look for structural renal anomalies. Regular monitoring for vision issues, hearing loss, scoliosis, high blood pressure, and abnormal thyroid function

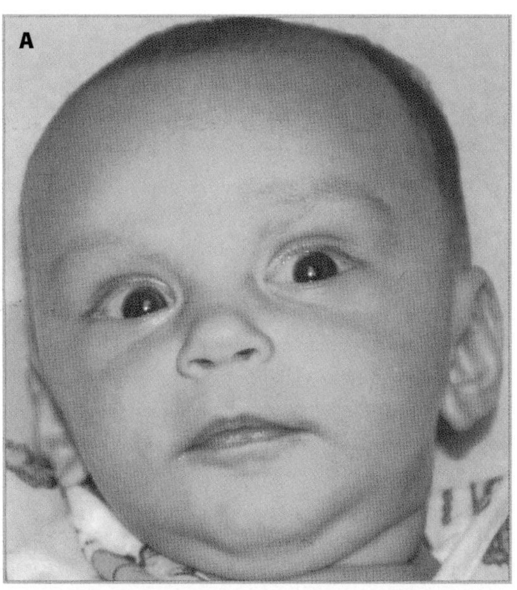

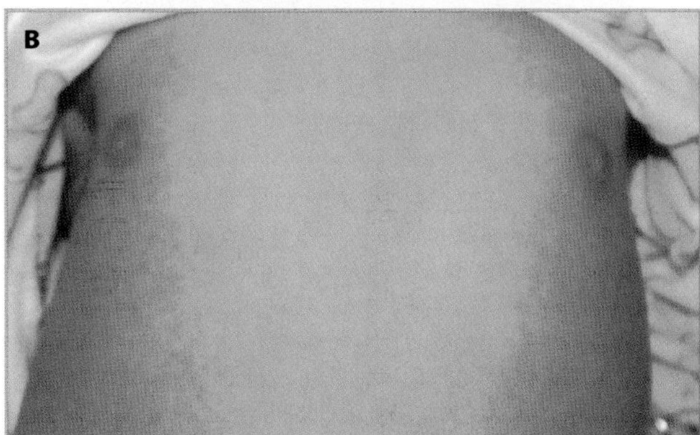

Figure 9-13A–D. Facial features, wide-spaced nipples, and lymphedema of the foot in a female with Turner syndrome.

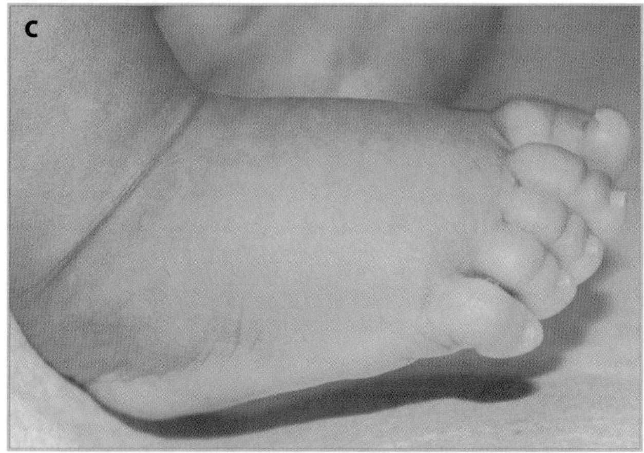
C

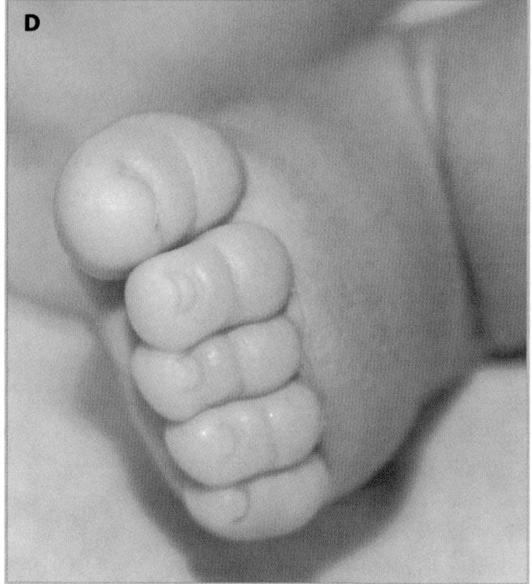
D

Table 9-15. Turner Syndrome Characteristic Features

Area	Feature
Cardiovascular	Coarctation of the aorta Bicuspid aortic valve Aortic root dilation/dissection Hypertension
Craniofacial	Epicanthal folds Excess nuchal skin Webbed neck Low posterior hairline
Dermatologic	Pigmented nevi
Endocrine	Hypothyroidism
Genitourinary	Gonadal dysgenesis—leads to delayed/absent puberty Streak ovaries (majority infertile) Renal malformations (horseshoe kidneys most common)
Growth	Short stature
Musculoskeletal	Lymphedema of hands and feet at birth Deep-set hyperconvex nails Short fourth metacarpals Cubitus valgus Broad chest with wide-spaced nipples Scoliosis
Neurodevelopment	Learning difficulties (typically normal intelligence)
Ophthalmologic	Strabismus
Otolaryngologic	Hearing loss

is recommended. She will be referred to endocrinology to discuss the possible use of growth hormone and sex hormone replacement therapy in the future.

Velocardiofacial Syndrome

Clinical Features

A 12-year-old male has a history of tetralogy of Fallot and developmental delays. A physical examination reveals hooded eyelids, small and cupped ears, bulbous nasal tip, and submucous cleft palate (Figure 9-14). The patient's clini-

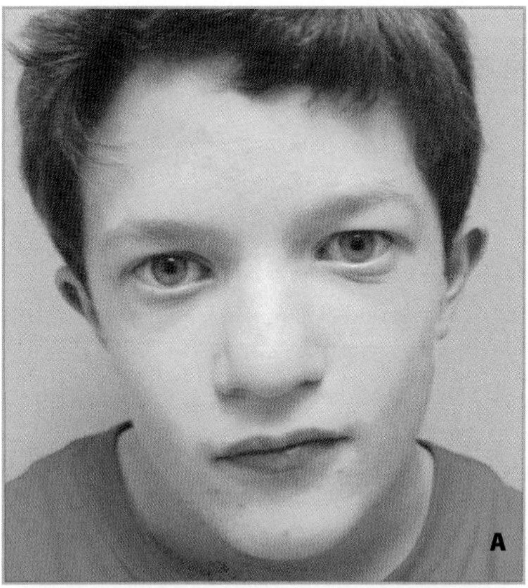

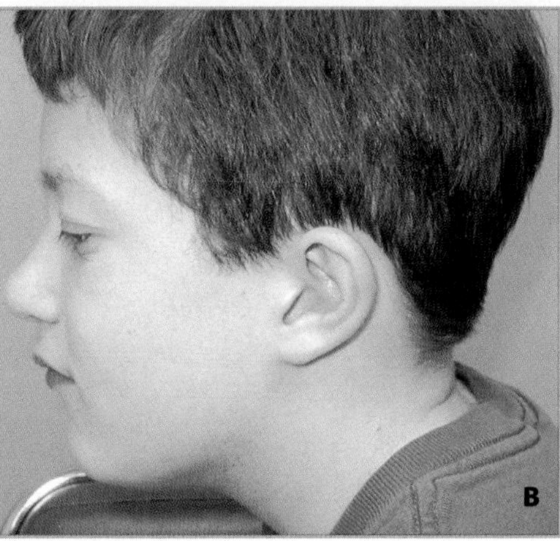

Figure 9-14A, B. Hooded eyelids, small and cupped ears, and a bulbous nasal tip in a male with velocardiofacial syndrome.

cal features are consistent with a diagnosis of velocardiofacial syndrome (Table 9-16). Individuals with velocardiofacial syndrome have a wide range of clinical features with variable expression between and within families.

Laboratory Diagnosis

Chromosome analysis is normal. FISH analysis to look for a 22q11.2 deletion is abnormal and consistent with a diagnosis of velocardiofacial syndrome. A deletion of 22q11.2 detectable by FISH analysis is

Table 9-16. Velocardiofacial Syndrome Characteristic Features

Area	Feature
Cardiovascular	Congenital heart defects (ventricular septal defect, interrupted aortic arch, tetralogy of Fallot, truncus arteriosus)
Craniofacial	Hooded upper eyelids Ocular hypertelorism Ear anomalies (overfolded helices, small and cupped ears) Nose anomalies (prominent nasal root, bulbous nasal tip, hypoplastic alae nasi) Asymmetrical crying facies
Endocrine	Hypocalcemia
Genitourinary	Renal anomalies
Growth	Short stature (majority have normal height)
Immunologic	Immune deficiency Autoimmune disorders
Musculoskeletal	Vertebral anomalies
Neurodevelopment	Developmental delay Learning difficulties Psychiatric illness
Ophthalmologic	Strabismus Posterior embryotoxon
Otolaryngologic	Palatal abnormalities (cleft palate, submucous cleft palate, velopharyngeal incompetence, hypernasal speech) Nasal regurgitation Hearing loss

identified in more than 95% of individuals with velocardiofacial syndrome. A common 3 megabase deletion is identified in 90% of affected individuals while a 1.5 megabase deletion is seen in approximately 7% to 8% of cases. Smaller, atypical deletions involving the critical region on 22q11.2 have also been detected and account for less than 5% of cases. Chromosome translocations involving 22q11.2 in individuals with features of velocardiofacial syndrome are rare. Some individuals with velocardiofacial syndrome have mutations in the *TBX1* gene, which is located in the commonly deleted regions.

Genetic Counseling

The family is counseled that velocardiofacial syndrome is a relatively common contiguous gene deletion syndrome with a prevalence of approximately 1:4,000. Other conditions, such as DiGeorge syndrome, due to a deletion of the same region on chromosome 22q11.2 are now felt to be the same disorder. Velocardiofacial syndrome is inherited in an autosomal dominant manner. FISH analysis of the parents to look for evidence of a 22q11.2 deletion is normal, indicating that this is a new deletion that occurred for the first time. New deletions account for approximately 93% of cases of velocardiofacial syndrome. As the patient has a new deletion, the recurrence risk is low for his parents to have another child with velocardiofacial syndrome. An affected parent is identified in approximately 7% of cases. Individuals with a 22q11.2 deletion have a 50% chance of passing the deletion to their children.

Management

Growth should be followed closely. Individuals with velocardiofacial syndrome should be monitored for developmental delay, learning difficulties, behavior problems, and psychiatric issues. The patient is followed by a craniofacial team to address palatal issues. A renal ultrasound and spine x-rays are recommended. The patient has had surgical correction of his congenital heart defect. After an initial diagnosis, individuals with velocardiofacial syndrome are screened for evidence of a congenital heart defect and managed by cardiology as needed. Calcium concentration is evaluated and abnormalities are treated as necessary. An evaluation for immunodeficiency is recommended. Individuals with abnormal lymphocytes should avoid live vaccines.

Williams Syndrome

Clinical Features

A 6-year-old female has developmental delay and pulmonic stenosis. A physical examination reveals short stature, curly hair, anteverted nares, wide mouth, long and smooth philtrum, and full cheeks (Figure 9-15). The patient's clinical features are consistent with a diagnosis of Williams syndrome (Table 9-17).

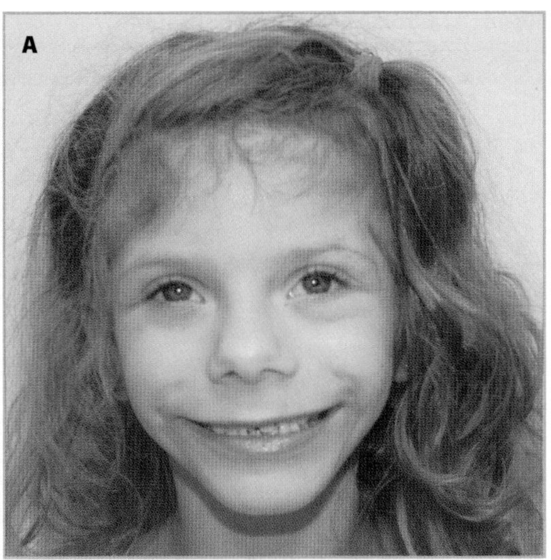

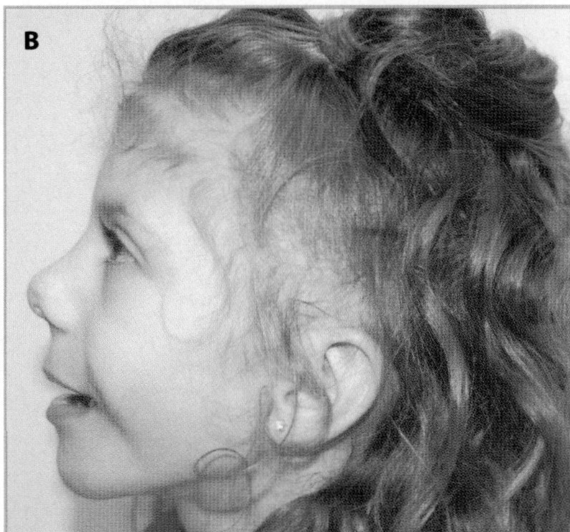

Figure 9-15A, B. Anteverted nares, wide mouth, long and smooth philtrum, and full cheeks in a female with Williams syndrome.

Laboratory Diagnosis

Chromosome analysis is normal. FISH analysis of chromosome 7q11.23 reveals a deletion consistent with Williams syndrome. More than 99% of individuals with Williams syndrome have a deletion of the Williams syndrome critical region. The commonly deleted region is 1.5 Mb and includes the *ELN* gene, which codes for the protein elastin. Many of the connective tissue problems associated with Williams syndrome are due to deletion of the *ELN* gene.

Table 9-17. Williams Syndrome Characteristic Features

Area	Feature
Cardiovascular	Supravalvular aortic stenosis Peripheral pulmonary artery stenosis Hypertension (may be result of renal artery stenosis)
Craniofacial	Bitemporal narrowing Epicanthal folds Periorbital fullness Short nose Full nasal tip Full cheeks Long philtrum Full lips Wide mouth Small jaw Long face and neck in adults
Endocrine	Hypercalcemia Hypercalciuria Hypothyroidism
Gastrointestinal	Diverticulosis Constipation
Growth	Short stature Failure to thrive
Musculoskeletal	Hernias Joint hypermobility or limitation
Neurodevelopment	Intellectual disability with visuospatial weakness Overly friendly Hypersensitive to sound Anxiety Attention problems Hypotonia
Ophthalmologic	Stellate iris pattern Strabismus
Otolaryngologic	Hoarse voice

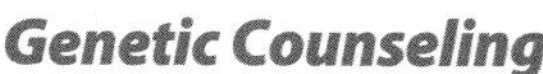

Genetic Counseling

The family is counseled that Williams syndrome is a contiguous gene deletion syndrome with a prevalence of 1:7,500 to 1:10,000. Williams syndrome is an autosomal dominant disorder. Most cases are new mutations that occur for the first time in a family with a low recurrence risk. Individuals with Williams syndrome have a 50% chance of passing the deletion to their children. There have been rare reports of familial cases with parent-to-child transmission. In 25% of Williams syndrome cases, a parent carries a chromosome 7 inversion, which involves the Williams syndrome critical region. The chromosome 7 inversion has been found in 6% of the general population. Testing for the chromosome 7 inversion is currently available only on a research basis.

Management

Growth should be closely followed. Growth charts specific for Williams syndrome are available. Regular monitoring of development, behavior, vision, hearing, and blood pressure is recommended. Early education planning and therapies are initiated, with attention paid to strengths in verbal skills and weaknesses in visuospatial skills typically seen in individuals with Williams syndrome. The patient is regularly followed by pediatric cardiology. A renal ultrasound is recommended for individuals with Williams syndrome. Renal function is monitored by regularly checking serum creatinine and a urinalysis. Calcium levels are followed by evaluating serum calcium and a spot urine for calcium/creatinine ratio. Thyroid function studies are evaluated on a regular basis to screen for hypothyroidism. Individuals with hypercalcemia can be treated with diet modification or medications. A referral to nephrology may be necessary to manage nephrocalcinosis and difficulties related to hypercalcemia. Pediatric multivitamins contain vitamin D and should be avoided in children with Williams syndrome. Individuals with Williams syndrome who require surgery should have a pediatric anesthesia consultation.

Bibliography

Achondroplasia

Horton WA, Hall JG, Hecht JT. Achondroplasia. *Lancet.* 2007;370(9582):162–172

Trotter TL, Hall JG; American Academy of Pediatrics Committee on Genetics. Health supervision for children with achondroplasia. *Pediatrics.* 2005;116(3):771–783

Angelman Syndrome

Williams CA. Angelman syndrome. In: Cassidy SB, Allanson JE, eds. *Management of Genetic Syndromes.* 2nd ed. Hoboken, NJ: Wiley-Liss; 2005:53–62

Williams CA, Driscoll DJ, Dagli AI. Clinical and genetic aspects of Angelman syndrome. *Genet Med.* 2010;12(7):385–395

Beckwith-Wiedemann syndrome

Weksberg R, Shuman C. Beckwith-Wiedemann syndrome. In: Cassidy SB, Allanson JE, eds. *Management of Genetic Syndromes.* 2nd ed. Hoboken, NJ: Wiley-Liss; 2005:101–115

Weksberg R, Shuman C, Beckwith JB. Beckwith-Wiedemann syndrome. *Eur J Hum Genet.* 2010;18:8–14

Down Syndrome

Bull MJ; American Academy of Pediatrics Committee on Genetics. Health supervision for children with Down syndrome. *Pediatrics.* 2011;128(2):393–406

Hunter AGW. Down syndrome. In: Cassidy SB, Allanson JE, eds. *Management of Genetic Syndromes.* 2nd ed. Hoboken, NJ: Wiley-Liss; 2005:191–210

Fragile X Syndrome

Hagerman RJ, Berry-Kravis E, Kaufmann WE, et al. Advances in the treatment of fragile X syndrome. *Pediatrics.* 2009;123(1):378–390

Hersh JH, Saul RA; American Academy of Pediatrics Committee on Genetics. Health supervision for children with fragile X syndrome. *Pediatrics.* 2011;127(5):994–1006

Klinefelter Syndrome

Simpson JL, Graham JM Jr, Samango-Sprouse C, Swerdloff R. Klinefelter syndrome. In: Cassidy SB, Allanson JE, eds. *Management of Genetic Syndromes.* 2nd ed. Hoboken, NJ: Wiley-Liss; 2005:323–333

Visootsak J, Graham JM Jr. Klinefelter syndrome and other sex chromosome aneuploidies. *Orphanet J Rare Dis.* 2006;1:42–46

Marfan Syndrome

American Academy of Pediatrics Committee on Genetics. Health supervision for children with Marfan syndrome. *Pediatrics.* 1996;98(5):978–982

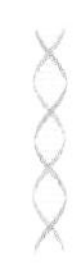

Schrijver I, Alcorn DM, Francke U. Marfan syndrome. In: Cassidy SB, Allanson JE, eds. *Management of Genetic Syndromes.* 2nd ed. Hoboken, NJ: Wiley-Liss;2005:335–349

Neurofibromatosis

Hersh JH; American Academy of Pediatrics Committee on Genetics. Health supervision for children with neurofibromatosis. *Pediatrics.* 2008;121(3):633–642

Viskochil D. Neurofibromatosis type 1. In: Cassidy SB, Allanson JE, eds. *Management of Genetic Syndromes.* 2nd ed. Hoboken, NJ: Wiley-Liss; 2005:369–384

Noonan Syndrome

Allanson JE. Noonan syndrome. In: Cassidy SB, Allanson JE, eds. *Management of Genetic Syndromes.* 2nd ed. Hoboken, NJ: Wiley-Liss; 2005:385–397

Van der Burgt I. Noonan syndrome. *Orphanet J Rare Dis.* 2007;2:4–9

Osteogenesis Imperfecta

Basel D, Steiner RD. Osteogenesis imperfecta: recent findings shed new light on this once well-understood condition. *Genet Med.* 2009;11(6):375–385

Marini JC, Letocha AD, Chernoff EJ. Osteogenesis imperfecta. In: Cassidy SB, Allanson JE, eds. *Management of Genetic Syndromes.* 2nd ed. Hoboken, NJ: Wiley-Liss; 2005:407–420

Prader-Willi Syndrome

Cassidy SB, McCandless SE. Prader-Willi syndrome. In: Cassidy SB, Allanson JE, eds. *Management of Genetic Syndromes.* 2nd ed. Hoboken, NJ: Wiley-Liss;2005:429–448

McCandless SE; American Academy of Pediatrics Committee on Genetics. Clinical report—health supervision for children with Prader-Willi syndrome. *Pediatrics.* 2011;127(1):195–204

Smith-Magenis Syndrome

Elsea SH, Girirajan S. Smith-Magenis syndrome. *Eur J Hum Genet.* 2008;16(4):412–421

Smith ACM, Gropman A. Smith-Magenis syndrome. In: Cassidy SB, Allanson JE, eds. *Management of Genetic Syndromes.* 2nd ed. Hoboken, NJ: Wiley-Liss;2005:507–525

Turner Syndrome

Bondy CA; Turner Syndrome Study Group. Care of girls and women with Turner syndrome: a guideline of the Turner Syndrome Study Group. *J Clin Endocrinol Metab.* 2007;92(1):10–25

Frías JL, Davenport ML; American Academy of Pediatrics Committee on Genetics and Section on Endocrinology. Health supervision for children with Turner syndrome [review]. *Pediatrics.* 2003;111(3): 692–702

Velocardiofacial Syndrome

Kobrynski LJ, Sullivan KE. Velocardiofacial syndrome, DiGeorge syndrome: the chromosome 22q11.2 deletion syndromes. *Lancet.* 2007;370(9596):1443–1452

Shprintzen RJ. Velo-cardio-facial syndrome. In: Cassidy SB, Allanson JE, eds. *Management of Genetic Syndromes.* 2nd ed. Hoboken, NJ: Wiley-Liss; 2005:615–631

Williams Syndrome

American Academy of Pediatrics Committee on Genetics. Health care supervision for children with Williams syndrome. *Pediatrics.* 2001;107(5):1192–1204

Morris CA. Williams syndrome. In: Cassidy SB, Allanson JE, eds. *Management of Genetic Syndromes.* 2nd ed. Hoboken, NJ: Wiley-Liss; 2005:655–665

Section 3: Genetic Testing

Chapter 10

Overview of Genetic Testing

Sarah L. Dugan, MD

Introduction

Genetic abnormalities often underlie chronic medical conditions, which produce a substantial percentage of the workload in primary care. Improved diagnostic technology has led to correspondingly improved diagnostic yield among affected individuals. Increasingly, primary care physicians (PCPs) are called on to initiate the diagnostic evaluation and to interpret complex genetic diagnoses. Understanding basic diagnostic techniques, their applications, and their limitations can increase the quality and efficiency of care.

Testing strategies covered in this chapter aim to detect 3 basic kinds of genetic disorders: genomic losses or gains, single-gene disorders, and epigenetic abnormalities. Although these categories overlap somewhat, they are useful for understanding diagnostic techniques and testing strategies. Metabolic testing (including mitochondrial testing and dried blood spot newborn screening) is covered in Chapters 7 and 17.

Testing for Genomic Disorders

Chromosomal disorders are caused by loss or gain of genomic material resulting in an excess or deficiency of multiple genes and are frequently encountered in primary care practice. They are often clinically recognizable, as in the case of Down syndrome (caused by trisomy 21) and Williams syndrome (caused by a microdeletion at 7q11.23). Other chromosomal disorders are less clinically distinct. Understanding the basic diagnostic modalities available to assess for chromosome differences is essential for a thoughtful approach to genetic testing.

Karyotype—Background and Technique

The karyotype, or the characterization of a cell's chromosome content, is routinely ordered as a simple blood test by both PCPs and specialists. The chromosomes are usually shown as the neatly arranged karyogram generated by the cytogenetics laboratory (Figure 10-1). The normal karyogram has 46 chromosomes arranged in pairs. The chromosomes are tightly condensed and are arranged by size, the location of the primary constriction or centromere, and the banding or staining pattern. Chromosomes 1 through 22 are autosomes and have a similar appearance in both males and females. The sex chromosomes (the X and Y chromosomes) are different between genders, with males having one X and one Y chromosome and females having 2 X chromosomes. The chromosomes adopt this configuration only during metaphase, which spans less than one-twentieth of the cell cycle. During most of the cell cycle, the chromosomes are loosely sprawled and appear as a dense jumble of chromatin in the nucleus.

Although the karyotype is often thought of as a basic test, it relies on meticulous technique and extensive training. It is the cornerstone of

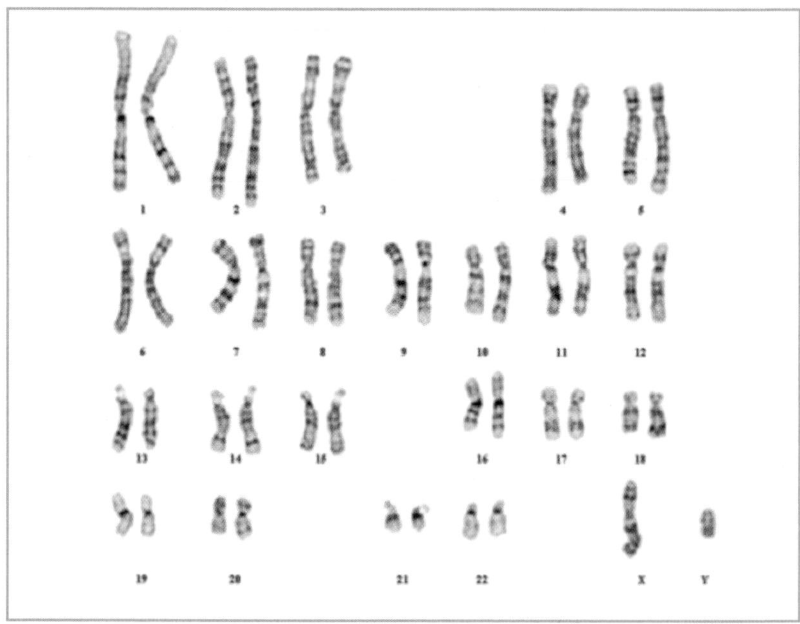

Figure 10-1. Karyogram of a normal male chromosome complement, corresponding to a karyotype of 46,XY.

all cytogenetic testing and has taken the better part of the past century to perfect. Establishing the correct number of chromosomes in a human diploid cell (46) was not possible until 1956, and it was not until 3 years later that trisomy 21 was identified as the cause of Down syndrome.

Refinement of cytogenetic technique makes the karyogram possible. Standard technique starts with culturing cells from peripheral blood or other tissue. The cultured cells are arrested in metaphase with colchicine or other mitotic spindle inhibitor and then exposed to a hypotonic solution that swells the cells, allowing the chromosomes to spread apart. The cells are then fixed with a methanol and acetic acid solution. The fixed cells are dropped onto slides, dried, and stained. A trained cytogenetic technician will examine the resulting slides, analyze the chromosomes on the slide, and then photograph representative metaphases (Figure 10-2). Specialized software helps the technician arrange the chromosome images into a karyogram. Finally, a cytogeneticist will review and interpret the karyogram and report this as a karytoype.

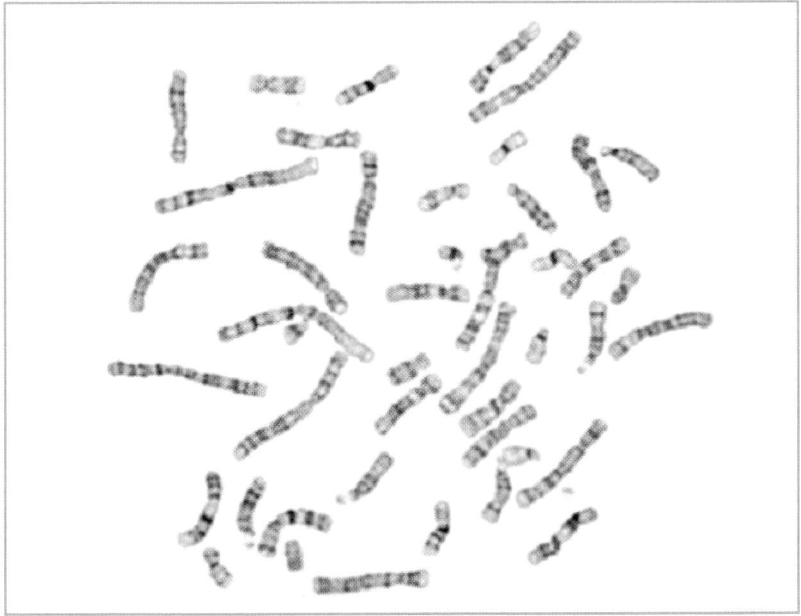

Figure 10-2. Metaphase chromosomes as they appear on the slide prior to construction of the karyogram.

Karyotype—Clinical Applications, Interpretation, and Limitations

Abnormalities detectable by karyotype analysis include polyploidy, genomic imbalance, and genomic rearrangements. Polyploidy refers to the presence of extra copies of the entire chromosome set (eg, triploidy, in which there are 69 chromosomes). Polyploidy is rare in liveborn individuals but may be seen in mosaic form. Chromosome imbalances, in which all or part of an entire chromosome has been deleted or duplicated, are much more common. Chromosome rearrangements refer to genetic material that is present but not in its expected position or orientation. For example, a piece of one chromosome may be translocated to another chromosome, or a segment of a chromosome may be inverted.

In most cases, the laboratory report will contain a karyotype, which is a shorthand notation stating the total number of chromosomes, followed by the sex chromosomes, followed by a description of any additional variants or abnormalities detected on the karyogram analysis. Most reports will expand the karyotype in plain language to explain any abnormalities detected, and many will discuss the clinical relevance of the change. Consultation with a geneticist or genetic counselor is indicated for any abnormality that is not considered a normal variant.

Normal karyotype analysis does not rule out a genomic imbalance. Some changes are simply too small to see on microscopic analysis. For example, chromosome deletion at 22q11.2 (associated with the condition velocardiofacial syndrome) is not usually detected by routine chromosome analysis. Other cryptic deletions, though large, may come from a chromosomal region with few bands and thus may not change the overall banding pattern of the chromosome. The study also analyzes a discrete number of cells in a single tissue and may therefore miss some mosaic chromosomal abnormalities (ie, abnormalities present in some but not all cells of the body).

Fluorescence in situ Hybridization (FISH)—Background and Technique

FISH is a technique that renders specific small genomic imbalances (deletions or duplications) easily visible at the microscopic level. This technology emerged in the 1980s but did not become clinically useful until the 1990s, following development of stable probes and techniques to minimize background fluorescence. Probe design is central to the process. The probe consists of a fluorescently tagged sequence of nucleotides (DNA) designed to bind (hybridize) only

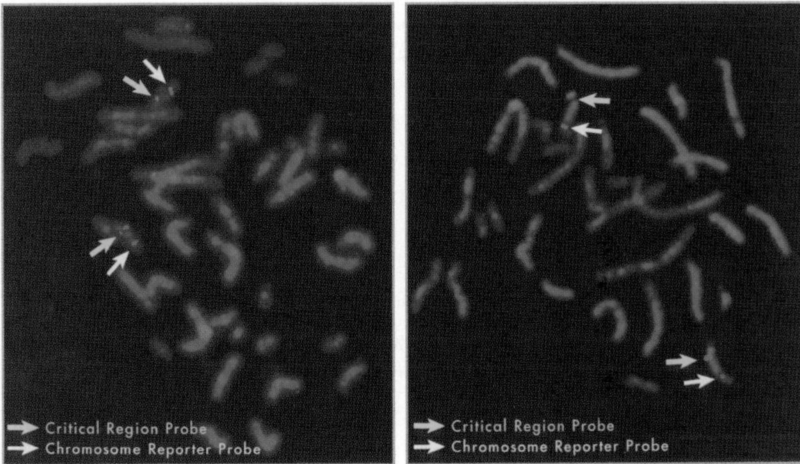

Figure 10-3. Fluorescence in situ hybridization for 22q11 in a typical individual and an individual with velocardiofacial syndrome. Both probes hybridize in the typical cell; there are 2 signals from the control probe but only 1 signal from the probe that hybridizes at 22q11 in the cells from a patient with the deletion. From *Genetic Counseling Aids,* Greenwood Genetic Center, 5th Edition.

to the locus of interest. In most clinical assays, a prepared metaphase spread (Figure 10-2) from the patient will be prepared to interrupt the double helix, resulting in single-stranded DNA, which is then incubated with the probe long enough for hybridization to occur. The excess probe is then washed away, and a technician reviews large numbers of cells under ultraviolet light to bring out the fluorescent signal of the probe for signal count. For autosomes, 2 probe signals are usually expected, since each normal cell has 2 copies of each chromosome. An extra signal in each cell suggests a duplication at the specific gene locus, while fewer signals than expected indicates a deletion. For example, performing a FISH assay at 22q11 in an individual with velocardiofacial syndrome should reveal only one signal at 22q11 per cell, because the site where the probe would ordinarily hybridize has been deleted from one chromosome but is still present on the other. Cells from an unaffected individual should display 2 signals: one corresponding to each copy of chromosome 22 (Figure 10-3).

Fluorescence in situ Hybridization—Clinical Applications, Interpretation, and Limitations

FISH is an invaluable tool for a clinician looking for a specific chromosome deletion. It is a fast, reliable test for deletions at the targeted locus. When a life-threatening form of aneuploidy (such as trisomy 13 or trisomy 18) is suspected, FISH technology can be applied to interphase nuclei for rapid confirmation of diagnosis. Because FISH allows large numbers of cells to be reviewed in a short time, mosaicism is less likely to be missed by FISH than by karyotype analysis. However, this technology is limited by its specificity. FISH is not a reasonable first-line approach in conditions such as Prader-Willi syndrome and Angelman syndrome, in which other diagnostic modalities detect not only the forms caused by genomic imbalance but also those caused by epigenetic factors. Furthermore, though many different probes are available, each one hybridizes to a specific site only and must be ordered individually based on clinical suspicion. Sending a FISH study requires significant confidence that a patient's presentation has been caused by a specific chromosome abnormality. If the differential diagnosis includes several different chromosome abnormalities, whole-genome analysis is probably a higher-yield approach.

Array-Based Genomic Analysis—History and Technique

Genomic microarray enables simultaneous assessment of thousands upon thousands of loci throughout the genome for deletions or duplications. Microarray analysis relies on both molecular and cytogenetic expertise and has rapidly become part of the standard genetics workup.

The concept of array-based testing arose out of attempts to design a FISH-based approach to genome-wide assessment. FISH technology can, in theory, be used across the genome. Whole-chromosome painting uses multiple FISH probes to assess multiple regions on each chromosome. It is still used occasionally to identify chromosomal fragments too tiny and nondescript to be recognized by banding pattern. However, using FISH in this way is limited by resolution and color perception of the human eye and by the logistics of probe design. Array-based testing addresses this issue by using a computer to quantify fluorescent signal and hybridizing free DNA from the patient to individual probes rather than hybridizing free probes to the patient's DNA. The array consists of numerous tiny segments of DNA, each corresponding to a specific part of the genome, and each fused to a specific area on a solid surface of a special slide or cartridge.

The most basic form of array-based testing uses a technology known as comparative genomic hybridization (CGH), in which arrays of thousands of oligonucleotide probes are individually fused onto a slide (called a "chip"). Each probe is produced based on the usual DNA sequence at a given locus,

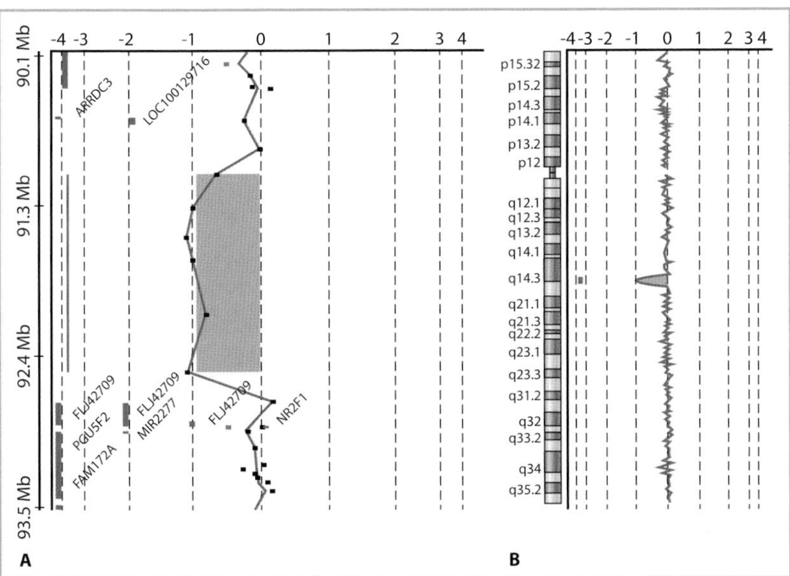

Figure 10-4. A. Microarray results showing a relative decrease in the patient's DNA signal. Relative fluorescent signal strength (horizontal axis) versus chromosome locus (vertical axis) indicates a deletion. **B.** Zooming out on the same results clearly demonstrates a deletion at 5q14. A cartoon of chromosome 5 is superimposed. Courtesy of Betsy Hirsch, PhD, FACMG.

and the resolution of an array depends on the number of oligonucleotide probes used. The patient's DNA and control DNA are each tagged with a different fluorescent marker. Flooding the slide with the DNA mixture allows them to compete at each probe locus, and their relative signal strength is measured at each probe to allow assessment of copy number change throughout the entire genome. If the patient has a chromosomal duplication, the patient's signal should be twice as strong as that of the control at that locus; if the patient has a chromosomal deletion, the control's signal should be twice as strong at that locus (Figure 10-5).

Array-based genomic testing has progressed to single-nucleotide polymorphism (SNP)-based arrays. These arrays use essentially the same technology as CGH-based arrays but use many more probes and yield more nuanced results. While CGH-based testing represents each small segment of the genome with only one probe, SNP-based arrays employ, at many loci, multiple probes that vary by only a single nucleotide. The alternative sequences, called polymorphisms, are considered normal variants. The patient's DNA will bind preferentially to its corresponding probe. Like typical oligonucleotide arrays, SNP arrays show regions of chromosomal loss or gain. However, they have the added ability to highlight regions of loss of heterozygosity for SNPs, as can be seen in consanguinity or uniparental disomy.

Microarray Testing—Clinical Applications and Interpretation

Aneuploidy, well-described duplication and deletion syndromes, and rare or novel chromosomal losses and gains are all detectable by CGH. Although microarray testing has helped uncover the cause of developmental and medical differences in many individuals, its emergence onto the clinical scene has also brought about confusion in some instances. Variations of unclear significance are common results of this test and should prompt referral to a geneticist or genetic counselor for investigation and discussion. Furthermore, not all array-based testing is equivalent. In other words, a "normal" array result should be interpreted in light of the resolution and type of array used. Finally, clinicians should remember that this technology evaluates only for DNA copy number variation and does not rule out or rule in structural chromosomal abnormalities. Array-based testing will not detect balanced genomic rearrangements, which rarely may disrupt a gene or regulatory region of a gene, leading to a clinical phenotype. Karyotype analysis is necessary to detect a balanced rearrangement.

Selecting a Cytogenetic Approach

Evaluating for genomic disorders generally occurs early in the genetic workup. When a physician strongly suspects a given genomic disorder, the least expensive or fastest approach should be taken to make that diagnosis. This may be a FISH study, as when velocardiofacial syndrome is suspected, or STAT karyotype (as when Turner [45,X] syndrome is suspected). If trisomy 13 or trisomy 18 is suspected, performing FISH on interphase nuclei as an adjunct to karyotype analysis can yield a diagnosis in 24 hours, allowing more definitive prognosis earlier in care. Where a syndromic diagnosis is suspected but the clinical picture is less clear, physicians may choose to evaluate in a stepwise process. Although karyotype analysis was traditionally the first-line study, sending array-based testing first is becoming more typical as this study is more sensitive for symptomatic genetic changes.[1] Array-based testing can be followed by routine karyotype to evaluate for structural changes.

Testing for Single-Gene Disorders

Although chromosome testing reveals a diagnosis for many families, it generally does not detect single-gene disorders. Uncovering these disorders requires targeted analysis of individual genes by a wide variety of molecular techniques. Understanding the scope and limitations of specific tests and discussing these issues with the family prior to testing aid in selecting a testing strategy and interpreting results.

Most single-gene disorders can result from a variety of different kinds of genetic changes, not all of which are assessed for in each genetic test. Testing laboratories often specify which parts of the gene are assessed. A genetic change in an exon may encode a truncated or structurally altered protein product, altering the function of the gene. Intronic mutations can lead to altered splicing of mRNA, leading to a change in the final protein product. Changes occurring in regulatory elements of a gene may also cause disease by increasing or decreasing gene expression. Ordering physicians should also be aware of the type of genetic change detectable by a molecular test. For example, sequence changes and large intragenic deletions and duplications are not necessarily detected by the same tests.

A genetic testing result generally is accompanied by explanation and discussion by the performing laboratory. Mutation type or incidence may have some bearing on clinical relevance and may therefore be described. Missense mutations, in which a single nucleotide substitution changes the amino acid encoded at that locus of the gene, may alter stability or activity of an encoded protein. Nonsense mutations, in which a single nucleotide substitution produces a stop codon in the gene, lead to a truncated protein product or to haploinsufficiency via nonsense-mediated decay.

While certain types of genetic changes can easily be interpreted as damaging to a gene, others may not be as obviously damaging. In some cases, pathogenicity of a change can be predicted based on the frequency with which it is reported in association with disease. A variant known not to be damaging is called a polymorphism. Some variants cannot be classified at the time of testing and are considered variants of unknown significance. Classification of these poorly understood variants may improve with time.

Mutation Scanning

When a specific single-gene disorder is suspected, certain situations call for a targeted approach, such as mutation analysis in which the presence or absence of only certain specific mutations is confirmed. In such situations, mutation analysis may be the cheapest, fastest, and most effective strategy to detect a mutation. Perhaps the most obvious example of an appropriate use of mutation analysis is the case of a known familial mutation. If the specific mutation is known, targeted testing is often available for other family members.

Other indications for targeted mutation scanning include conditions in which a single mutation or handful of mutations is responsible for the overwhelming majority of disease. More than 99% of individuals with achondroplasia have the $G^{1138}A$ mutation (substitution of adenine for guanine at nucleotide 1138) in the fibroblast growth factor receptor 3 *(FGFR3)* gene, making mutation scanning a more cost-effective testing strategy than sequencing the entire gene. This strategy uses a variety of molecular techniques. The ordering physician should be aware of whether mutation scanning is available as a testing strategy because of its potential to save money and time—and because of its limitations. Mutation scanning will detect only the specifically queried genetic changes and will miss other changes within and around the gene that might cause the disease in question.

DNA Sequencing

DNA sequencing, in which the nucleotide progression of a strand of DNA is determined, emerged as a laboratory technique in the 1970s and has gradually become faster, cheaper, and more reliable. In 1975 Frederick Sanger developed chain termination-based sequencing, the basis for most clinical sequencing performed today. The process relies on primers designed to specifically bind to various target sequences within the gene. In chain terminator sequencing, the patient's DNA, along with a specific primer, is incubated with a nucleotide mix and allowed to undergo polymerase chain reaction (PCR) in order to amplify the DNA sequences. The nucleotide mix contains not only the bases adenine, thymine, cytosine, and guanine, but also fluorescently tagged dideoxyribonucleotide triphosphates (ddNTPs), special nucleotide bases that, though structurally analogous to regular nucleotides, have no 3'-OH group, rendering them unable to bind other nucleotides at that terminus. Once a ddNTP binds, the strand terminates at that position. By the end of the reaction, each nucleotide in the patient's gene should be represented by a DNA molecule terminating in a ddNTP at that position. In the dye-based sequencing method, each of the 4 types of ddNTPs (corresponding to A, T, C, and G) has a unique fluorescent signal, which can be detected during separation by capillary electrophoresis (Figure 10-5).

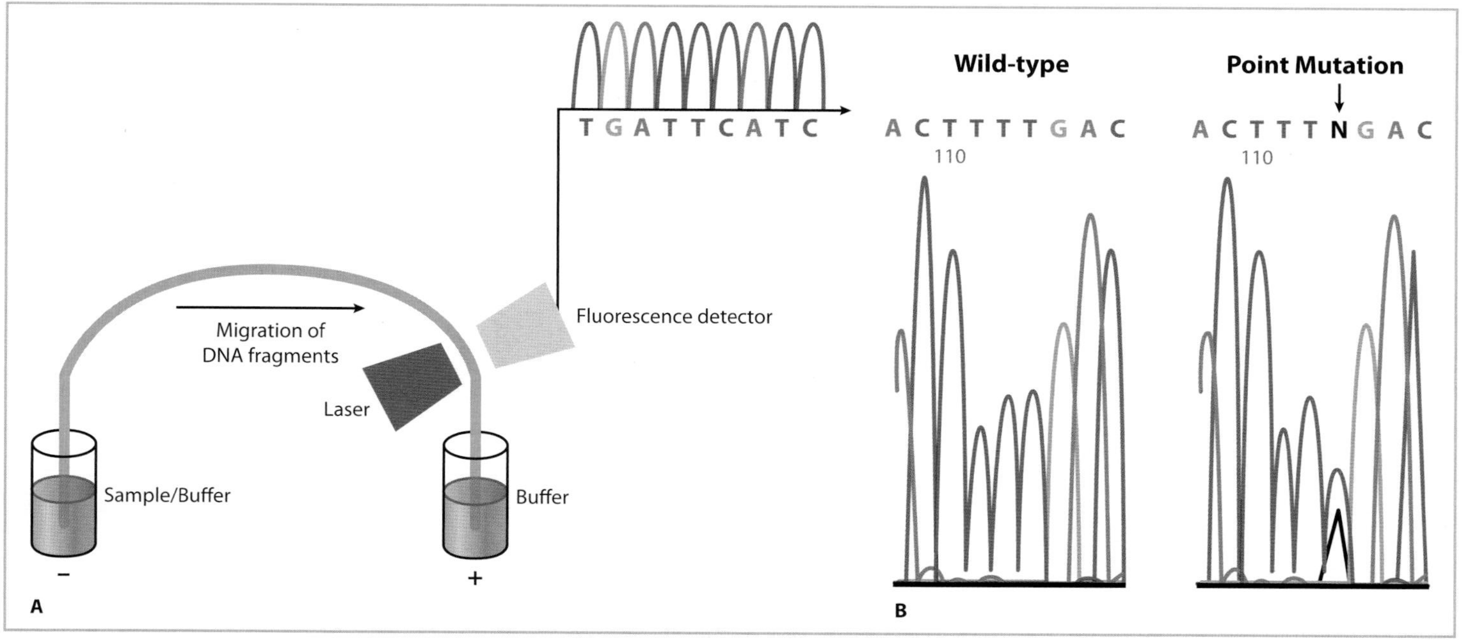

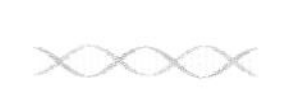

Figure 10-5. A. Chain terminator sequencing. DNA fragments terminating in a fluorescent nucleotide are separated by length using capillary electrophoresis. Each emits a fluorescent signal corresponding to its terminating fluorescent dye. **B.** An example of a single nucleotide substitution detected by this method. Two different fluorescent signals are detected at one locus, corresponding to heterozygosity for a thymine-to-cytosine substitution.

Although it continues to be widely used, chain terminator–based sequencing has certain technical limitations. Each gene sequenced requires multiple reactions because a primer is reliable only for a short segment of the gene. Array-based sequencing uses a chip housing numerous oligonucleotide probes representing all targeted regions of the gene. Fluorescently labeled DNA from the patient binds some probes and not others, allowing ascertainment of the sequence. Parallel sequencing technologies also decrease the steps required to sequence a given gene. They involve binding DNA fragments to a surface and interrogating nucleotides one by one. All methods continue to rely on amplification of the target gene, a time-consuming step. Eliminating this amplification step may be the next breakthrough in high-throughput sequencing.

Deletion and Duplication Scanning

Most conventional sequencing technologies have another major drawback in that they can easily miss deletions and duplications. Conventional sequencing misses deletions when the deleted segment includes the site at which the primer was expected to bind. Amplification and sequencing occur on the homologous chromosome only, and results reflect only the sequence of the gene not containing a deletion. Duplications may not prevent primer binding, but they would not necessarily lead to an abnormal sequence, as sequencing does not detect copy number variation. High-resolution karyotype will typically not detect deletions and duplications smaller than 4 million base pairs (compared with the typical gene length of several hundred to several thousand base pairs). Microarray analysis occasionally detects deletions or duplications leading to single-gene disorders—but only when the array platform targets the gene in question. The performing laboratory will usually be able to find out whether their platform would detect deletions or duplications within a specific gene. If the deletion would not be detected by array-based testing, another modality should be used. The molecular techniques most frequently used to detect small deletions and duplications include Southern blot, real-time quantitative PCR, and multiplex ligand-dependent probe assay (MLPA).

Southern blotting, developed in the 1970s, relies on the use of targeted probes that aid in amplifying the region of interest. The amplified DNA is cut with restriction enzymes and run on a gel to separate the fragments by size. This process yields a characteristic band pattern that is altered by intragenic deletions or duplications. It is time-consuming and requires a large amount of DNA, but it is a widely accessible and versatile technique.

Southern blotting will pick up not only large intragenic deletions and duplications, but also all other mutations that affect restriction fragment size, including trinucleotide repeat expansion, as seen in fragile X syndrome, and certain point mutations.

Real-time quantitative PCR (RT-PCR) requires expensive supplies and equipment but is a fast, reliable method for detecting intragenic deletions and duplications. This technique couples amplification via a set of targeted primers with generation of a fluorescent signal. One variation uses a probe designed to hybridize to the targeted sequence between the 2 primers. The probe contains a fluorescent dye at the 5' end and a proximity-dependent quencher molecule at the 3' end. As the targeted primer set amplifies the region of interest, the fluorescent dye is freed from the probe and can give off its signal. In another variation of RT-PCR, the fluorescent signal is produced by a dye that fluoresces after binding to double-stranded DNA. In either variation, measuring signal intensity allows for copy number analysis.

MLPA requires multiple pairs of half-probes, each designed to target a specific region within the target gene. Each pair consists of one half-probe bound to a universal primer sequence and another half-probe bound to both a universal primer sequence and a "stuffer sequence." The half-probe pairs bind immediately adjacent to each other and are ligated to form one whole fragment (consisting of the 2 half-probes, a stuffer sequence, and universal primers at either end) (Figure 10-6). Multiple sets of probes are then amplified using the universal primers. The "stuffer sequence" length is different in each probe pair, allowing separation of the amplified fragments by gel electrophoresis. Intragenic deletions and duplications can then be detected by variations in band intensity. MLPA is a generally reliable technique but requires meticulous probe design. For example, the technique can give a false-positive result when a probe does not bind because of a non-deleterious polymorphism in the target region.

Diagnostic Alternatives to Genetic Testing for Single-Gene Disorders

Genetic testing may not be a useful diagnostic option for all families. The most obvious example of this issue is when testing is not clinically available, or when clinically available testing does not detect the causative mutation in a specific family or individual. In such cases, research-based testing may be available. In kindreds containing multiple living affected individuals, linkage analysis may also be an option. Linkage might also

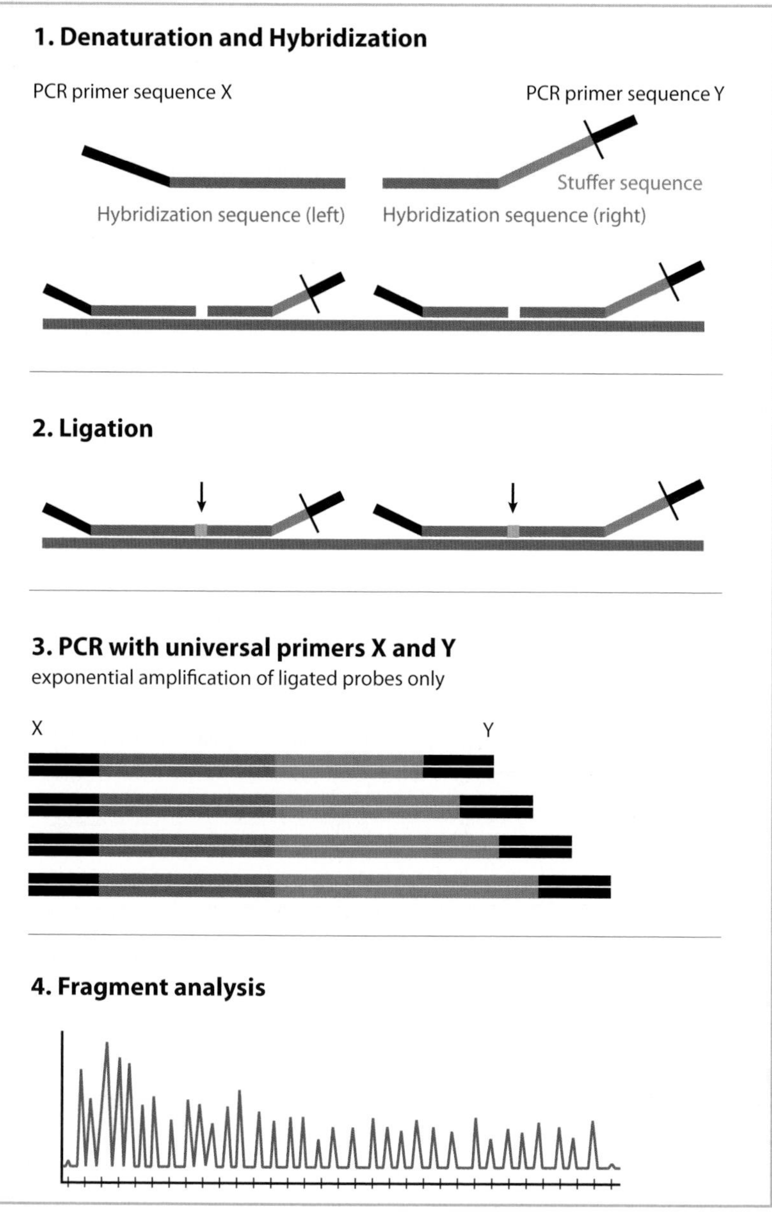

Figure 10-6. Multiplex ligation-dependent probe amplification (MLPA) is a technique for determining genomic dosage of up to 50 genes or regions of interest using semi-quantitative amplification of select representative DNA sequences. The 4 steps of MLPA are 1) A sample of DNA from the patient is initially denatured followed by hybridization of sequence-specific adjacent probes targeting the genes or regions of interest; 2) Properly hybridized probes are then ligated with a ligase-dependent polymerase; 3) Multiplex polymerase chain reaction (PCR) is then used to amplify multiple copies of the correctly paired probes. Incorrectly targeted or paired probes (secondary to an abnormality in the gene sequence) will not hybridize and thus cannot serve as viable template for PCR; 4) The fragments of interest generated by multiplex PCR are separated by electrophoresis with the resulting peak intensities electronically translated into genomic dosage based on a comparison to reference controls. This information allows the sequences of interest to be interpreted as normal, deleted, or duplicated relative to the expected genomic dosage.

be an alternative to genetic testing when certain family members wish to know their genetic diagnosis without revealing the affected or unaffected status of other family members. Clinical diagnosis or secondary laboratory diagnosis (eg, enzyme activity levels) may also be an option in certain conditions. Referral to a geneticist or genetic counselor is indicated in all of the above scenarios.

The Future of Testing for Single-Gene Disorders

As understanding of genetic disorders expands, so do the testing options. To simplify testing strategies, many laboratories now offer panel-based testing. Panel-based testing is easy to order, but ordering physicians should be aware of whether it is more cost-effective than selecting individual tests. Testing panels that sequence multiple genes in parallel may be very expensive. Consultation with a specialist may hone the diagnostic approach.

Even a specialist, however, must acknowledge the extensive clinical over-lap among conditions caused by changes in different genes. Multiple genes, for example, lead to familial hypertrophic cardiomyopathy and can be clinically indistinguishable. Array-based sequencing of multiple associated genes addresses this issue in an ultimately cost-effective and time-efficient manner. This diagnostic approach is increasingly available and is a harbinger of even broader approaches to genetic diagnosis of single-gene disorders. Sequencing of the entire protein-coding portion of the genome (exome sequencing) is an emerging option to identify the genetic cause of single-gene disorders. Many laboratories will perform this exhaustive testing only in patients with multiple affected family members or who have very clear manifestations of a specific, well-described condition. Result interpretation is challenging, as exome sequencing may identify dozens of variants in each patient. The test may lead to more questions than answers in some patients, particularly during its first few years of clinical application. However, it seems likely that exome sequencing will become a routine part of clinical genetics evaluation. Whole-genome sequencing, which once seemed like science fiction, may be just around the corner as a diagnostic option.

Summary: Testing Strategy for Single-Gene Disorders

A few years ago, physicians had to order tests for each target gene individually, but panel-based testing is increasingly available, and exome sequencing is on the rise. Testing for specific genes can be very expensive, and consultation with a geneticist or genetic counselor is indicated in cases of unclear clinical diagnosis, high genetic heterogeneity, or complex testing strategies. Above all, the ordering physician should be aware of the diagnostic approaches available for the condition in question and of the sensitivity, limitations, and expense of the various options. Discussing these issues with the patient and family prior to ordering the testing can facilitate the testing and interpretation process.

Testing for Epigenetic Disorders

Epigenetic disorders are those conditions that involve chemical modification of a gene without change of the base pair sequence. These chemical modifications, primarily methylation and acetylation, alter a gene's ability to be transcribed. Physicians should be aware of whether epigenetic factors are likely to play a role in a condition's pathogenesis, as this feature of a condition may influence the ideal diagnostic strategy. Methylation analysis can be performed to assess for conditions with an epigenetic component.

Clinical Indication of Methylation Analysis

In an epigenetic process known as imprinting, which takes place early in embryonic development, certain regions of the genome take 1 of 2 distinct methylation patterns: one specific to the paternally inherited copy of the region and one specific to the maternally inherited copy. In these imprinted regions, both copies are necessary for normal development. Prader-Willi syndrome and Angelman syndrome, 2 clinically distinct conditions, both generally result from deletion of material from 15q11 to 15q13. When the material is deleted from the maternal chromosome, Angelman syndrome occurs; the same segment deleted from the paternal chromosome results in Prader-Willi syndrome. Although the syndromes are generally clinically distinct, clinical presentations overlap in young infants. Furthermore, the conditions can be caused by intrinsic imprinting abnormalities and uniparental disomy, in which an individual has 2 copies of chromosome 15 from a single parent rather than having one copy from each parent. In uniparental disomy or in cases where diagnosis is unclear, methylation analysis is necessary. If either condition is suspected, microarray or FISH alone is insufficient to rule the condition out.

Methylation analysis is necessary in a handful of other conditions, including the overgrowth disorder Beckwith-Wiedemann syndrome and the growth failure disorder Russell-Silver syndrome, both of which can be caused by abnormal imprinting. Southern blot analysis alone will detect most cases of fragile X syndrome, which is caused mainly by expansion of a trinucleotide repeat within the *FMR1* gene. However, manifestation of the condition also depends on methylation of the expanded gene, which prevents transcription. Methylation analysis is therefore also an essential step in molecular diagnosis of this condition.

Methylation Analysis: Technique

Methylation analysis exploits basic molecular techniques to make them depend on the presence of a specific methylation pattern. Methylation-specific restriction enzymes cut only at sequences that are methylated, yielding a product only when that specific methylation pattern was present. Methylation-specific PCR first chemically modifies methylated cytosine residues to transform them into uracil residues. Specifically designed primers can then bind to the modified base sequences, binding only when the targeted methylation pattern was present at the locus.

Key Points

- Options for genetic testing have expanded greatly over the past half-century.
- Genetic testing options have become more complex and can be difficult for both physicians and patients to understand.
- Testing options screen for 3 categories of abnormalities—genomic, single gene, and epigenetic disorders.
- Initial evaluation in the primary care setting is reasonable as long as both the physician and patient (or family) are comfortable with the testing strategy.
- Consultation with a genetic specialist should be obtained for any individual with a confirmed or suspected genetic condition.

Suggested Readings

Levsky JM, Singer RH. Fluorescence in situ hybridization: past, present, and future. *J Cell Sci.* 2003;116(pt 14):2833–2838

Nussbaum R, McInnes RR, Willard HF. *Thompson & Thompson Genetics in Medicine.* 7th ed. Philadelphia, PA: Saunders; 2007

Pettersson E, Lundeberg J, Ahmadian A. Generations of sequencing technologies. *Genomics.* 2008;93:105–111

Sellner LN, Taylor GR. MLPA and MAPH: new techniques for detection of gene deletions. *Hum Mutat.* 2004;23:413–419

Reference

1. Manning M, Hudgins L; Professional Practice and Guidelines Committee. Array-based technology and recommendations for utilization in medical genetics practice for detection of chromosomal abnormalities. *Genet Med.* 2010;12(11):742–745

Chapter 11

Genetic Testing in Children: The Need for Caution

Leah Weyerts Burke, MD

Genetic testing in children has long been the subject of ethical and legal debate. Pediatricians should be aware of the ethical and legal ramifications of genetic testing in children. The primary applications for clinical genetic testing include (1) diagnostic testing, to make or confirm a diagnosis of a genetic condition in an affected or symptomatic individual; (2) presymptomatic evaluation for a specific familial condition with adult or adolescent onset of symptoms; (3) susceptibility testing for common disorders with a familial predilection to determine disease predisposition; (4) carrier testing to determine reproductive risk; and (5) pharmacogenetic analysis.

Informed Consent in Genetic Testing

Geneticists and genetic counselors have traditionally followed the approach that any genetic testing should be undertaken only after informed consent has been obtained. This informed consent includes the sensitivity of the test, the implications of a positive or negative result for the individual and other family members, as well as the legal and insurance implications of a positive test result. Some state statutes governing informed consent for genetic testing make a distinction between genetic testing that is done for diagnostic purposes and genetic testing done for non-diagnostic reasons. Written informed consent is often not required for the former but is for the latter. In contrast to many other diagnostic tests, the results of diagnostic genetic testing can have serious implications for other family members; therefore, many geneticists and genetic counselors go through an informed consent process even for diagnostic genetic testing. Children or minors cannot give informed consent in a legal sense; therefore, genetic testing in minors poses a particular dilemma for the practitioner. The American Academy of Pediatrics (AAP) Committee on Bioethics has reviewed the issues of informed consent and assent in general pediatric practice as well as in the area of genetic testing. It is recommended that assent be obtained in older children and adolescents, although there is some controversy about the age of assent. The committee report suggested that the age of assent may depend on the procedure or test being undertaken. Because of the complexity of genetic testing, assent may not be appropriate.

The AAP also encouraged newborn screening programs to evaluate informed consent procedures. In reality, informed consent for newborn screening tests is rarely implemented, although newborn screening panels are mandatory in all 50 states. This practice is defended by the American College of Medical Genetics and Genomics (ACMG) because the considerable benefits are thought to greatly outweigh the minimal risks involved.

In 1995 the American Society of Human Genetics (ASHG) and the ACMG advised against predictive genetic testing in children for adult-onset diseases, unless there are established medically useful therapies available that could be offered in the case of a positive test.[1] The AAP reviewed the ethical issues with genetic testing in 2001 and outlined the differences between genetic testing and other medical testing. The AAP concluded that genetic testing should receive special consideration and recommended that "detailed counseling, informed consent, and confidentiality should be key aspects of the genetic testing process." They also recommended that carrier testing in children and testing for adult-onset conditions be deferred until adulthood.[2,3] The consensus opinion from these 2 sets of guidelines on genetic testing in children is summarized in the algorithm in Figure 11-1.

Ethical Considerations

Adults have the right to refuse to have genetic testing just as they have the right to refuse other medical testing or therapeutics. In the case of children, parents are given rights for the medical decision-making unless it is shown that the decisions they make are not in the best interest of the child. Parents may enroll their child in research studies as long as the risk does not outweigh the benefit to either the child or others. Institutional review boards govern research studies to determine the risk to children in research, uphold participant rights and welfare, and ensure that federal regulations are followed. In the case of predictive genetic testing for

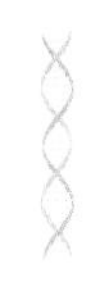

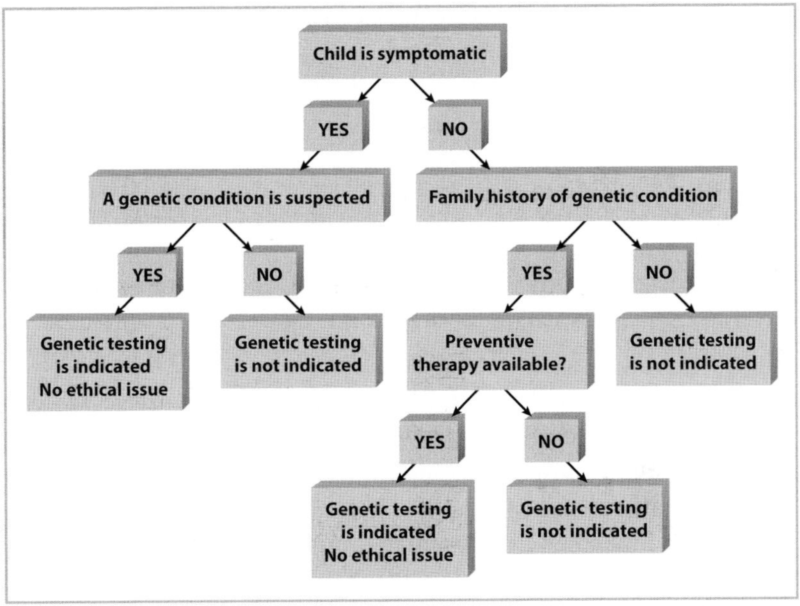

Figure 11-1. Decision tree for performing genetic testing in children.

adult-onset conditions, if there is no potential therapy that has been shown to prevent or significantly improve the future outcome of the condition, the right to decide whether or not to be tested is protected and the decision is deferred until the child becomes an adult to preserve the child's autonomy in that decision-making process.

The right to privacy is also an issue in decision-making regarding genetic testing. In many families, the individual members prefer to keep their testing results to themselves and not share their personal results with other family members. This decision may be based on some family disagreement or estrangement. However, it may also be based on a more beneficent desire not to inflict survival guilt, parental guilt, or other feelings on loved family members. An individual should have the right to keep their genetic testing results private, something that would be impossible if the testing were done at the request of a parent while the individual was still a child.

False-positive screening may identify carrier status. This is the case with sickle cell disease and with some of the recent additions to the newborn screening panel, including cystic fibrosis. Further, with the advent of molecular reflex testing being done for some of the metabolic conditions, such as galactosemia and cystic fibrosis, more and more carriers are being identified. In studies that assess the psychological effect of a positive newborn screen for cystic fibrosis that identifies a carrier status, there certainly can be a negative effect on the family in the form of anxiety and stress. However, studies generally show that the early identification of affected newborns still outweighs the negative effect.[4]

Genetic Testing and Developmental Delay or Autism Spectrum Disorders

There has been an explosion of molecular genetic testing in the areas of developmental delay and autism. The consensus recommendation of the ACMG is that a diagnostic workup for children with unexplained developmental delay or autism spectrum disorder should include genetic testing.[5–8] The first tier of genetic testing should be a whole genome chromosomal microarray followed by confirmation testing of any abnormal findings.[8] If the microarray testing is negative, the second tier should include DNA testing for fragile X syndrome and other single gene tests that are appropriate for the clinical findings.[4] The results from this genetic testing do not necessarily provide any improvement in the treatment of the condition, although sometimes can suggest further testing to uncover unappreciated medical conditions and subsequently provide information to qualify the child for additional services. A genetic diagnosis can give a presumed cause and information for reproductive planning, but can bring with it a stigma. In some cases, the stigma of a label outweighs the positive benefits of the diagnosis; however, appropriate genetic counseling should help allay many fears the family may have.

Often the primary motivation for doing genetic testing in children with developmental delay or autism is to decrease the ambiguity of the diagnosis and to suggest a cause. With the introduction of whole genome microarray testing, the ambiguity may not be decreased at all. The microarray often reveals a result for which there is limited information or understanding. The results may state that it is a "variant of unknown significance." Despite having informed consent prior to the testing as well as posttest counseling, these results are not easily explained or understood by the parents. Therefore, rather than decreasing the ambiguity with a clear cause, the result may cause more confusion and ambiguity. Many pediatricians are not prepared to offer assistance in these situations and need to rely on the geneticist or genetic counselor for explanations. Parental blood samples

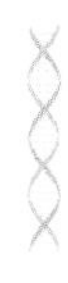

may be requested to try to predict whether or not the copy number variant is pathogenic and whether or not the variant is de novo or inherited. This can be traumatic for the family because there can be feelings of blame and guilt in these situations.

The pediatrician should be aware of the ambiguous nature of the newer genetic testing and make sure that not only is there sufficient pretest and posttest genetic counseling, but that there is also consideration made to whether or not the testing will be helpful at all to the family. In the medical home, it is important that the interests of the child as well as the family as a whole are considered before diagnostic or predictive genetic testing is undertaken.

Clinical Genetic Testing and Familial Cancer

Genetic testing of children and adolescents for familial cancers is primarily predictive, and in most cases the genes are susceptibility genes. That is, the presence of a familial cancer gene mutation indicates an increased susceptibility rather than the presence of a disease. As with adult-onset conditions, the guidelines from the AAP and from American Society of Clinical Oncology (ASCO) recommend that testing only be performed in those situations in which there is clear evidence that earlier screening or surveillance testing will affect the severity or outcome of the cancer.[9] For some familial cancer syndromes, such as familial adenomatous polyposis, Li-Fraumeni syndrome, or von Hippel-Lindau syndrome, the testing of children or adolescents can be performed to provide early testing for those who are found to carry the predisposing gene mutation or for reassurance and avoidance of other invasive testing procedures for those who are mutation negative. The ASCO guidelines specifically prohibit testing in children for cancer conditions in which there is no medical value to early information about the child's status.

This prohibition on predictive testing in children for late-onset familial cancer genes was virtually unanimous in the 1990s. More recently, however, studies of at-risk adolescents and young adults indicate that for some, the positive effects of certainty may in fact outweigh the negative effects of adverse psychological reaction to the news.[10–12] Clearly more studies are needed to address these issues, and current guidelines may need to be revised. Parents will look to their pediatrician for guidance with respect to genetic testing in their children as well as guidance about how to discuss the family history of genetic conditions.

Direct-to-Consumer Testing

Direct-to-consumer (DTC) genetic testing by definition does not involve the intermediary of a health care provider. There is a debate in the genetics community and the medical community in general concerning the ethics and usefulness of such testing. This testing is largely unregulated by the usual quality assurance testing required for certification of clinical laboratories. Although most of these companies have a disclaimer that emphasizes the fact that their results should not be used to make medical decisions, there is no requirement that they address the issue of testing of minors. The ACMG recently suggested 5 criteria that should be satisfied before DTC testing is done: (1) testing is ordered and interpreted by a knowledgeable professional; (2) the consumer is fully informed about what the test can and cannot say about their health; (3) the testing is based on sound scientific evidence, and this is clearly stated; (4) the laboratory is accredited; and (5) privacy concerns are addressed.[13] These criteria in conjunction with AAP policy[2,3] provide a sound basis for refraining from DTC testing for children in most circumstances. It should be noted that a test ordered by a parent from the privacy of one's home may not protect the rights of the child. Should a parent decide to test their child through a DTC site, the parents may call their pediatrician for assistance in interpreting the results. Pediatricians should understand the basics of DTC testing that are available and should offer genetic counseling to these families to assist in this effort.

The types of genetic testing that are offered by the DTC companies include such testing as paternity and ancestry testing, and susceptibility testing for common complex genetic disorders such as cardiovascular disease, diabetes, and osteoporosis. Other DTC testing includes testing for drug responsiveness and nutritional genetic predispositions. Some companies offer testing for a variety of single nucleotide polymorphisms (SNPs) that are said to provide personal health and susceptibility information. These SNPs are not causative but simply indicate a possible higher susceptibility to certain diseases based on population studies. Finally, there are DTC companies that offer very specific genetic testing for single gene disorders for which there is testing available through a certified clinical laboratory.

Direct-to-consumer genetic testing does not meet the recognized standards for protection of autonomy and privacy of the child. Proponents state that increased knowledge of genetic risk factors will allow individuals to exercise greater control over their lives. Knowledge of family history has proven to

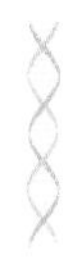

be a much more universally useful tool for assessing risk thus far. Pediatricians can encourage parents to inform their children about the family medical history.

Special Challenges in Newborn Metabolic Screening

The most common genetic test is the newborn metabolic screen. This panel of tests was initiated and has been expanded to include new conditions, largely through the efforts of patient advocacy groups and public health legislation. With the introduction of tandem mass spectrometry, the ability to do many more tests on the same blood spots has opened the door to increasing numbers of tests. In 2005 a uniform newborn screening panel was recommended as a result of a report by the ACMG commissioned by the federal Health Resources and Services Administration.[14] There are movements to continually expand the panel of tests that are done through newborn screening. Much of the push for this expansion has been by patient advocacy groups. The recent practice of rapid addition of new conditions to the newborn screening panel has, in some cases, led to the inclusion of disorders for which data on screening effectiveness in improving health outcomes are limited. In the case of the metabolic disorder known as 3-MCC, or 3-methylcrotonyl-coenzyme A carboxylase deficiency, for example, a positive newborn screen may represent the mother's condition rather than the baby's because the condition can be completely without symptoms.[15]

The AAP guidance concerning newborn screening includes a recommendation for informed consent for refusal of newborn screening. In the event of refusal, specific information should be shared with the family to inform them of the potential grave risks to the infant. The primary care physician should post a notice in the patient's chart about the non-screening status in the event that problems develop in the future.[16]

Additional blood spots are usually left over after the initial screening tests. Those specimens are often used to develop new testing techniques without the express informed consent of either the parent or the child. It is argued that the social value in such cases outweighs the individual rights. Should this waiver of consent extend into perpetuity, and what are the limitations on their use? These questions are being debated in the newborn screening arenas. Pediatricians need to know the newborn screening regulations in their states[16] and be able to counsel their patients and patients' parents (http://genes-r-us.uthscsa.edu/). (See Chapter 17.)

Genetic Testing in Adoption

In 2000 the ASHG/ACMG addressed the issue of genetic testing in adoption through a joint policy statement,[17] stating genetic testing of children during the adoption process should only be performed for diseases that can be prevented or the outcome improved through early treatment and for serious childhood illnesses. They also stated that other tests might be indicated because of information that may be available about the health of their birth siblings. The statement relied on the principle of equity to justify limitations of testing that are similar to those recommended for children who are not adopted. This consensus view is primarily to protect the rights of the child being considered for adoption.

Some believe that the issue of genetic testing must also include the rights of the adoptive parents. They argue that birth parents not only have the benefit of a more complete family history in most cases, but also have the option of doing prenatal testing that has a much wider scope. This argument is the right to know argument for the adoptive parents. In an article reviewing the ethics of pre-adoption genetic testing, Jansen and Ross[18] point out that there is a significant difference between the moral authority of birth parents and the moral authority of adoptive parents. The birth mother has moral authority over her child from the time of conception. The adoptive parents only have moral authority of their child after the adoption is complete.[18]

The principle of equity is in direct conflict with the concept of matching children with potential adoptive parents. Family history information is often gathered in order to better match the child with a family or parents, and some believe that genetic testing is an extension of this practice. Opponents of extensive pre-adoption genetic testing would argue that the results of genetic testing would lead to discrimination of that child, making it more difficult to match them with an adoptive family. For now, the consensus view remains that of the ASHG/ACMG policy statement.

National Biobank Initiatives

In recent years the development of national biobanks, repositories of biological materials, has increased. Some of them, such as those associated with the cancer registries, are disease specific, while others, like the National Children's Study, are population based.[19] The purpose of the National Children's Study is to examine the effects of environmental influences on the health and development of children. Biological samples are collected from participants, both adults and children. Although informed consent is a part of the study, the longitudinal nature of this study and ones like it raise the question about informed consent for children as they mature. It is not clear whether there will be or should be any mechanism for obtaining informed consent from the children when they reach majority age.

Key Points

- Genetic testing is a rapidly expanding field.
- Pediatricians need to understand not only the scientific, but also the ethical, social, and legal implications of genetic testing.
- Genetic testing in children and adolescents is a unique challenge that requires balancing the needs of the child with the needs of the family.

References

1. American Society of Human Genetics (ASHG) Board of Directors and American College of Medical Genetics (ACMG) Board of Directors. Points to consider: ethical, legal, and psychosocial issues with genetic testing in children and adolescents. *Am J Human Genet.* 1995;57:1233–1241
2. American Academy of Pediatrics Committee on Bioethics. Informed consent, parental permission, and assent in pediatric practice. *Pediatrics.* 1995;95(2):314–379
3. American Academy of Pediatrics Committee on Bioethics. Ethical issues with genetic testing in pediatrics. *Pediatrics.* 2001;107:1451–1455
4. Southern KW, Merelle MM, Dankert-Roelse JE, Nagelkerke AD. Newborn screening for cystic fibrosis. *Cochrane Database Syst Rev.* 2009;(1):CD001402
5. Shen Y, Dies KA, Holm IA, Bridgemohan C. Clinical genetic testing for patients with autism spectrum disorders. *Pediatrics.* 2010;125(4):e727–e735
6. Moeschler JB, Shevell M; American Academy of Pediatrics Committee on Genetics. Clinical genetic evaluation of the child with mental retardation or developmental delays. *Pediatrics.* 2006;117(6):2304–2316
7. Schaefer GB, Mendelsohn NJ; Professional Practice and Guidelines Committee. Clinical genetics evaluation in identifying the etiology of autism spectrum disorders. *Genet Med.* 2008;10(4):301–305
8. Miller DT, Adam MP, Aradhya S, et al. Consensus statement: chromosomal microarray is a first-tier clinical diagnostic test for individuals with developmental disabilities or congenital anomalies. *Am J Human Genet.* 2010;86:749–764
9. American Society of Clinical Oncology. Policy statement update: genetic testing for cancer susceptibility. *J Clin Oncol.* 2003;21(12):2397–2406
10. Ross LF. Ethical and policy issues raised by heterozygote carrier identification and predictive genetic testing of adolescents. *Adolesc Med State Art Rev.* 2011;22(2): 251–264, ix
11. McConkie-Rosell A, Spiridigliozzi GA, Melvin E, Dawson DV, Lachiewicz AM. Living with genetic risk: effect on adolescent self-concept. *Am J Med Genet C Semin Med Genet.* 2008;148C(1):56–69

12. Duncan RE, Gillam L, Savulescu J, Williamson R, Rogers JG, Delatycki MB. "You're one of us now": young people describe their experiences of predictive genetic testing for Huntington disease (HD) and familial adenomatous polyposis (FAP). *Am J Med Genet C Semin Genet.* 2008;148C(10):47–55
13. American College of Medical Genetics. ACMG Statement on Direct-to-Consumer Genetic Testing. http://www.acmg.net/StaticContent/StaticPages/DTC_Statement.pdf. Accessed June 8, 2012
14. Maternal and Child Health Bureau of Health Resources Services Administration, American College of Medical Genetics. Newborn screening: toward a uniform screening panel and system. *Genet Med.* 2006;8(5)1s–250s. http://mchb.hrsa.gov/programs/newbornscreening/screeningreportpdf.pdf
15. Koeberl DD, Millington DS, Smith WE, et al. Evaluation of 3-methylcrotonyl-CoA carboxylase deficiency detected by tandem mass spectrometry newborn screening. *J Inherit Metab Dis.* 2003;26(1):25–35
16. American Academy of Pediatrics Newborn Screening Authoring Committee. Newborn screening expands: recommendations for pediatricians and medical homes—implications for the system. *Pediatrics.* 2008:121(1):191–217
17. American Society of Human Genetics (ASHG) Social Issue Committee and American College of Medical Genetics (ACMG) Social, Ethical and Legal Issues Committee. Genetic testing in adoption. *Am J Human Genet.* 2000;66:761–767
18. Jansen LA, Ross LF. The ethics of preadoption genetic testing. *Am J Med Genet.* 2001;104:214–220
19. National Institute for Child Health and Human Development. The National Children's Study. http://www.nationalchildrensstudy.gov/Pages/default.aspx

Chapter 12

Population-Based Genetic Screening

James Flory, MD, MSCE
Hakon Hakonarson, MD, PhD

Introduction

Genetics, the study of inheritance and variation in living organisms, has important applications in screening for disease risk (eg, newborn screening for cystic fibrosis). Genetic testing can be used to explain disease once it is present (diagnosis of inherited immune deficiencies in children with repeated infections). Genetic tests can further help define treatment and prognosis in disease (eg, testing for homocystinuria). They can also predict beneficial versus adverse reactions to treatment (eg, testing for risk of Stevens-Johnson syndrome from carbamazepine therapy).

Definitions

Population-level screening is defined as testing a usually asymptomatic group to detect individuals with a high probability of having or developing a particular disease. Most examples given here of established screening tests are taken from newborn screening programs, but the scope of the discussion here includes screening performed at later stages in childhood. Most often genetic tests are used when a patient is already symptomatic or is at particularly high risk for disease. This chapter includes some examples of these kinds of test to explore whether they can be adapted into useful screening tests.

While the narrowest definition of a genetic test would refer just to variations in the nucleotide sequence of DNA that manifest as variations in phenotype, modern genetics overlaps with other concepts and potential assays. One example is epigenetics, defined here as persistent alteration of gene expression through mechanisms other than changes in the actual genetic sequence, including DNA methylation and histone deacetylation.

(See Chapter 2.) Unlike classic genetic variation, epigenetic variation can occur during the life of an organism, yet can still be inherited by offspring.[1] As more assays of mRNA and protein expression are used, such proteomic assays will also become important in clinical genetics.

Genetic testing includes any test that directly assesses genetic variation, as well as tests that do not directly assess genetic variants but still effectively detect them, such as the sweat-chloride and immunoreactive trypsinogen tests for cystic fibrosis. Closely related technologies like epigenetic assays are also included by this definition, although epigenetics is an emerging field and has yet to prove itself for clinically relevant tests, much less population-level screening tests. This definition of genetic testing is similar to one used in recent legislation (Genetic Information Non-Discrimination Act of 2008), referring to "an analysis of human DNA, RNA, chromosomes, proteins, or metabolites, that detects genotypes, mutations, or chromosomal changes."[2]

Screening Technology

Most existing genetic screening tests do not look directly at DNA but are actually tests for chemical markers that result from genetic variation with established role in disease.[3] However, DNA tests already have applications in screening, such as follow-up testing for cystic fibrosis once an initial test is positive. In the future, we will likely see a shift toward technologies that read the genome directly. The current generation of genotyping chips sample a selection of single nucleotide polymorphisms (SNP), essentially providing a lower resolution view of the genome compared to the high-resolution picture provided by complete DNA sequencing. These chips, also called tag-SNP arrays, can also be used in some cases to assess for copy number variations (CNVs) in the form of deletions or duplications. Both SNPs and CNVs have been associated with various diseases. Private companies already use these chips and these associations to provide prognostic information, and this model could easily develop to the point where it is used in clinical applications, possibly including newborn screening or other population-level screening programs.[4,5]

Whole genome sequencing remains expensive, but the price is rapidly dropping.[6] If prices continue to fall, even routine genetic screening may involve actual sequencing of all or part of the genome. However, it is impossible to predict when or if this approach will be important clinically, both because the technology has not quite arrived and because whole-genome sequencing may provide far more information than is clinically relevant. Progress and debate are focused around the cheaper and more limited tag-SNP arrays.

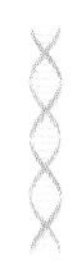

The essential feature of all of these technologies is that they may identify inherent traits that have profound prognostic implications, not just for the patient, but potentially for the patient's relatives. Because of this, genetic tests raise technical, ethical, and policy questions. If they are to be used as population-level screening tests, these questions are particularly important because a screening test applied to a whole population typically has a fairly small potential benefit to each child, which means that the risks must also be low.

Newborn Screening

Pediatrics is one of the few areas in medicine where population-level genetic testing has been practiced for many years in routine newborn screening panels. These began with screening for phenylketonuria (PKU) in 1963 (although screening has historically used a bacterial inhibition assay to detect phenylalanine levels, it effectively diagnoses a group of autosomal recessive mutations in the *PAH* gene). Subsequently, newborn screening has expanded to the point where it commonly includes many other diseases, including sickle cell disease, cystic fibrosis, galactosemia, biotinidase deficiency, congenital adrenal hyperplasia, and maple syrup urine disease, to name a few.[3] (See Chapter 17.)

Most of these disorders are detected now using techniques that do not directly assess the genome. Instead tests generally look at biomarkers, like mass-spectrometric assays for amino acid and acylcarnitine levels. But these assays are considered genetic tests because the diagnosis of the biomarker abnormality also demonstrates that the patient has a relevant genetic mutation.[3] In some cases, this practice of looking at biomarkers has advantages over looking directly at genetic variation.

For example, in patients with cystic fibrosis, there are many potential genetic mutations at the CFTR locus that can lead to the disease, and short of sequencing the locus in every newborn (which is not yet cost-effective), it would not be practical to detect them all. However, tests like the immunoreactive trypsinogen test provide simple proxies for a wide range of functional mutations.[7] A positive immunoreactive trypsinogen test can be followed up by mutation analysis to identify which specific genetic variation the screening test has detected.

New genetic tests are more likely to directly assess a patient's genetic material. But in spite of changes in technology, many of the issues raised by the new tests have already come up in the development of newborn screening. There has been a long debate over which genetic tests are appropriate for use as population-level screening tests. (See Choosing to Use Tests.) The existence of multiplex tests that assess for multiple traits at the same time, and evolution in our understanding of carrier states and their clinical implications, has prefigured similar but more dramatic issues likely to arise with new tests. (See New Tests on the Horizon.) Likewise, experiences developing policies around informed consent for newborn screening will remain applicable as population-based genetic screening evolves. (See Implications for Public Policy and Primary Care.)

Much, if not all, population-level genetic screening can be done in newborns, since the germline genome does not change over the course of a life. However, somatic mutations can take place at any point, and DNA can also be modified through epigenetic mechanisms. There may also be ethical reasons to wait until later in life to decide whether to perform some genetic tests. (See Choosing to Use Tests.) Hence, while newborn screening is the best-established paradigm for population-level genetic screening, there may be a place for genetic screening done at older ages.

Rare Versus Common Genetic Diseases

The distinction between rare and common disease is fundamental both in genetics and in screening, but for different reasons. In genetics, the major difference is that some (but not all) rare diseases have a clearly defined cause that relates to a particular locus where defined mutations will result in a disease. Examples include cystic fibrosis, sickle cell disease, and PKU. No common disease (incidence >1 in 500 persons) has ever been shown to have a single genetic cause. Instead the common diseases seem to be multifactorial, with contributions from many different genes and from the environment. A possible reason for this is that a common genetic variant that typically resulted in a disease would likely be deleterious enough to be eliminated by natural selection. In fact, one of the major findings from the recent burst of genome-wide association studies has been that complex disorders seem to have even more different contributing genetic variations than originally expected.[8]

From a clinician's perspective, this means there are a number of excellent genetic tests for rare disorders like cystic fibrosis, with high sensitivity and specificity, but no sensitive or specific tests for common genetic disorders. For example, there is not one single genetic mutation that leads to asthma.

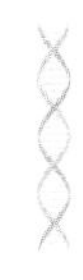

Researchers are attempting to develop genetic tests for common disease risk that could potentially be used as population-level screening tests. These screening tests employ dozens of different genetic markers and eventually may use hundreds or thousands of such markers to zero in on the complex contribution of genetics to an individual's disease risk.[4,9]

In screening, the distinction between rare and common diseases is important because screening for rare diseases is harder. A screening test for a rare disease needs to be extremely specific (even 99% is often not good enough), otherwise the ratio of false-positive to true-positive tests will be prohibitively high. This problem can be expressed with the concept of a positive predictive value, which represents the probability that a person has a disease if a test for that disease is positive:

$$PPV = \frac{(sensitivity)\ (prevalence)}{(sensitivity)\ (prevalence) + (1 - specificity)\ (1 - prevalence)}$$

where prevalence is the percentage of the population with a disease at any given time, sensitivity is the probability that a test will yield a positive result in a person who has the disease, and specificity is the probability that a test will yield a negative result in a person who does not have the disease.

In most clinical scenarios, a test with 100% sensitivity and 99% specificity would be valuable. But suppose a screening program for healthy newborns applies such a test to look for a devastating condition with an incidence of 1 in a million. With 99% specificity, the positive predictive value is only 0.0001. This means that if a million newborns were screened there would be 10,000 false-positive results to go along with a single true-positive. Depending on the parental stress involved in each false-positive result and the kinds of further testing involved, such a test might not be worthwhile. So tests that screen for rare diseases need to be extremely specific, and the benefits of early detection must be high enough to justify the cost and risks of screening thousands of children to identify a single case.

Screening for common diseases is less problematic. High specificity is desirable but not as critical, and the benefits need not be as great because with any reasonable sensitivity one expects to correctly diagnose many cases without having to screen an inordinate number of children. For example, asthma has approximately a 10% incidence; if the test described above were used to screen a million children for asthma susceptibility, the positive predictive value would be a respectable 0.91. There would 9,000 false-positive results to go along with 100,000 true-positives, performance that is much more likely to be clinically useful (provided, of course, that there is some useful clinical intervention to be done for children who test positive).

Unlike any other area of diagnostic screening, genetic testing is at its best for rare diseases, where the tests perform so well that they make up for the problems inherent in screening for something rare. Thus we have useful, well-established screening tests for cystic fibrosis but nothing clinically meaningful yet for asthma, obesity, or depression. This reflects the technical challenges of developing genetic tests for common diseases.

Standards for a Good Screening Test

Wilson and Jungner[10] proposed criteria for screening programs that were published by the World Health Organization in 1968 and remain relevant (Box 12-1). An examination of each of these rules in the context of genetic testing may prove useful in both showing how some genetic tests fail to be good screening tests, and in showing minor ways in which these criteria might be updated to apply better to genetic screening methods.

Rule 1: The condition to be screened must be an important health problem.

This rule remains clearly applicable. It should be noted that it does not preclude screening for very rare diseases. For example, PKU has an incidence of only 1 in 15,000 and medium-chain acyl-CoA dehydrogenase deficiency (MCAD) about 1 in 17,000.[3] This societal decision reflects the

Box 12-1. Wilson and Jungner's Criteria for Screening Tests[10]

1. The condition to be screened must be an important health problem.
2. The natural history of the disease must be well-known.
3. There must be an identifiable early stage.
4. Early treatment must provide greater benefits than at later stages.
5. An appropriate test must be developed for the early stage.
6. The test must be acceptable to the population.
7. Intervals must be defined for repeating the test.
8. Health care service provision must be adequate for the extra clinical work resulting from screening.
9. The risks, both psychological and physical, should be less than the benefits.

severity of these disorders, the efficacy of early treatment, and the low cost of the screening test.

Rule 2: The natural history of the disease must be well-known.
In general, the diseases included in newborn screening panels have had well-understood natural histories. Genetic research that searches for causal genes in less clearly characterized disorders may yield functional genetic tests before the underlying causal pathways are fully understood. However, it is likely in such cases that it will be more difficult to meet other criteria on Wilson and Jungner's list—if, for example, there is no effective intervention available for children who test positive. (See rules 3–5.)

Rules 3–5: There must be an identifiable early stage, early treatment must provide greater benefits than at later stages, and an appropriate test must be developed for the early stage.
These rules capture the idea that testing is not useful if there is no prodrome to the disease in which useful preventive measures can be taken. Hypothetically, there might be little utility in a screening test for attention-deficit/hyperactivity disorder (ADHD) if there were no effective preventive intervention to take before ADHD declared itself clinically. This idea is very important and explains why many genetic tests may not belong in a screening program.

Rule 6: The test must be acceptable to the population.
This is a key issue with genetics. Overall, public attitudes toward genetic testing are fairly positive,[11] but this has the potential to change, especially if policy does not handle the potential downsides of the technology well. Some recent media commentary has suggested that parents may be uncomfortable with aspects of DNA testing, particularly when they are not aware that it might be done or that detailed genetic information and genetic samples may be held by the state. This issue is addressed more thoroughly later in this chapter.

Rule 7: Intervals must be defined for repeating the test.
This issue is less important in genetic testing, because the genome does not generally change over the lifetime of an individual. Epigenetic tests might be an exception, since epigenetic modification can occur later in life, but the clinical implications of this principle are not clear yet.

However, a related issue is determining at what point in a child's life testing is best performed. If it is important to know about a disease as early as possible in order to treat it, newborn screening for the disease may be appropriate. For some other conditions it may still make sense to screen early just to ensure that screening takes place for everyone. However, if there is any substantial risk to the test, it may be appropriate to wait longer to give the child an opportunity to decide whether they want to be tested.

Rule 8: Health care service provision must be adequate for the extra clinical work resulting from screening.
In some cases, like PKU, the preventive method (eg, dietary modification to prevent phenylalanine intake) is very cheap and very effective. But for other tests, the effective intervention may be intensive screening regimens that are very expensive and only gradually become feasible as technology progresses. For example, if elevated risk for some childhood malignancy were identified on a genetic test, and indicated that some population of children would have a slight benefit from annual contrast magnetic resonance imaging, it might not be clear that the test would be useful given the high ratio of cost to benefit.

Rule 9: The risks, both physical and psychological, must be less than the benefits.
For genetic screening this is a significant concern. The physical risks of genetic testing are generally negligible, but the psychological risks should be considered carefully.[12] These risks do not simply apply to the newborn child, but to parents, siblings, and other relatives who may be identified as carriers or high-risk individuals based on the test. Other risks to consider include social stigma and the risk of losing insurance or access to insurance based on genetic information.

Choosing to Use Tests

The benefits of testing for certain rare genetic diseases that can be caused by a single, highly penetrant genetic mutation, like PKU and MCAD, are generally accepted. These tests are widely felt to meet criteria similar to those outlined by Wilson and Jungner. At present the American College of Medical Genetics and Genomics has identified a panel of 29 (generally rare and monogenic) diseases for which it suggests that neonatal screening should be a public responsibility (Table 12-1).[3] Tests were rated using systematically collected data and expert opinion on a set of criteria similar to Wilson and Jungner's rules, and scores were normalized to give the expert group rank were reported in the right-hand column. MCAD scored the highest of all tests and received a rank of 1; by comparison, cystic fibrosis was relatively low-ranked at 0.57, which the authors said reflected ongoing debate about whether screening had been convincingly shown to benefit patients. In the United States, the average number of disorders screened for at birth was actually 43 (with a range of 14–57 disorders nationwide).[3]

So far there are no tests for complex genetic diseases (eg, asthma or type 1 diabetes) that made this list or meet Wilson and Jungner's criteria well. In a systematic study of potential newborn screening tests, the major arguments against inclusion of type 1 diabetes included identifying an effective screening test, but the absence of an effective intervention was a key consideration.[3]

As new tests are developed, it may be useful to look at the history of cystic fibrosis testing to illustrate the challenges involved in introducing a new genetic test. Cystic fibrosis testing did not immediately become a universal form of newborn screening. In 2002 only 10% of newborns with the disease were screened.[13] The slow rollout of cystic fibrosis screening was in part due to concerns about psychological risk and no clear benefit. Randomized clinical trials that demonstrated that screening resulted in better clinical outcomes helped to promote the widespread use of cystic fibrosis screening.[7,13]

This story illustrates a scenario that is likely to recur as tests for other common diseases become feasible. A number of disorders, like asthma, inflammatory bowel disease (IBD), and diabetes, meet a few of Wilson and Jungner's criteria easily: They are important and their natural history is fairly well understood. The question is whether these diseases have an early stage in which clinical interventions might be useful. In cystic fibrosis this was never self-evident—it was possible that the burdens of the screening test were not counterbalanced by any real benefit compared with waiting for cystic fibrosis to declare itself clinically. This is likely to be a difficult empirical question for many diseases.

Oncologic screening tests have received special attention in the past. The *BRCA* screening tests have never been extended to the general population.[14] In pediatrics, oncologic screening tests are even less likely to become widely used, because for many oncologic risks, including breast/ovarian cancers, it is currently acceptable to wait until a person is old enough to make an informed decision about whether or not they want testing.[14]

Table 12-1. Conditions in the Core Panel Recommended by American College of Medical Genetics and Genomics[a3]

Abbreviation	Disease	Expert Group Risk
HMG	3-hydroxy 3-methylglutaric aciduria	0.82
3-MCC	3-methylcrotonyl-CoA	0.75
ASA	Argininosuccinic aciduria	0.64
BKT	Beta-ketothiolase	0.66
BIO	Biotinidase	0.95
CUD	Carnitine uptake deficiency	0.69
CIT	Citrullinemia type I	0.65
CAH	Congenital adrenal hyperplasia	0.93
CH	Congenital hypothyroidism	0.99
CF	Cystic fibrosis	0.57
GAI	Glutaric acidemia type I	0.83
HEAR	Hearing loss	0.73
HCY	Homocystinuria	0.76
IVA	Isovaleric acidemia	0.89
LCHAD	Long-chain 3-hydroxyacyl CoA dehydrogenase	0.84
MSUD	Maple syrup urine disease	0.89
MCAD	Medium-chain acyl-CoA dehydrogenase	1.00
Cbl-A,B	Methylmalonic acidemia	0.72
MUT	Methylmalonic acidemia	0.77
MCD	Multiple carboxylase	0.8
PKU	Phenylketonuria	0.98
PROP	Propionic acidemia	0.71
Hb S/A	S-beta thalassemia	0.87
Hb S/C	Sickle C disease	0.86
Hb S/S	Sickle cell	0.94
GALT	Transferase deficient galactosemia	0.88
TFP	Trifunctional protein deficiency	0.81
TYR-1	Tyrosinemia type 1	0.63
VLCAD	Very long-chain acyl-CoA dehydrogenase	0.89

[a] Numerical ranks reflect consensus among a large panel of experts on the utility of these screening tests using criteria similar to Wilson and Jungner's; 1.0 represents best results.

New Tests on the Horizon

In several areas (notably IBD and type 1 diabetes), preliminary tests based on multiple markers have been developed.[9,15] An important feature of these tests is that they may be effective only when they take into account large numbers (hundreds or thousands) of genetic markers.[9] As these tests incorporate large panels of SNPs (potentially in combination with other biomarkers, CNV assays, and epigenetic measures), they may eventually become accurate enough to be used in population-level screening.

Why type 1 diabetes and IBD specifically? These are both conditions where a fairly large set of independent genetic risk factors have been identified and can be combined into one test.[9,15] For other complex diseases, even those where there is certainly a significant genetic component to risk, there are not yet enough well-characterized risk loci. Interestingly, as more risk factors are found and more carefully characterized, some genetic tests may also help to identify interventions that will be useful once the disease risk is identified. For example, one of the few known susceptibility loci for asthma *(ORMDL3)* raises the risk of asthma more strongly when an individual is exposed to tobacco smoke.[16] If more similar loci were found, they might be used in a genetic test that did not simply identify newborns at risk of asthma, but identified children who needed to be kept away from certain environmental stimuli to keep them from developing asthma.

Infectious disease may be a particularly interesting area for new screening tests. This is one type of common disease where on occasion there may be very strong genetic associations as well as robust predictors of disease severity. These tests could work to triage children for vaccination, particularly in years when supplies of vaccine are scarce and genetic factors may predict either the effectiveness of a vaccine[17] or the likelihood of severe disease if the child is infected.

For example, most children are exposed to respiratory syncytial virus (RSV), but a small minority becomes extremely ill from the virus. There are potentially genetic variants that may predict this variable response.[18] Such a genetic test could be of value in guiding emergency department triage of a child or the use of therapies for RSV.

In addition to asthma, type 1 diabetes, infectious disease, and IBD, genome-wide association studies have been completed for a variety of pediatric conditions, including ADHD, mathematical ability, obesity, autism, juvenile idiopathic arthritis, cystic fibrosis severity, acute lymphocytic leukemia, conduct disorder, young onset hypertension, celiac disease,

Kawasaki disease, atopic dermatitis, neuroblastoma, and sickle cell anemia severity.[19] These are all traits with substantial heritability for which multimarker tests might eventually be developed. But at this point, there have not been nearly enough susceptibility loci identified for any of these conditions—new genetic associations and new methodologies are needed before genetic tests are feasible in most of these areas.

Efforts to screen children for polygenic diseases will increase the complexity of the screening process. If tests use a panel of different genetic markers, and the panel is frequently updated as new discoveries are made, these constantly changing tests are likely to require changes in current regulations. Multi-marker tests will also require direct assessment of an individual's genetic code, probably through use of tag-SNP arrays or even sequencing. They may also require collection of large amounts of genetic information—if a test requires collection of several thousand genetic markers, it would mean collecting enough genetic information to uniquely identify the subject of the test, and perhaps to assess risk for numerous diseases, not just the one intended for screening.

This is not an entirely new issue. Tests to assess for a single genetic disorder have historically often given information on a range of related disorders. For example, screening for sickle cell disease can yield information on a wide range of other hemoglobinopathies, including sickle cell trait. Testing for cystic fibrosis and many other recessive traits can also reveal carrier status for the child and even some relatives.[3] Although a screening program may only be intended to identify a handful of severe diseases, if it uncovers milder related diseases or carrier status, policies need to be in place to govern reporting and management of that information. This issue stands to become much more important as technology develops.

For example, if a screening panel for IBD, asthma, type 1 diabetes, and a few other common disorders involved assessment of 20,000 different genetic markers, such a panel might permit an even wider-ranging assessment of a child's genetic risk and carrier status for other diseases, as well as the child's ancestry. This would blur the line between population screening—which in newborns has been closely focused on a discrete list of carefully selected conditions—and the types of comprehensive genetic risk assessment packages now offered by private companies.

These companies offer individuals the opportunity to be genotyped using a tag-SNP array that assesses anywhere from hundreds of thousands to millions of SNPs, at a cost of a few hundred dollars. This product differs radically from conventional screening tests in several ways. First, it is nearly unregulated and even described as "recreational genomics."[20] Doctors are not currently gatekeepers for this technology, and nor at present is the US Food and Drug Administration (FDA), although the FDA's role in this kind of test is an area of active debate. Second, instead of asking focused questions about carefully selected diseases, these panels identify modest increases or decreases in risk for a wide range of conditions. This is done regardless of whether there is any clinical utility to the information. Instead it is essentially being provided because the consumer is interested in it. (Also see Chapter 11.)

These direct-to-consumer (DTC) products could be adapted, in theory, into newborn screening tests for genetic risk. Their use would challenge many of the assumptions made in this article up to this point. Suppose that instead of screening newborns for a specific list of genetic conditions, large arrays of genetic data (even complete genome sequencing) were used to make a broad range of prognostic judgments with varying degrees of certainty. Adults are already free to embrace this model of genetic risk prediction, and even this is considered ethically problematic. In the pediatric population these issues are more pronounced.[5]

Applications of DTC technology to newborns would set up a tension between 2 different models. The first would be the existing model of newborn screening: state mandated, standardized, and focused on conditions where the benefits of screening are clear and risks are low. This model is exemplified by cystic fibrosis screening, which took years of study, including randomized controlled trials, before it was widely accepted. The new model would be newborn (or early childhood) testing that is driven by consumer demand and uses technology to gather the widest possible range of prognostic information, even if its quality and clinical utility are not totally clear. How much to regulate such testing may be a policy debate in the future. Pediatricians will need to decide what role to play in that debate and, assuming that DTC genetic testing of newborns is legal, will need to help parents make a complicated choice well.

Implications for Public Policy and Primary Care

A variety of special ethical and policy issues surround genetic testing and the idea of using it widely. Genetic information is often thought of as special (genetic exceptionalism) because it could theoretically reveal information that profoundly affects patients' access to care, access to employment, social status, and even sense of identity.[21] Genetic data also may affect relatives of the study subject.

Pediatricians may find themselves in a position to shape fundamental policies and public attitudes about genetic screening for diseases. Although levels of public trust in genetic testing are fairly high,[11] anxiety about the potential downsides of any genetic test are a staple in public debate about health technology.

One rational and fundamental fear is of insurance discrimination based on the results of genetic testing. Children diagnosed at an early age with a severe genetic disorder or a significant predisposition to common diseases might face higher insurance premiums from the very beginning of life. The recent history of legislation in the United States suggests growing protection against genetic discrimination. The Health Insurance Portability and Accountability Act, passed in 1996, took some steps to prevent genetic discrimination in group health insurance policies (although not in individual policies). A complex network of state laws has provided additional protections since then. A key event in protection against genetic discrimination was passage of the Genetic Information Nondiscrimation Act of 2008 (GINA).[22]

GINA forbids insurers from discriminating against potential policyholders based on genetic risk factors. It prohibits employers from requesting, requiring, or purchasing genetic information; requiring employees to take genetic tests; or discriminating on the basis of genetic information. It also prevents health insurance companies from denying or canceling coverage, or adjusting premiums, based on genetic information. However, GINA does not apply if an individual has "manifestation of a disease, disorder, or pathological condition," which creates a possible loophole, since many genetic conditions may have some clinical manifestation even at the time of screening.[22]

There is not yet a body of law that clarifies how thorough the protections offered by these laws are. In his 2009 column "Dad's Life or Yours," Nicholas Kristof captures at least one strain of fear when he tells the story of a man with polycystic kidney disease whose children are advised not to be tested for the potentially preventable disorder because it could impact their chances of getting health insurance. He cites GINA but does not reassure readers that it solves the problem.[23]

A recent survey of experts in genetic counseling for cancer patients showed that 94% considered the risk of genetic discrimination to be low to theoretical, and 64% expressed confidence in already existing federal laws that protect against genetic discrimination. Compared with a similar survey conducted in 2000, more genetic counselors felt confident enough in the legal protections to bill insurance for genetic testing for cancer risk. However, the survey also uncovered some evidence that even genetic counselors are not fully versed in the legal implications of genetic information; for example, only 42% knew whether relevant state legislation applied to individually purchased insurance policies or only to group policies.[22]

Navigation of these complex issues will increasingly fall to pediatricians as more genetic tests become available for newborns and are considered for inclusion in newborn screening panels. In 2001 the American Academy of Pediatrics (AAP) issued a policy statement that "pediatricians need to provide parents the necessary information and counseling about the limits of genetic knowledge and treatment capabilities; the potential harm that may be done by gaining certain genetic information, including the possibilities for psychological harm, stigmatization, and discrimination; and medical conditions and disability and potential treatments and services for children with genetic conditions. Pediatricians can be assisted in managing many of the complex issues involved in genetic testing by collaboration with geneticists, genetic counselors, and prenatal care providers."[24]

In addition to working with patients on an individual level, pediatricians may want to participate in several major policy decisions. These include deciding what new tests belong in standard newborn screening panels, whether such panels should be mandatory for all children, and whether there should be regulation or even banning of some types of genetic testing of newborns.

A key issue is whether screening of newborns with any consensus test panel should be mandatory or voluntary. The term mandatory tends to confuse the issue somewhat, since in reality a mandatory approach can be declined if parents so wish. The real meaning of a mandatory approach is that in a mandatory system informed consent is not required, and screening may occur without necessarily notifying parents that the testing is taking place.[24]

In its policy statement, the AAP makes the point that routinely obtaining informed consent for newborn screening may be a good model, particularly since it would make it more practical to incorporate new and experimental tests into newborn screening. In a study of newborn screening in Maryland, most women preferred that they be asked for permission before screening, and rates of informed refusal were very low (<1%).[25] The AAP recommendation is that states mandate the *offering* of the appropriate panel of newborn screening tests.[24]

The ethical complexity of genetic testing suggests that offering such panels, with explanation of how the testing works, may be important. Even now, when genetic testing in newborn screening is still in its infancy, state practices in performing genetic analysis and storing newborns' genetic samples vary considerably. CNN reported that parents in Texas and Minnesota have filed lawsuits out of concern that not only did their states perform newborn screening without obtaining informed consent, they stored the DNA samples for a period (indefinitely in some states) and even made them available for research in certain contexts.[26] A more complete informed consent process might help to prevent this kind of controversy.

Finally, the advent of DTC genetic testing and its potential application to children and neonates means that there will be some level of demand for testing of healthy newborns far beyond what is appropriate for inclusion in a screening program. Because the broad range of prognostic tests in DTC packages will probably outstrip available clinical evidence on how useful the tests are, pediatricians may face difficult choices about whether to help parents obtain genetic tests that will not clearly benefit a child and may impose risks. One clear point raised by the AAP is that genetic testing for late-onset disease (like the *BRCA* breast and ovarian cancer susceptibility variants) is probably not appropriate in children, since these conditions can safely be tested for later in life, and some children might decide later in life that they did not want to be screened for those conditions.[24]

However, much more liberal attitudes toward genetic testing of children exist, and include essentially recreational activities, like one company's suggestion that its customers can "Add some excitement to your family reunion by comparing the DNA of children with other relatives."[5] Obtaining the kinds of broad-ranging genetic information (hundreds of thousands of SNPs) used in DTC genetic testing means creation of a dataset that not only can provide very wide-ranging prognostic information about a child, but will also be uniquely identifiable as belonging to that child. A recent policy article on this subject essentially held off on making policy recommendations and recommended more research on the risks of DTC testing in children and newborns.[5] This is an unformed policy area that pediatricians may wish to help shape.

Key Points

- Technology for population-based genetic screening is evolving rapidly and will soon include tag-SNP arrays and whole- or part-genome sequencing.
- Population-based genetic screening has been practiced in newborns since the 1960s. It now includes nearly 60 commonly used tests, many of which offer very good sensitivity and specificity for rare monogenic diseases.
- There are 9 well-established criteria for an established screening test, including the principle that the screening test must identify a stage of the disease where a useful intervention can be performed.
- As a general rule, existing successful genetic tests address rare monogenic diseases.
- Tests exist that use many genetic markers to test for susceptibility to complex diseases, including some common diseases, but they do not yet meet criteria for a useful population-level screening test. Examples include tests for asthma, type 1 diabetes, and IBD.
- In some cases, like cystic fibrosis screening, randomized trials of the effect of testing on clinical outcome have been feasible and useful.
- The future is likely to bring a proliferation of complicated screening tests of questionable clinical benefit.
- Pediatricians need to help parents make informed choices about what types of screening to use.

References

1. Francis DD. Conceptualizing child health disparities: a role for developmental neurogenomics. *Pediatrics.* 2009;124(suppl 3):S196–S202
2. Pub L No. 110-233, 122 Stat 881.
3. Watson MS, Lloyd-Puryear MA, Mann MY, Rinaldo P, Howell RR. Newborn screening: toward a uniform screening panel and system. *Genet Med.* 2006;8(5):1s–250s
4. Kuehn BM. Risks and benefits of direct-to-consumer genetic testing remain unclear. *JAMA.* 2008;300(13):1503–1505
5. Tabor HK, Kelley M. Challenges in the use of direct-to-consumer personal genome testing in children. *AJOB* 2009;9(7):32
6. Pool JE, Hellmann I, Jensen JD, Nielsen R. Population genetic inference from genomic sequence variation. *Genome Res.* 2010;20(3):291–300
7. Southern KW, Mérelle MM, Dankert-Roelse JE, Nagelkerke AD. Newborn screening for cystic fibrosis. *Cochrane Database Syst Rev.* 2009;(1):CD001402
8. Manolio TA, Collins FS, Cox NJ, et al. Finding the missing heritability of complex diseases. *Nature.* 2009;461(7265):747–753

9. Wei Z, Wang K, Qu HQ, et al. From disease association to risk assessment: an optimistic view from genome-wide association studies on type 1 diabetes. *PLoS Genet.* 2009;5(10):e1000678
10. Wilson JMG, Jungner G. *Principles and Practice of Screening for Disease.* Geneva: World Health Organization; 1968
11. Etchegary H, Cappelli M, Potter B, et al. Attitude and knowledge about genetics and genetic testing. *Public Health Genomics.* 2010;13(2):80–88
12. Hamilton JG, Lobel M, Moyer A. Emotional distress following genetic testing for hereditary breast and ovarian cancer: a meta-analytic review. *Health Psychol.* 2009;28(4):510–518
13. Wilcken B. Cystic fibrosis: refining the approach to newborn screening. *J Pediatr.* 2009;155(5):605–606
14. US Preventive Services Task Force. Genetic risk assessment and *BRCA* mutation testing for breast and ovarian cancer susceptibility: recommendation statement. *Ann Intern Med.* 2005;143:355–361
15. Imielinski M, Baldassano RN, Griffiths A, et al. Common variants at five new loci associated with early-onset inflammatory bowel disease. *Nat Genet.* 2009;41(12): 1335–1340
16. Bouzigon E, Corda E, Aschard H, et al. Effect of 17q21 variants and smoking exposure in early-onset asthma. *N Engl J Med.* 2008;359:1985–1994
17. Li Y, Ni R, Song W, et al. Clear and independent associations of several HLA-DRB1 alleles with differential antibody responses to hepatitis B vaccination in youth. *Hum Genet.* 2009;126(5):685–696
18. El Saleeby CM, Li R, Somes GW, Dahmer MK, Quasney MW, Devincenzo JP. Surfactant protein A2 polymorphisms and disease severity in a respiratory syncytial virus-infected population. *J Pediatr.* 2010;156(3):409–414
19. National Human Genome Research Institute. www.genome.gov/gwastudies/. Accessed June 14, 2012
20. Kaye J. The regulation of direct-to-consumer genetic tests. *Hum Mol Genet.* 2008;17(R2):R180–R183
21. Wasson K. Direct-to-consumer genomics and research ethics: should a more robust informed consent process be included? *Am J Bioeth.* 2009;9(6-7):56–58
22. Huizenga CR, Lowstuter K, Banks KC, Lagos VI, Vandergon VO, Weitzel JN. Evolving perspectives on genetic discrimination in health insurance among health care providers. *Fam Cancer.* 2010;9(2):253–260
23. Kristof N. Dad's life or yours, *New York Times.* October 4, 2009. http://www.nytimes.com/2009/10/04/opinion/04kristof.html. Accessed February 8, 2010
24. American Academy of Pediatrics Committee on Bioethics. Ethical issues with genetic testing in pediatrics. *Pediatrics.* 2001;107(6):1451–1455
25. Faden R, Chwalow AJ, Holtzman NA, Horn SD. A survey to evaluate parental consent as public policy for neonatal screening. *Am J Public Health.* 1982;72(12):1347–1352
26. Cohen E. The government has your baby's DNA. February 4, 2010. CNN Web site. http://www.cnn.com/2010/HEALTH/02/04/baby.dna.government/index.html. Accessed June 14, 2012

Section 4: Counseling, Community, and Ethics

Chapter 13

Genetic Counseling Principles

Dinel Pond, MS, CGC
Lori Terry, MS, CGC

Introduction

Genetic counseling is a process of communication, education, and support to individuals or families affected by genetic or suspected genetic-related disease. The principles of genetic counseling[1] (Box 13-1) acknowledge the patient's ability to participate in the decision-making process and highlight that the psychological aspects of genetic disease are as important as education and risk-assessment components.[2] The practice of genetic counseling may require greater experience or time commitment than the primary care physician (PCP) may have, depending on the latter's degree of training and the complexity of the patient's problems.[3]

Genetic counseling can be defined as the process of helping people understand and adapt to the medical, psychological, and familial implications of genetic contributions to disease.[4] This process integrates the interpretation of family and medical histories to assess the chance of disease occurrence or recurrence; education about inheritance, testing, management, prevention, resources, and research; and counseling to promote informed choices and adaptation to the risk or condition. Genetic counseling is usually performed by clinical geneticists and genetic counselors for complex issues, but PCPs and other subspecialists are often well-suited and able to perform such roles also.

Genetic counseling involves all stages of the human life cycle, from preconception to the postnatal environment and infancy, through childhood and adolescence and adulthood, and finally to the diagnosis of an elderly individual with an inherited disorder such as dementia.[5] Genetics plays a role in most aspects of medicine, including complex disorders such as

Box 13-1. Principles of Genetic Counseling

- Educate the patient about what to expect in a genetic counseling session.
- Recognize the aspects of "crisis" inherent in the diagnosis of a genetic or potentially genetic condition.
- Cooperate with other medical personnel and specialists to ensure the correctness of the diagnosis and that accurate information is given to the patient.
- Address the patient's concerns about reproductive decisions and options and planning for child rearing.
- Provide support for the patient who is dealing with situations outside his/her previous range of experience.
- Recognize and explore the emotions inherent in the genetic counseling process.
- Facilitate decision-making.
- Respect the autonomy and decision-making capacity of the patient.
- Respect the patient's experience, knowledge, and values as valid bases for decision-making.
- Adapt the giving and gathering of information to the individual needs of the patient.
- Act as an advocate for the patient.
- Work consistently toward empowering patients to make autonomous decisions and to advocate on their behalf.
- Maintain surveillance over one's own biases and values.

From Marks J, Heimler A, Reich E, Wexler N, Ince S. Genetic counseling principles in action: a casebook. *Birth Defects Orig Artic Ser.* 1989;25(5):1–142.

cardiovascular disease, cancer, diabetes, asthma, and even drug metabolism (pharmacogenetics). Because of its ubiquitous role in medicine, most physicians, including those in both primary and specialty care, are confronted with the genetic aspects of medicine in the care of their patients. Genetic counseling translates advances and their effects on health care for patients and their families and, often, for the PCPs involved in their care. Parents and pediatricians have increasing exposure to genomic and proteonomic analyses, and geneticists and genetic counselors are integral to the process of educating the families and the PCPs.

Genetic counseling is a communication process that aims to provide the most applicable and accurate genetic information in an understandable manner such that patients can make individualized, educated, and informed decisions regarding their genetic health care. Genetic counseling facilitates the decision-making and adaptation processes of health care decision-making by recognizing and addressing the associated psychological and social factors while at the same time providing empathy and support (Figure 13-1). Nondirective counseling is the guiding principle of the genetic counseling process, yet each situation is unique, and the key to communication is nonjudgment.

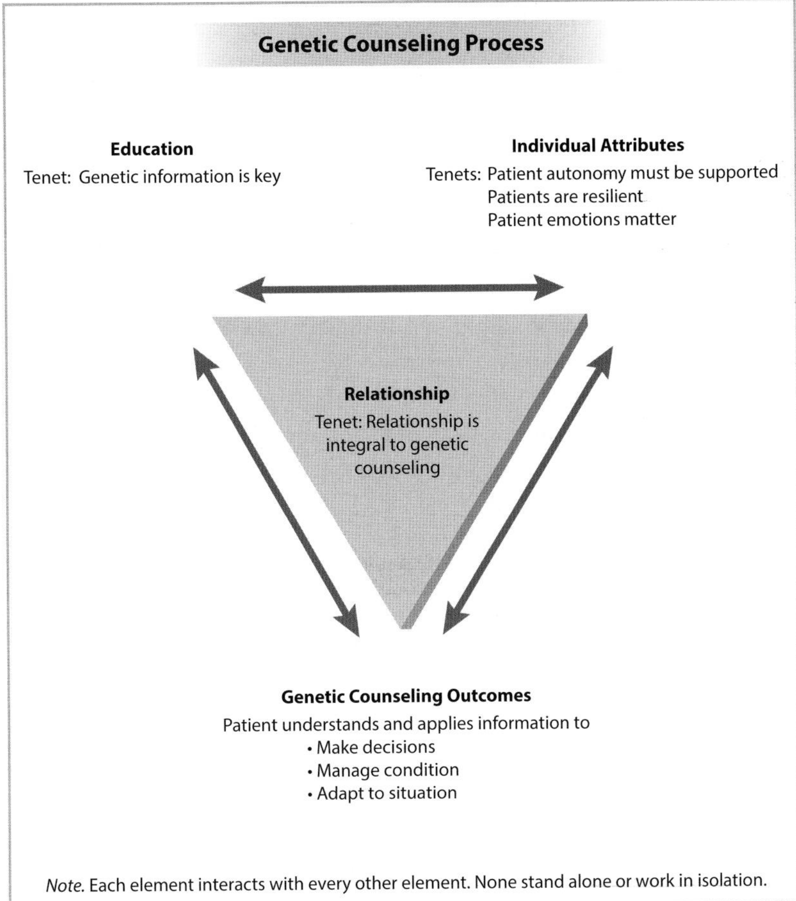
Genetic Counseling Process
Education
Tenet: Genetic information is key
Individual Attributes
Tenets: Patient autonomy must be supported
Patients are resilient
Patient emotions matter
Relationship
Tenet: Relationship is integral to genetic counseling
Genetic Counseling Outcomes
Patient understands and applies information to
• Make decisions
• Manage condition
• Adapt to situation
Note. Each element interacts with every other element. None stand alone or work in isolation.

Figure 13-1. The genetic counseling process. From Veach P, Bartels D, LeRoy B. Coming full circle: a reciprocal-engagement model of genetic counseling practice. *J Genet Counsel*. 2007;16:713–728. Reprinted with permission from Springer Business + Science Media.

Genetic Counseling Providers

The provider of genetic counseling can vary depending on the clinical situation. Often multiple providers in the same clinic or institution provide genetic counseling, or at least different elements of genetic counseling. Clinical geneticists and other pediatric subspecialists evaluate patients with known or suspected genetic conditions, make genetic diagnoses, and manage the clinical care of their patients. They have a significant role in educating and supporting the patient and family and, as part of their practice, provide genetic counseling.

Obstetricians and gynecologists often provide genetic counseling, especially in the context of prenatal screening and prenatal diagnosis. As recommendations for screening for genetic conditions have become more widespread, obstetricians often discuss availability of carrier testing for conditions such as cystic fibrosis, diagnostic testing prenatally for Down syndrome and other conditions, or even testing for cancer susceptibility genes such as *BRCA1/2*.

Because a nurse's role in a genetics clinic involves frequent interaction with patients with genetic conditions, many nurses also provide genetic counseling.[6] Advanced practice nurses are increasingly being used in the genetics clinic to care for patients with specific genetic conditions. Genetic counselors have a master's degree with specialized training in human genetics, counseling skills, and the psychosocial issues encountered during a genetics consultation.

Genetic Counseling in Pediatrics

Information gathering is an important part of the genetic consultation (Box 13-2). Often one of the primary responsibilities of the genetic counselor is obtaining a detailed family history. The family history may provide clues to a potential diagnosis, and focused questions regarding

Box 13-2. Primary Roles of Genetic Counseling in Pediatrics

- **Information gathering**
  - Family history
  - Medical history, including previous test results and consultations
- **Testing information**
- **Recurrence risk counseling**
- **Psychosocial support**

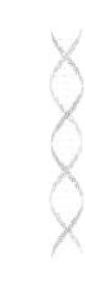

symptoms of potential differential diagnoses are often asked. In the pediatric genetics clinic, the genetic counselor is part of a team involved in evaluating children and adolescents for genetic conditions that present after birth or develop over time. Depending on the setting, the specific roles of the genetic counselor vary. In general, however, many of the activities of the genetic counselor have an educational component and a supportive component. In the pediatric setting, genetic counselors may be asked to educate a variety of people, including parents, extended family members, other health care professionals, and the general public.

The genetic counselor may also be involved in gathering records or reports of other evaluations that may be pertinent to the genetics evaluation. When a patient is referred for genetic counseling regarding a particular diagnosis, the genetic counselor must first establish the validity of the diagnosis. This typically involves obtaining test results and may involve talking to other providers or to laboratory personnel to determine the significance of the findings. When working with the clinical geneticist in the process of evaluating a patient, the genetic counselor explains the testing being recommended and obtains informed consent.

If a specific diagnosis is established with a known inheritance pattern, such as an autosomal recessive condition, genetic counseling is needed to explain the inheritance pattern and the recurrence risk to the family. In cases without a specific diagnosis or when the inheritance pattern is not certain, other methods of risk assessment may be used, including empiric risks, Bayesian analysis, or pedigree-based analysis. Risk assessment also extends to discussing the potential for specific complications to occur. Genetic counseling helps families and individuals understand risk analysis and helps patients and their families understand and assess their own perception of risk.[7]

Another role for genetic counseling is to provide support, both emotional and educational, to families. This may include identifying condition-specific support and advocacy groups, referring to other providers, or finding local resources to assist the family in navigating systems, such as the school system or financial systems. The genetic counselor often is the individual who serves as the primary contact person for the family in the genetics clinic; someone they can easily reach with questions about their child's diagnosis or about where to go for help with a particular issue. Finally, the genetic counselor helps the family to adjust to the medical problems or diagnoses in the family and addresses issues regarding uncertainty.

Benefits of Genetic Counseling

Several studies have found that patients and families believe the information obtained during a genetic counseling session, the manner in which the information was delivered, and the assistance they received with decision-making were beneficial factors of genetic counseling.[8,9] Bernhardt and colleagues also found unanticipated benefits of genetic counseling included patient or family satisfaction with development of an interpersonal relationship with the genetic counselor because of their understanding, attentiveness, time, expertise, and long-term commitment.[8] Patients report the genetic counseling process helped improve communication about genetic issues within the family, provided anticipation of feelings or experiences stemming from future events, and helped clarify the values underlying their decisions or attitudes. The education, understanding, and support that is incorporated into the process of genetic counseling serves to empower a patient or family and provides them with an increased sense of control over their situation. Ultimately, this helps reduce the anxiety, stress, and feelings of uncertainty often induced by genetic issues and gives patients and families a more positive outlook on their health care. Informed and empowered patients and parents will serve as advocates for themselves and their children not only in a complicated medical system but also in their families and communities. It should never be assumed that genetic counseling with the family has eliminated all potential confusion. The counseling process is an ongoing one throughout the medical professional's interactions with the patient and family.

The benefits of genetic counseling can also extend to PCPs. Physicians, including pediatricians, can rely on those providing genetic counseling services as a source of help and assistance in dealing with genetic concepts and issues. Just as genetic counselors specialize in translating the complexities of these issues to patients, they can also provide similar services to physicians who may not be as familiar with the concepts. In addition, by establishing communication and relationships with the genetics team, a PCP can ensure that the highest quality of care is provided to their patients and that the genetic needs of their patients are met.

Payment for Genetic Counseling

Genetic counseling services are typically paid quite variably based on the state, medical center, and genetics unit. Genetic counselors usually bill under the auspices of a medical geneticist. Even though genetic counseling *Current Procedural Terminology* codes are available, payment from private

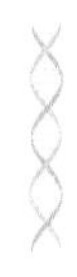

and public payers for these services is usually lacking. Even genetic counseling provided by medical geneticists is paid inconsistently, depending on the insurance provider and the location.[10]

Key Points

- Genetic counseling provides genetic information to individuals and families so they can make informed decisions about their genetic health care.
- Genetic counseling may be provided by geneticists, pediatric subspecialists, obstetricians/gynecologists, nurses, or genetic counselors.
- Genetic counselors gather information from other providers and from the patient and family in a nondirective and nonjudgmental manner. They also provide emotional and educational support.
- For the genetic evaluation and follow-up care, genetic counselors are often the primary point of contact for the family and other health care professionals, including the PCP.
- For genetic-related conditions often cared for by pediatric subspecialists, genetic professionals (clinical geneticists and genetic counselors) are available to assist as needed.

References

1. Marks JH, Heimler A, Reich E, Wexler NS, Ince SE. Genetic counseling principles in action: a casebook. *Birth Defects Orig Artic Ser.* 1989;25(5):1–142
2. American Society of Human Genetics Ad Hoc Committee on Genetic Counseling. Genetic counseling. *Am J Hum Genet.* 1975;27:240–242
3. Walker A. The practice of genetic counseling. In: Baker D, Schuette J, Uhlmann W, eds. *A Guide to Genetic Counseling.* Wilmington, DE: Wiley-Liss, Inc;1998:1–20
4. National Society of Genetic Counselors' Definition Task Force. A new definition of genetic counseling: National Society of Genetic Counselors' Task Force report. *J Genet Counsel.* 2006;15(2):77–83
5. Bennett R, Hampel H, Mandell J, Marks J. Genetic counselors: translating genomic science into clinical practice. *J Clin Invest.* 2003;112:1274–1279
6. Visovsky C. Genetics counseling: a basic competency for nurses? *Nurs Leadersh Forum.* 1999;4(2):40–43
7. Smith A. Patient education. In: Baker D, Schuette J, Uhlmann W, eds. *A Guide to Genetic Counseling.* Wilmington, DE: Wiley-Liss, Inc; 1998:99–122
8. Bernhardt B, Biesecker B, Mastromarino C. Goals, benefits, and outcomes of genetic counseling: client and genetic counselor assessment. *Am J Med Genet.* 2000;94:189–197
9. Veach P, Truesdell S, LeRoy B, Bartels D. Client perceptions of the impact of genetic counseling: an exploratory study. *J Genet Counsel.* 1999;8(4):191–216
10. Harrison TA, Doyle DL, McGowan C, et al. Billing for medical genetics and genetic counseling services: a national survey. *J Genet Counsel.* 2010;19:38–43

Chapter 14

Genetics and the Community: A Commentary

Robert A. Saul, MD
Frances Edwards Rushton Jr, MD

Pediatricians, apart from their professional practice, are often called on to support and participate in various child-focused initiatives in their communities. Pediatricians are passionate and committed to the overall well-being of children. Their training and their relationships over time with children and families enable them to have a unique vantage point from which to guide community policies. They are often called on by local governmental authorities, volunteer agencies, schools, and civic groups to render an opinion in regard to initiatives and policy proposals. Until recently genetic expertise has not been a traditional factor in these deliberations. With the explosion in genetic information, genetics is assuming an increasingly more important role in the repertoire of the community pediatrician. This chapter will explore potential issues with the assimilation of genetics into traditional community pediatrics expertise and reflect the personal viewpoint of the authors.

Genetics and Community Pediatrics

The intersection between pediatrics and other local services for children is often defined as community pediatrics. Community pediatrics is a perspective that expands the pediatrician's activities from one child to all children. The pediatrician must recognize that genetic, family, cultural, social, spiritual, and environmental factors all impact the health and function of children. Community pediatrics is a synthesis of clinical practice and public health principles and implies a commitment to use community resources on behalf of children. Working with the community is an integral part of the professional responsibility of pediatricians and an important tool in dealing with the genetic revolution.[1]

Community health initiatives are multifaceted. They involve many entities such as agencies (governmental, volunteer, public health, social services, and others), schools, churches, parent groups, business groups, civic groups, physicians, medical societies and, most importantly, families and their children. This list just touches the surface of the interrelated systems that interact to improve the lives of children through community health initiatives. These services, along with the informal relationships that families call on in time of crisis, can be referred to as social capital.

Social capital responds to and affects the environment within which we all work and live. Community environmental factors can include pollution, drugs and violence, significant socioeconomic disparities, teen pregnancy, and overcrowded neighborhoods. Not all environmental factors are negative. They can represent community assets, such as industrial and business resources, the arts, parks, libraries, festivals, community good will, and virtually anything that happens to reflect positively on the life of a community. The boundaries between what constitutes an environmental factor and what is social capital may be somewhat blurred. Good schools, for example, could provide both positive social capital relationships through teachers and an ideal learning environment for the child. Social capital can alter our environment, and our environment can alter social capital to affect positive change.

Maximizing social capital enables patients and families to deal with illness in a positive way. A positive environment lays the foundation for good health. These factors are critical considerations for community initiatives aimed at the improvement of child health. There is another factor also to be considered—genetics. Patients and families almost always recognize that kinship (close genetic relationships) is a key factor in health care. Families' recognition of the increased risk of certain common multifactorial disorders (such as heart disease, hypertension, obesity, cancer, and diabetes) is common. One might argue that social capital and environmental factors are the potentially malleable or changeable factors in this triad. Genetic factors are less susceptible to change. But we also need to understand that perception of genetic issues (real or imagined) will affect the ability to achieve positive change. Education about genetic factors and any possible misperceptions can be essential in promoting health. The primary care physician plays a vital role in the dissemination of accurate genetic information to patients, their families, and the community at large. Genetic understanding is a factor in the development of community initiatives and needs to be thoroughly explored before significant initiatives are proposed or undertaken.

Community pediatricians thus have the opportunity to address genetic factors in a manner that maximizes the use of available social capital and environmental factors to promote health. Genetic issues can positively or negatively influence the community improvement process and need to be considered throughout any attempts at community improvement. Genetic predispositions for many common disorders should help drive the policy debates and social initiatives designed to improve the lives of our children. Box 14-1 lists the proposed responsibilities of the community pediatrician for the use of genetic information for such initiatives. Pediatricians must use their genetic knowledge to help lead the way.

Genetics and Public Policy

Social capital, genetics, and the environment all interact with social policy. Social policy makers (public health officials, social service officials, local hospitals, and state legislators), local governments, school officials, and medical practitioners can alter environmental factors that impact the lives

Box 14-1. Responsibilities of the Community Pediatrician for the Use of Genetic Information for Community Improvement

- Is a source of knowledge and advice in the genetic basis of disease
- Provides critical screening for common genetic-based diseases in a given community (including newborn screening)
- Coordinates care for individuals with complex medical needs related to their disease complexes
- Promotes optimal wellness for all individuals in their community regardless of genetic factors
- Ensures that appropriate wraparound services for patients with genetic-based services are available
- Helps provide community awareness of certain genetic-based services so that the disease burden of the community is diminished
- Advocates on a community and state level for genetics and related issues (privacy issues, equity in screening and prevention, and the availability of services)
- Recognizes the impact of epigenetic factors on disease and helps diminish their impact over time

of children. Good health, an excellent education, and sound financial well-being are all tied to our ability as a community to set policy and initiate programs that help children and their families.

Pediatricians are often called on for expertise regarding community projects aimed to help children at the local, state, and federal level. The interplay of social capital, the environment, and genetics are important determinants of individual and public health. Policy makers and legislators often lack the expertise and experience for most children's health initiatives. Social capital, environment, and genetics are all worthy of consideration as local and state officials confer with children's health experts (pediatricians and the American Academy of Pediatrics) to improve the health of children.

Knowledge of genetic information can be helpful, but frequently there are unintended negative consequences for the individual and the community. Genetic information can be a deterrent to change.[2] Families often have a "perceived helplessness" about their life circumstances based on their understanding of their metabolism or genetic makeup. They foresee a lack of control about their future, that there is nothing that they can do to improve the inevitable outcome of genetic problems that are intrinsic in their families. These problems might include rare or unusual disorders but are more likely to be common ailments with some genetic component, like hypertension, diabetes, cancer, or obesity. This perceived helplessness potentially clouds the thinking of some of our medically fragile citizens (like low-income groups) and can also affect the thinking of the health care professionals.[3] This sense of futility can unfortunately provide a rationalization for continued negative behaviors and the reason for the lack of the ability or desire to change such behaviors. Pediatricians must be aware of the potential negative effects (like perceived helplessness) genetics can have on both the individual and the community.

The recently passed Genetic Information Non-Discrimination (GINA) Act of 2008 (PL 110-233) provides federal protection for genetic information.[4] Genetic information cannot be used to discriminate against individuals for the provision of their health care or regarding their employment. But this information can still be used or interpreted in a negative way by families and their health care professionals. In addition to the perceived helplessness mentioned previously, genetic information can lead to stigmatization of individuals or groups of individuals and affects their ability or willingness to be engaged in community outreach efforts. These folks might be

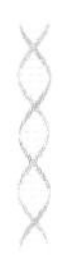

"labeled" because of their genetic predisposition and be perceived as incapable of change based on the inaccurate perception of their innate makeup. GINA minimizes but does not remove the potential for genetic stigmatization. Pediatricians must be mindful of this in their professional practices.

Genetics, Family, and the Community

Most common diseases managed in primary care pediatrics have some genetic component. Susceptibility to infectious agents, differences in metabolism, response to pharmaceuticals, body habitus, and multiple other factors are all influenced by the constitutional makeup of the individual, but the response of the individual to these factors occurs always within the context of the family. This family unit can include siblings, parents, aunts/uncles, grandparents, and maybe even more. When children are sick, families often recognize and care for their ailments based on how other family members responded to the same illness. These responses might be appropriate or inappropriate for a specific illness in a child. Pediatricians must recognize that the past and current responses of other family members to illness might affect how this family now treats an acute, subacute, or chronic illness in their current patient. Family belief systems are often influenced by the family's experience with a particular genetic-based condition and sometimes by impairments within other family members because they share the same genetic deficit. The family needs to be instructed to consider genetic factors with the usual childhood illnesses. Family illnesses can indeed be a helpful window into the future health of our children, and we should use that information to the best of our ability. Chapter 5 discusses the tools for acquiring that information, and Chapter 21 explores the future integration of this information electronically into primary care.

Genetic diseases in a family can have a significant impact on the nurturing of a child. If a parent or a caregiver develops a debilitating disease, the family usually provides extended care for the parents and then assists with the care of the child. Often the community is called on to assist in this care by fundraising or other nurturing activities. Unfortunate circumstances such as these often lead to opportunities to come together and care for one another. Family belief systems are also influenced by their cultural norms and the communities in which they reside. Discussing cultural, social, and religious beliefs and attitudes toward genetically based conditions with the family is essential in the management of disease. Alternative therapies based on individual cultural beliefs should be considered nonjudgmentally by the health care provider. The appropriate information as to potential benefits and risks should be shared honestly. Cultural norms and attitudes are often held in aggregate by the community in general and impact both the disease course and the ability of communities to provide supportive social capital.

Communities also differ profoundly in their abilities to support children and families based on socioeconomic conditions, the burden of genetically based disease present, political activism, and social institutions. Enlarging the perspective of the pediatrician to the community level frequently assists the management of groups of children with similar genetic conditions. It is at this community level that the pediatrician can frequently have the greatest success impacting disease outcome. A commitment to fight for appropriate public health interventions, Title V programs, home visiting programs, and other community resources is an integral part of the responsibility of the pediatrician.[1]

Certain ethnic groups have an increased propensity for particular genetic disorders (Ashkenazi Jews [Tay-Sachs disease], African Americans [sickle cell disease], Danish [α-1-antitrypsin deficiency], and US Caucasians [cystic fibrosis]).[5] It is very important for pediatricians to be aware of such associations. Since members of ethnic groups tend to live in proximity to one another, pediatricians also need to lend their expertise to community efforts and education (dissemination of medical information or screening clinics) that can have a positive impact for the specific group and the community. Community-based systems should be developed or enhanced to meet the disproportionate needs of the affected groups and to learn how to assist without the inappropriate stigmatization of the individuals, families, and groups.

Socioeconomic distress, incidence of substance abuse, and lack of availability of care impact many communities and their ability to support illness. Some studies have shown that the greater the heterogeneity in a community in socioeconomic status, the less healthy the community is and the less likely there are to be social capital supports.[6] Children of all backgrounds, especially the poor, racial minorities, and those from different religious backgrounds, require equal consideration as part of social justice. Only when all children have equal rights can we significantly impact health disparities in genetically based disease. Pediatricians must help ensure that health disparities that occur in communities based on socioeconomic

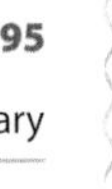

differences are minimized. Services for all children should include analysis of genetic information and incorporation of its use into patient care. All health care tools should be available to all. One specific example will help illustrate the interaction of genetics and the dynamics of health care.

Sickle cell disease, hemoglobin SS, is clearly genetically determined and now diagnosable in the newborn period via newborn screening. (See Chapter 17.) Yet there is marked variation in the expression of this disorder from family to family and even within affected siblings. Some of the factors affecting the expression of the disease include access to health care, availability of appropriate antibiotics and vaccinations, mental health status of the patient and family, social capital, nutrition, socioeconomic status, and knowledge of the disease. The genetic needs of the family must be addressed, including delineation of carrier status in relatives. Consideration of local African American cultural beliefs and their impact on care must be weighed. Socioeconomic factors, racial attitudes, and community acceptance of affected individuals will affect outcome. And finally, the impact of the burden of sickle cell disease on the community and its ability to respond should be considered.

Epigenetics and Long-term Community Effects

One of the startling revelations during the recent revolution of genetic discoveries is that altered genetic information can be passed on from generation to generation, yet this can occur in the absence of any intrinsic change in the DNA base pair sequence. This phenomenon is known as epigenetics. (See Chapter 2.) There are several epigenetic mechanisms currently known. The primary one appears to occur when extra methyl groups ($-CH_3$) are added to the cytosine bases in DNA in a process called methylation. It is now recognized that methylation changes can function like an on-off switch, affecting the gene or DNA transcription. Too much methylation will lead to genes being switched off, and too little methylation can leave genes switched on. This methylation process is even postulated to fine-tune the on-off switch so that variable changes in gene regulation (like a rheostat or variable light switch) can occur.

Broader areas of methylation on a chromosome have been found to affect the paternal or maternal chromosome of a chromosome pair differently. Each chromosome of an autosome pair comes either from the father or the mother. If, for example, a certain region of paternal chromosome 15 is differentially methylated compared with the corresponding region of maternal chromosome 15, the paternal chromosome is said to have undergone imprinting. That region would most likely be "turned off." Imprinting is most likely to be silent in most cases, but in certain situations the imprinting phenomenon can lead to the expression of specific disease states. Thus the mechanism of imprinting explains that certain disorders are expressed independent of the methylation status of the paternal or maternal chromosome. (See Chapter 2.)

How does epigenetics affect the community? There is an increasing body of evidence that epigenetic changes can occur in germ cells (sperm or ovum), and it appears that these changes could be secondary to an environmental influence and be passed on to subsequent generations. The most striking feature is that the transgenerational effects might not be noticed until the next generation or even the following one.[7–12] Swedish harvest data is significantly compelling.[8,10] If during a certain period a group of young males (probably preteen) were exposed to an abundance of food (based on harvesting information dating back into the 19th century), their grandchildren had an increased risk of developing cardiovascular disease or diabetes. In contrast, if a group of young males were exposed to a paucity of food (based on harvesting information), their grandchildren had a decreased risk of developing cardiovascular disease or diabetes. This study has remarkable implications for the impact of diet and the environment on transgenerational health. Data from the Dutch famine of World War II and the Chinese famine in the 20th century also demonstrate the presumed effects of environmental factors on subsequent generations.[9]

Epigenetics, therefore, is a genetic factor to be recognized and considered from a community standpoint. While we do not currently understand its total impact or how to change our behaviors to diminish its potential negative impact, we need to be mindful that what we do today will have an influence on subsequent generations. It is naïve to think that this influence will only be positive. For example, is it possible that the obesity epidemic currently affecting our children will have a detrimental effect in future generations?[13] Will communities, such as those in Appalachia, burdened by disproportionate incidence of obesity take generations to recover? How will the widespread presence of disease impact community structure and social capital for decades? What effects will epigenetics have on health disparities in our society?[11] What is apparent is that just as the community environment and social capital impact the disease outcome of genetically based conditions, genetic factors impact the structure and future of the communities themselves. As further information regarding epigenetic phenomena becomes available, pediatricians will need to help disseminate the appropriate information and advice to the community and to advocate for effective change. Our great, great grandchildren's lives depend on it!

Key Points

- An understanding of genetic information is important for pediatricians as they carry their responsibility for children and their families out of their offices and into the community.
- Genetic information can impact children both positively and negatively depending on a multitude of factors within the community.
- Environmental and other community factors can impact children for generations through epigenetic mechanisms.
- Child health functioning is the end result of a complex interplay between social capital, the environment, and genetics. The more the pediatrician understands this interaction, the better his or her ability will be to impact the outcomes of patients in the community.
- Pediatricians should advocate at all levels for appropriate treatment and supportive care for children and families impacted by genetic, genetically related, or epigenetically related diseases.

References

1. American Academy of Pediatrics Committee on Community Health Services. The pediatrician's role in community pediatrics. *Pediatrics.* 2005;115:10:92–94
2. Withall J, Jago R, Cross J. Families' and health professionals' perceptions of influences on diet, activity and obesity in a low-income community. *Health Place.* 2009;15:1078–1085
3. Seham M. Poverty, illness, and the Negro child. *Pediatrics.* 1970;46(2):305–311
4. Erwin C. Legal update: living with the Genetic Information Nondiscrimination Act. *Genet Med.* 2008;10(12):869–873
5. Nussbaum R, Innes R, Willard H. Genetic variation in individuals and populations: mutation and polymorphism. In: *Thompson and Thompson Genetics in Medicine.* 7th ed. Philadelphia, PA. Saunders-Elsevier; 2007:175–205
6. Rushton F, Greenberg R. The relationship between standard of living and physical development. In: Andrews AB, Kaufman NH, eds. *Implementing the U.N. Convention on the Rights of the Child: A Standard of Living Adequate for Development.* Westport, CT: Greenwood Publishing Co (Praeger); 1999:59–68
7. Beaudet A. Is medical genetics neglecting epigenetics? *Genet Med.* 2002;4(5):399–402
8. Kaati G, Bygren L, Edvinsson S. Cardiovascular and diabetes mortality determined during parents' and grandparents' slow growth period. *Eur J Hum Genet.* 2002;10:682–688
9. St Clair D, Xu M, Wang P, et al. Rates of adult schizophrenia following prenatal exposure to the Chinese famine of 1959–1961. *JAMA.* 2005;294:557–562

10. Kaati G, Bygren L, Pembrey M, et al. Transgenerational response to nutrition, early life circumstances and longevity. *Eur J Hum Genet.* 2007;15:784–790
11. Francis D. Conceptualizing child health disparities: a role for developmental neurogenomics. *Pediatrics.* 2009:124(suppl):S196–S202
12. Pembrey M. Time to take epigenetic inheritance seriously. *Eur J Hum Genet.* 2002;10:669–671
13. Benson L, Baer H, Kaelber D. Trends in the diagnosis of overweight and obesity in children and adolescents: 199–2007. *Pediatrics.* 2009;123(1):e153–e158

Chapter 15

Genetics and Ethics in Pediatrics

Michelle Huckaby Lewis, MD, JD
Ellen Wright Clayton, MD, JD

Advances in technology are fostering the increased use of genetic testing in clinical practice. The current workforce of medical geneticists and genetic counselors, however, is not sufficient to address the informational needs of pediatric patients and their families. Consequently, pediatricians are obligated to expand their knowledge about genetics and the risks and benefits of genetic testing to promote the health and well-being of their patients.

Genetic testing is challenging in part because the allocation of decision-making authority in the care of children is different than in the care of adults. Ideally adult medicine involves a patient-physician partnership, in which there is some degree of shared decision-making. Competent adults have the right to decide what medical care they receive. The physician's obligation is to provide the patient with the information necessary for an informed decision. The only options available to the physician who disagrees with her patient's choice is to continue to discuss how to proceed, accede to the patient's preferences, or transfer the patient's care to another clinician.

In caring for children, the allocation of decision-making authority is not as clear. Parents are presumed to act in the best interests of their children, and parents have broad, but not unfettered, authority to make medical decisions on their children's behalf.[1] According to many, the extent to which children may participate in decisions about their medical care varies with the age and maturity of the child and the nature of the medical intervention.[2] The pediatrician has an obligation not to follow blindly the wishes of either parent or the not yet legally competent minor, but to consider independently what is in the best interests of the child. When the pediatrician considers a proposed medical intervention to be contrary to the child's best interests, she has an obligation to advocate on behalf of the child.

The questions of whether and when to consider genetic testing in children highlight some of the ethical dilemmas pediatricians may face as a result of advances in genetic technology. The cases that follow illustrate how some of these issues should be addressed in the context of pediatric medicine.

Case 1: 5-Year-Old With Possible Duchenne Muscular Dystrophy

A family brings their 5-year-old son, Johnny, to see their pediatrician. The parents relate that Johnny is increasingly clumsy. He seems to fall a lot and he has a hard time getting up from the floor. On examination, he has proximal muscle weakness and very prominent calves. When asked to get up from the floor, he exhibits a classic Gower sign, using his arms to "walk up" his legs. The pediatrician strongly suspects that he has Duchenne muscular dystrophy (DMD), which is caused by a genetic mutation. The pediatrician will make a referral to a pediatric neurologist, but knows that obtaining an appointment will take months. The pediatrician would like to order a genetic test so that the neurologist will have that information in hand, and is happy to talk with the neurologist about which test to order.

Discussion: Case 1

When considering genetic testing in a child, the primary goal is to promote the well-being of the child.[3,4] In Case 1, a genetic test for DMD is warranted to provide diagnostic information about the child. Since there may be a significant delay between the time the pediatrician sees the patient and when the child may be seen by a subspecialist, in this case a pediatric neurologist, it is not appropriate to simply refer the child to the subspecialist for genetic testing without providing the family with at least some information.

The 2 main difficulties in Case 1 are that (1) the pediatrician may not know how to find out which test to order and (2) test results, if ordered, may come back before the pediatric neurologist can see the family to discuss the results. The pediatrician may be uncomfortable discussing the results of the genetic test with the family.

Nevertheless, deferring testing until after the child has seen the subspecialist entails further delay in diagnosis. A telephone call by the pediatrician to the

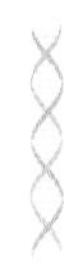

pediatric neurologist can provide the pediatrician with information about the appropriate test to order and additional sources of information, such as Web sites, that may be helpful to the family. If that consultation is not available, the physician may want to speak with the local geneticist or go to Web sites like www.genetests.org. Before ordering the test, education and counseling should be offered to the parents, and their permission to perform the test should be sought. If the pediatrician is concerned she cannot provide appropriate interpretation of any tests or up-to-date information about the disease, she may want to tell the family that although the results of the test may be sent to the pediatrician before the family sees the pediatric neurologist, the pediatrician feels that it would be best if the pediatric neurologist is the one to discuss the test results with them.

Case 2

Johnny (from Case 1) has DMD, and his mutation has been defined. The family returns to their pediatrician with their 8-year-old daughter Elizabeth, their newborn son Dan, and their 16-year-old daughter Sally, seeking testing for all 3.

Discussion of Case 2: Testing Dan, the Newborn

The parents want to test Dan because they want to know if he too has DMD. The ethical issues with testing the siblings of a child with DMD are complex. There has been a longstanding official policy consensus that children should not receive genetic tests unless the results affect their immediate care.[3] This is the justification for newborn screening for phenylketonuria and galactosemia, disorders for which immediate intervention averts serious harm. This is also the ethical warrant for testing Johnny, since making the diagnosis in a child who is already symptomatic affects his care.

Because genetic information is familial, test results from one person may have direct health implications for others who are genetically related. Since their older son is affected by DMD, the parents are concerned that their newborn son may have the condition as well. Dan is at increased risk of having DMD because of his family history, but increased risk by itself when there is no known effective preventive intervention is not a sufficient basis to justify performing genetic testing in an asymptomatic child.

In this case, the effect of potential benefits and harms, which are typically psychosocial rather than physical, to the child and his family should be considered. The potential benefit to Dan of detecting a mutation for DMD in this case is limited in the strictly medical sense. Since no preventive medical interventions to reduce the morbidity or mortality associated with the condition are available, there is no medical benefit to this child of identifying the condition before he becomes symptomatic. The potential benefit of eliminating the "diagnostic odyssey" is of limited value, since DMD would be high on the differential diagnosis list based on family history if he were to become symptomatic. The issue of benefit and harm for the child is inextricably tied up with the benefit and harm to the parents. Genetic testing would provide the parents with a definitive answer whether their newborn son also has DMD. Whether the test results are positive or negative, this reduction in uncertainty would be a psychological benefit to the parents. If Dan is affected, his parents can take the necessary steps to ensure that they have the financial and emotional support in place to care for a second child with this condition.

Most, but not all, experts argue against presymptomatic genetic testing in cases such as this on the grounds that a positive test result may affect the way the parents treat the baby while he is asymptomatic. This knowledge by his parents may deprive him of the childhood he otherwise would have had before he became symptomatic. The parents' uncertainty if testing is not done, however, may also adversely affect the way they treat their child. Some assert simply that parents are more intimately involved with the child's care and so are better situated to decide what information they need.[1] While the potential harm of presymptomatic testing typically outweighs the benefits for the child, even when considered in the context of the family, the pediatrician should be prepared to address parents' questions and potential anxiety.

Discussion of Case 2: Testing Elizabeth, the 8-Year-Old

When considering testing for Elizabeth, the 8-year-old sibling, most experts urge that carrier testing of a preadolescent female is inappropriate on the grounds that this is a decision that she should have the opportunity to make for herself once she is sufficiently mature or reaches the age of majority. The delay before she is tested may be relatively minimal since many adolescents have the capacity to make ethically valid choices well before legal majority, even if the parents' permission may still be legally required. Two practical factors also counsel against carrier testing at this time. One is that the parents still have the opportunity to counsel their daughter about the potential implications of being a carrier for DMD even

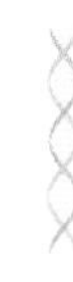

without testing. The test is not a prerequisite for parental guidance. The only potential benefit to testing her now is the 50-50 chance that she is not a carrier. The other is that young teenagers often do not take reproductive genetic risk into account when having unprotected sex.

The fact that 10% to 20% of carrier females develop some musculoskeletal symptoms or cardiomyopathy themselves, albeit usually not until adulthood,[5] does not change this analysis unless presymptomatic intervention during childhood makes a difference in outcome. Noting that many adults, when given the opportunity, choose not to pursue predisposition genetic testing—only about 50% at risk for inheriting mutations in *BRCA1,* for example, obtain the test—counsels for allowing Elizabeth to make her own decision once she matures.

Discussion of Case 2: Testing Sally, the 16-Year-Old

Sally may want to know if she is a carrier for DMD. She may also be direct enough to say that if she were pregnant she would pursue prenatal diagnosis for either the mutation or at least to determine the sex, planning to terminate the pregnancy depending on the results. Many health care providers, however, are opposed to abortion, and some of these argue that even discussing carrier testing or referring the patient to another provider for counseling would intrude too greatly on their beliefs. The question, then, is whether the legal protection of providers' conscientious objection to abortion (42 USC § 300a-7) extends to refusing to provide carrier testing or even to discussing the issue. While some commentators urge that clinicians should never be required to compromise their own beliefs,[6] a more nuanced approach weighs the burden on the clinician, who after all chose to become a physician, against the needs of the patient, who did not choose her condition. Even though information about carrier testing, in this case for DMD, is available on the Web (www.ornl.gov/sci/techresources/Human_Genome/medicine/genetest.shtml), such tests typically must be ordered by a physician. Elizabeth, in any event, is entitled to knowledgeable counseling about her decision. Thus a strong argument can be made that the conscientiously objecting physician has an obligation at least to help her find a physician who is qualified to help her.[7]

Case 3

A family in a pediatric practice has a strong history of medullary thyroid carcinoma. The mother was diagnosed in her early 30s, which was subsequently found to be due a mutation in the RET oncogene. The children are teenagers who inherited the mutation and are now undergoing periodic screening for early detection of tumors. The family history reveals the mother has a brother and a sister, neither of whom she has seen since she graduated from college. The pediatrician counsels her that she should talk with her siblings because they and their children may also have inherited this mutation, but she refuses. The pediatrician is concerned about the mother's nieces and nephews, who could benefit from periodic screening if they have the mutation as well.

Discussion of Case 3

The fact that genetic information is simultaneously personal and familial raises questions about whether physicians are permitted or even required to disclose genetic information to at-risk relatives. For the pediatrician, conflict can arise between the duty to maintain confidentiality and the possible duty to warn at-risk relatives if the patient or family refuses to disclose the relevant information. A conflict might be avoided with a thorough pretesting discussion about the implications of the testing for the patient, the immediate family, and other family members (such as aunts, uncles, and cousins).

Genetic information should be considered as medical information. Consequently, patient confidentiality regarding genetic information generally should be respected. The duty to maintain confidentiality, however, is not absolute. In some circumstances, health care providers have a legal duty to breach patient confidentiality. For example, there is a statutory requirement that evidence of child abuse or neglect be reported. Similarly, an affirmative duty to breach confidentiality and warn at-risk individuals exists under certain, exceptional circumstances. For example, a legal duty to warn was created in *Tarasoff v Regents of the University of California* (551 P2d 334 Ca 1976) after a psychiatrist failed to warn his patient's intended victim of his patient's intention to kill her. The court held that a duty to warn exists if (1) the physician held a special relationship with either the person who may cause the harm or the potential victim, (2) the person at risk is identifiable, and (3) the harm to the person at risk is foreseeable and serious. Subsequent courts, however, have been reluctant to extend this holding. It should also be noted that the duty to warn about a patient's specific threat to kill another can be distinguished from a possible duty to warn at-risk relatives about genetic risk in that in

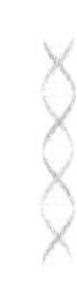

the former situation, it is the patient's actions that are likely to cause harm. Murder has been condemned for millennia. In contrast, in the case of increased genetic risk, the patient's actions do not increase risk to relatives. The relatives either have the mutation or they do not.

Case law in the United States is not settled with respect to this issue. In one case, the court held that a physician had a duty to warn his patient regarding the genetic risks associated with medullary thyroid carcinoma but no duty to warn her daughter, saying that this duty would place too heavy a burden on physicians (*Pate v Threlkel,* 661 So2d 278 Fla 1995). Another court held that a physician had a duty to warn those "known to be at risk of avoidable harm from a genetically transmissible condition" (677 A2d 1188 NJ App. 1996) when a daughter sued the estate of her father's physician for failing to inform her of the hereditary nature of her father's colon cancer, a ruling subsequently called into question by the enactment of the Privacy Rule of the Health Insurance Portability and Accountability Act (HIPAA) (45 CFR Part 160, and subparts A, E of part 164 [2012]). Although much attention was paid to these cases after they were handed down, there have been few or no lawsuits addressing this issue since.

According to the American Society of Human Genetics,[8] disclosure of genetic information to at-risk family members against a patient's wishes may be permissible if the following criteria are met:

1. Attempts to encourage disclosure by the patient have failed.
2. The harm is highly likely to occur.
3. The harm is serious and foreseeable.
4. The at-risk relative(s) is identifiable.
5. Either the disease is treatable/preventable or early monitoring will reduce the genetic risk.

In this case, since the criteria have been met, it may be *permissible* to disclose the information to the mother's relatives despite her objections. Whether the pediatrician in this case has a legal or ethical *obligation* to breach patient confidentiality and inform her patient's relatives about their increased risk of disease is at best unclear. The optimal course, in any event, is for the pediatrician to inform her patient's mother that the etiology of her condition means that her relatives may be at increased risk of disease. The doctor then should either offer to help the mother talk with her relatives or, if the mother still does not want to talk, ask her permission

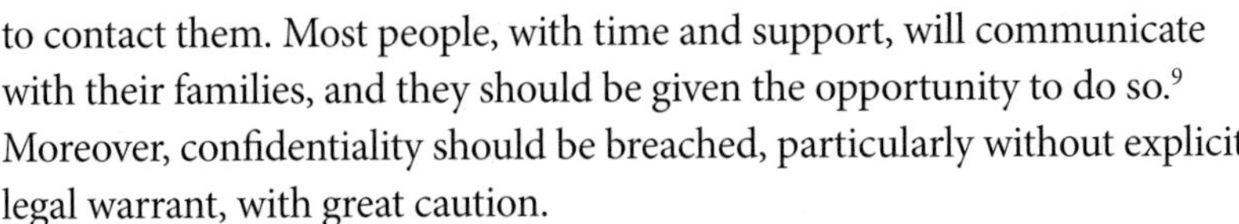

to contact them. Most people, with time and support, will communicate with their families, and they should be given the opportunity to do so.[9] Moreover, confidentiality should be breached, particularly without explicit legal warrant, with great caution.

Direct-to-Consumer (DTC) Genetic Tests

In the past, genetic testing was only available through health care providers. Today, due to the proliferation of DTC marketing through the Internet or other forms of advertising, genetic testing can be ordered by consumers without the involvement of a health care provider. If a consumer chooses to purchase a genetic test from one of the DTC companies, a test kit is mailed to the consumer, rather than the test being ordered by a physician. A DNA sample is obtained, usually through a buccal swab or collection of saliva, and mailed back to the company. Results may be obtained by mail, over the telephone, or online.

Among the most common concerns raised by professional organizations about DTC genetic testing[10–12] is that without the guidance of a physician or other health care provider, individuals may make important decisions about their health care based on inaccurate, incomplete, or misunderstood information about their health, although there is little evidence that this is occurring.[13,14] Direct-to-consumer genetic testing, however, currently is subject to little federal oversight because they purport not to provide clinical results.[15] Consumers who purchase these tests are at risk of harm if the testing is performed by laboratories that are not of high quality, if the tests are not accurate,[16] if the claims made about the tests are misleading, or if inadequate counseling is provided to permit the consumer to make informed decisions about the appropriateness of testing and what actions should be taken based on the test results.

While pediatricians cannot resolve these issues with DTC genetic tests, they should familiarize themselves with these tests and their strengths and weaknesses. (See Chapter 19.) Then when parents bring in test results for their children, the physicians will be prepared to deal with them, drawing on the same skills they use when parents bring in information from the Internet or other media, or even concerns raised by the child's grandparents and other relatives.

Key Points

- While the increasing capacity to identify genetic contributions to disease in children presents ethical challenges for pediatricians, guidance and experience, both specific to genetics and more generally to the practice of pediatrics, informs care.
- Advances in technology increase the use of genetic testing, and primary care physicians need to expand their knowledge of these tests.
- Genetic testing of children has a unique set of challenges due to the physician's obligation to provide a large amount of information and because of the parent's decision-making authority.
- The parent's decision-making authority should be tempered by the pediatrician's obligation to advocate on behalf of the child.
- Adolescents can and should have significant input into the decision-making process for their own genetic testing.
- Genetic testing might reveal information that has broad implications for the extended family, and pretesting discussions could potentially avoid post-result conflicts.
- Confidentiality is essential. Genetic information is protected medical information subject to the exception provided by HIPAA.

References

1. Ross LF. Children, families, and health care decision making. New York, NY: Clarendon Press; 1998
2. American Academy of Pediatrics Committee on Bioethics. Informed consent, parental permission, and assent in pediatric practice. *Pediatrics.* 1995;95(2):314–317
3. American Society of Human Genetics Board of Directors, American College of Medical Genetics Board of Directors. Points to consider: ethical, legal, and psychosocial implications of genetic testing in children and adolescents. *Am J Hum Genet.* 1995;57(5):1233–1241
4. American Academy of Pediatrics Committee on Bioethics. Ethical issues with genetic testing in pediatrics. *Pediatrics.* 2001;107(6):1451–1455
5. Soltanzadeh P, Friez MJ, Dunn D, et al. Clinical and genetic characterization of manifesting carriers of DMD mutations. *Neuromuscul Disord.* 2010;20(8):499–504
6. Curlin FA, Lawrence RE, Chin MH, Lantos JD. Religion, conscience, and controversial clinical practices. *N Engl J Med.* 2007;356(6):593–600
7. American Academy of Pediatrics Committee on Bioethics. Physician refusal to provide information or treatment on the basis of claims of conscience. *Pediatrics.* 2009;124(6):1689–1693
8. American Society of Human Genetics Social Issues Subcommittee on Familial Disclosure. ASHG statement. Professional disclosure of familial genetic information. *Am J Hum Genet.* 1998;62(2):474–483
9. Clayton EW. What should the law say about disclosure of genetic information to relatives? *J Health Care Law Policy.* 1998;1(2):373–390

10. ACOG Committee Opinion No. 409: direct-to-consumer marketing of genetic testing. *Obstet Gynecol.* 2008;111(6):1493–1494
11. American College of Medical Genetics. ACMG statement on direct-to-consumer genetic testing. April 2008. American College of Medical Genetics Web site. www.acmg.net/StaticContent/StaticPages/DTC_statement.pdf. Published April 7, 2008. Accessed March 13, 2013
12. Hudson K, Javitt G, Burke W, Byers P. ASHG statement on direct-to-consumer genetic testing in the United States. *Obstet Gynecol.* 2007;110(6):1392–1395
13. Bloss CS, Ornowski L, Silver E, et al. Consumer perceptions of direct-to-consumer personalized genomic risk assessments. *Genet Med.* 2010;12(9):556–566
14. McBride CM, Wade CH, Kaphingst KA. Consumers' views of direct-to-consumer genetic information. *Annu Rev Genomics Hum Genet.* 2010;11:427–446
15. McGuire AL, Evans BJ, Caulfield T, Burke W. Science and regulation. Regulating direct-to-consumer personal genome testing. *Science.* 2010;330(6001):181–182
16. Kuehn BM. Inconsistent results, inaccurate claims plague direct-to-consumer gene tests. *JAMA.* 2010;304(12):1313–1315

Section 5: Trends in Genetics

Chapter 16

Treating Genetic Disorders

Gustavo H. B. Maegawa, MD, PhD
Robert D. Steiner, MD

Introduction

Managing genetic diseases aims to relieve the symptoms of specific inherited conditions in patients. When managing patients with genetic diseases, physicians should consider that patients' family members may also be affected and take a careful family history. (See Chapter 5.) Management includes providing information about the disease and its risk to the patient and family members through appropriate genetic counseling. This chapter offers a brief historical perspective and discusses the current status of selected therapeutic interventions for specific genetic diseases.

Strategies for Treating Genetic Disorders

Nutritional Therapy

Phenylketonuria

Initially, the inborn errors of metabolism were considered untreatable. The first successful dietary control treatment was achieved with phenylketonuria (PKU), an autosomal recessive disease caused by mutations in the *PAH* gene encoding the enzyme L-phenylalanine hydroxylase (PAH).[1] Left untreated, PKU causes profound intellectual disability. A phenylalanine (Phe)-restricted diet prevents elevated blood Phe levels in individuals with PKU, resulting in substantial improvement in cognitive function.[1] Phenylketonuria represents the first genetic condition for which an effective therapy based on rational modification of environment was successfully applied. However, despite intensive research and treatment advances in PKU,[2] the pathophysiology by which defective PAH and resulting Phe accumulation lead to impairment of brain function and development remains unclear.[3] Despite strict dietary control, children with PKU often develop subtle learning disabilities and behavioral disturbances detected in neuropsychological tests.[4] Further, overtreatment leading to very low blood Phe levels leads to severe intellectual disability.

The children of women with PKU are at high risk for microcephaly, intellectual disability, and cardiac malformations if the mothers are no longer following a Phe-restricted diet and have high blood Phe levels during pregnancy.[5] Maternal PKU illustrates that treating genetic diseases requires long-term observation to provide detailed evidence of its efficacy and adverse effects.

Galactosemia

Galactosemia, which is caused by mutations in the gene encoding galactose-1-phosphatase uridyl-transferase, is treated with some efficacy with dietary restriction. Galactose-1-phosphatase uridyl-transferase catalyzes the interconversion of galactose and glucose. Therefore, the disease is associated with accumulation of galactose and its metabolites. The disease frequently presents in infancy with feeding difficulties, jaundice, and lethargy. Hepatocellular dysfunction is common, and coagulopathy, renal tubulopathy, cataracts, encephalopathy, and death from *Escherichia coli* sepsis may occur if treatment is delayed. Symptoms usually appear after the introduction of galactose in the diet, typically in the form of breast milk or lactose-containing infant formulas. The control of diet, essentially eliminating ingestion of galactose, is a fairly simple approach and remains the principal focus of therapy in galactosemia.[6] Despite adherence to the galactose-restricted diet, patients typically develop learning disabilities, especially speech-language impairments that can be severe.[7] In addition, most female patients develop ovarian failure likely caused by galactose toxicity. Galactosemia treatment illustrates that the pathology of a particular condition may not be manifested in different organs until patients survive long term on the standard therapy.

Nutritional therapy is the earliest example of rational effective treatment for genetic disorders. Other approaches, including toxin removal, cofactor replacement, enzyme replacement therapy, organ transplantation, and gene therapy, have also been developed. In general, inborn errors of metabolism provided an easy target for therapeutic development because typically the biochemical pathophysiology is understood. However, despite knowing the biochemical pathways disturbed in these conditions, the development of

specific therapies has proven to be much more complex, and only some of inborn errors of metabolism have specific therapeutic agents.

Enzyme Replacement Therapy

The initial concept that enzyme replacement (ERT) could be a potential therapy for lysosomal storage diseases (LSDs) came from early experiments carried out by Fratantoni et al[8] in cultured skin fibroblasts from mucopolysaccharidosis (MPS) patients, in which the metabolic defect was shown to be corrected with addition of lysosomal enzymes. Surprisingly, only about 5% of the wild type cellular enzyme activity was required to correct the metabolic defect. These pivotal studies suggested that administering intact normal lysosomal enzyme (eg, ERT) was a strategy to treat LSDs. The development of ERT dramatically alters some aspects of the disease phenotype in some LSDs with non-neuronopathic presentation. When the therapeutic agent is a large molecular weight recombinant enzyme, it is unable to cross the blood-brain barrier. ERT is therefore limited to treatment of non-neurologic symptoms, such as the visceral and hematologic complications seen in Gaucher disease (GD). Delivery of the active enzyme to the central nervous system remains a significant obstacle.

Chemical Inducers

Another treatment approach for genetic disorders arises from the management of hemoglobinopathies. The observation that HbF fetal hemoglobin (HbF; $\alpha_2\gamma_2$) has a protective effect in young patients with sickle cell anemia triggered the study of chemical inducers of the expression of genes responsible for the subunits of HbF.[9] These chemical inducers, such as hydroxyurea and butyrate, increase HbF levels as treatment for sickle cell disease (SCD) and β-thalassemia.[10] This type of treatment of the latter hemoglobinopathies manifesting with severe anemia was developed to avoid the frequent transfusions that can lead to iron overload after long-term treatment. More recently pharmacological iron chelators, such as desferrioxamine, have been developed to ameliorate the long-term adverse effects of repeated transfusions. Thus treatment of thalassemias is based on at least 2 prolonged therapeutic approaches.

Current Status of Treatment

Treatment for genetic diseases has advanced substantially in recent years. In a meta-analysis of 351 genetic disorders catalogued in the Mendelian

Inheritance in Man (now OMIM, www.ncbi.nlm.nih.gov/omim/), 1 in 7 disorders showed significant response to treatment. Among the 65 inborn errors of metabolism studied, 12% were successfully treated, 40% had a partial response, and 48% showed no response to the treatment at that time.[11] More than 10 years later, when analyzing 571 genetic disorders, Treacy et al[12] described the same proportion of genetic disorders (12%) as fully responsive to treatment; however, 54% were now partially responsive, and the group of poorly or nonresponsive was reduced to 34%. The advances in treating genetic disorders observed in this study has been related to the better understanding of the pathogenesis and natural history of the diseases, along with the development of different therapeutic strategies.

Most genetic diseases still lack specific management that corrects the pathophysiology of the condition. Unfortunately, because these conditions affect a small proportion of the population, it has been less appealing for scientists and industry to devote substantial investments of resources toward the understanding of fundamental biological disease mechanisms and, most importantly, in the development of novel therapeutic strategies.

Genetic counseling is a critical aspect of disease management (Chapter 13). When medical treatment is not available, supportive treatment may significantly improve the quality of life of patients.

Levels of Intervention in Genetic Diseases

The treatment of genetic diseases can be approached from different levels, from the mutated gene up to the level of the family of the affected patient. Table 16-1 illustrates the several levels where treatment can be designed to ameliorate the phenotype of the condition. Some of the treatment strategies are still experimental, such as those listed in the gene therapy and the RNA level. Symptomatic treatment is at the phenotype level, which is currently the mainstay of therapy for most patients with genetic diseases, especially with diseases causing congenital malformations.

Treatment of Lysosomal Storage Diseases

Much progress has been made in the treatment of LSDs during the past few years. The challenges faced in developing treatments for LSDs are shared with most other groups of genetic conditions, which makes this group of conditions a good example to illustrate the status of treatment development in the genetic diseases. Lysosomal storage diseases consist of a group of

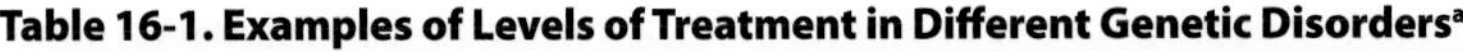

Table 16-1. Examples of Levels of Treatment in Different Genetic Disorders[a]

Treatment	Genetic Disease
Level of Mutant Gene	
Modification of Mutant Gene	
a. Organ transplantation	
– Bone marrow	Adenosine deaminase deficiency—severe combined immunodeficiency β-thalassemia major Fanconi anemia MPS-IH (Hurler disease) X-linked adrenoleukodystrophy
– Kidney	Fabry disease Nephropathic cystinosis Primary hyperoxaluria type I
– Heart	Fabry disease Mitochondrial ETC defects
– Liver	α-1-antitrypsin deficiency Crigler-Najjar type I Homozygous familial hypercholesterolemia GSD-I and -IV Hereditary hemochromatosis Primary hyperoxaluria type I Mitochondrial ETC defects MSUD Organic acidopathies Tyrosinemia type I (nonresponsive to NTBC) Urea cycle defects Wilson disease PFIC
b. Pharmacological modification of gene expression	
– Butyrate, hydroxyurea, and decitabine[b]	Sickle cell disease and β-thalassemia
c. Single-gene transfer with gammaretrovirus	X-linked severe combined immunodeficiency (CD34 cells) Adenosine deaminase deficiency (CD34 cells) Chronic granulomatous disease (CD34 cells) Epidermolysis bullosa (skin stem cells)
Level of Mutant mRNA	
a. Ribozyme gene transfer	Autosomal dominant retinitis pigmentosa
b. Exon-skipping therapy	Duchenne muscular dystrophy[c]

Table 16-1. Examples of Levels of Treatment in Different Genetic Disorders[a] *(cont)*

Treatment	Genetic Disease
Level of Mutant Gene *(cont)*	
Level of Mutant Protein	
a. Protein replacement	Enzyme replacement therapy in Gaucher disease (non-neuronopathic), MPS-I, -II, -VI; Fabry disease; Pompe disease[d] Hemophilia A, growth hormone deficiency
b. Protein enhancement therapy	Pharmacological chaperones in Fabry disease, Gaucher disease, GM2 and GM1 gangliosidosis, Pompe disease[e], PKU[f]
Substrate Restriction	
Dietary restriction	Phe—PKU Branched-chain amino acids—MSUD Galactose—galactosemia
Alternative pathway enhancement—toxic by-product management	Benzoate and phenyl acetate/phenylbutyrate—urea cycle defects Glycine—isovaleric acidemia Carnitine—organic acidemias Cysteamine—cystinosis
Metabolic inhibition	NTBC—tyrosinemia type I
Substrate reduction therapy—inhibition of substrate biosynthesis	Miglustat (inhibition of glucosylceramide transferase)—Gaucher disease Statins (inhibition of HMG CoA reductase)—familial hypercholesterolemia
Manipulation of metabolic pathways	Uridine—orotic aciduria Biotin—biotinidase deficiency Carnitine—carnitine transporter defect
Drug avoidance	G6PD deficiency—antimalarial drugs Acute intermittent porphyria—barbiturates and others
Depletion	Dialysis—hyperammonemia in urea cycle defects and organic acidurias LDL apheresis—homozygous familial hypercholesterolemia

Table 16-1. Examples of Levels of Treatment in Different Genetic Disorders[a] *(cont)*

Treatment	Genetic Disease
Level of Clinical Phenotype	
Medical and surgical procedures	Phlebotomy—hemochromatosis Cardiac surgery—tetralogy of Fallot in 22q11 deletion syndrome β-blockers and angiotension II blockade (losartan)—Marfan syndrome Phototherapy—Crigler-Najjar syndrome
Avoidance of drugs	5-fluoruracil—dihydropyrimidine dehydrogenase deficiency Irotecan—UDP-glucuronosyltransferase variants (TA_7)
Environmental—avoidance of sun exposure	Albinism, xeroderma pigmentosa
Trauma prevention	Osteogenesis imperfecta
Level of Family	
Genetic counseling	All genetic conditions
Carrier screening	For specific ethnic backgrounds such as Gaucher disease, Tay-Sachs disease, hereditary familial dysautonomia
Prenatal diagnosis	Family with previous child with infantile GM1 gangliosidosis
Presympomatic diagnosis	Huntington disease and autosomal dominant spinal cerebellar ataxias

Abbreviations: ETC, electron transport chain; G6PD, glucose-6-phospate dehydrogenase; GSD, glycogen storage disease; HMG CoA, 3-hydroxy-3-methylglutaryl coenzyme A; LDL, low-density lipoprotein; MPS, mucopolysaccharidosis; MSUD, maple syrup urine disease; NTBC, 2-[2-Nitro-4-(trifluoromethyl)benzoyl]-1,3-cyclohexanedione; Phe, phenylalanine; PKU, phenylketonuria; PFIC, progressive familial intra-hepatic cholestasis; UDP, uridine diphosphate.

[a] Some of the treatments are still in preclinical stage.

[b] Fathallah H, Atweh GF. Induction of fetal hemoglobin in the treatment of sickle cell disease. *Hematology Am Soc Hematol Educ Program.* 2006:58–62.

[c] Yokota T, Pistilli E, Duddy W, et al. Potential of oligonucleotide-mediated exon-skipping therapy for Duchenne muscular dystrophy. *Expert Opin Biol Ther.* 2007;7(6):831–842.

[d] Burrow TA, Hopkin RJ, Leslie ND, et al. Enzyme reconstitution/replacement therapy for lysosomal storage diseases. *Curr Opin Pediatr.* 2007;19(6):628–635.

[e] Fan JQ. A counterintuitive approach to treat enzyme deficiencies: use of enzyme inhibitors for restoring mutant enzyme activity. *Biol Chem.* 2008;389(1):1–11.

[f] Hegge KA, Horning KK, Peitz GJ, et al. Sapropterin: a new therapeutic agent for phenylketonuria. *Ann Pharmacother.* 2009;43(9):1466–1473.

almost 60 inherited metabolic conditions caused by defects in specific lysosomal and a few non-lysosomal proteins that result in lysosomal dysfunction. Most of these proteins are lysosomal hydrolases, which are responsible for degradation of complex molecules, such as glycosaminoglycans, glycosphingolipids, and oligosaccharides in cells of the body. Many LSDs lead to severe and progressive neurodegeneration with onset of symptoms ranging from the neonatal period to adulthood. Others are also progressive and ultimately fatal without treatment, but with predominantly somatic manifestations, sparing the central nervous system. Lysosomal storage diseases are individually rare, but collectively, the incidence is approximately 1/7,000 live births, making them a significant health problem worldwide.[13] Recent pilot newborn screening studies have shown a higher incidence (1,200–1,300 live births) of LSDs mostly due to the detection of late-onset forms.[14] Since ERT was introduced for GD type I (GD-1), other novel and exciting therapy modalities have been developed based on the benefits and principles of ERT but, also and most importantly, on its limitations. For these reasons, we will comment more in depth in the current and future therapies for LSDs as genetic diseases in which several therapies have been tested, with some of them successfully shown to alter the natural course of the disease.

Enzyme Replacement Therapy

In studies in skin fibroblasts from patients with different LSDs, Fratantoni et al[8] initially conceptualized ERT as the treatment modality for LSDs. The first clinical trial of ERT was performed in 12 patients with GD-1 (non-neuronopathic) who received enzyme extracted from human placenta (Ceradase· Genzyme-Sanofi Corp).[15] The recombinant enzyme produced in Chinese hamster ovarian (CHO) cells (Cerezyme, Genzyme-Sanofi Corp) was approved in 1994. No significant differences were found in terms of efficacy between the 2 preparations. Enzyme replacement therapy results in dramatic reduction of liver and spleen volumes and improvement of hematologic parameters typically in the first 12 months of therapy in patients with GD-1. The effect of ERT on bone disease is not as rapid.[16] In a large cohort of patients in long-term follow-up, ERT induced degradation of Gaucher cell deposits, reconversion of fat marrow, and increased bone mineral density.[17] Enzyme replacement therapy has been shown not to be effective for the chronic (type 3) and severe (type 2) forms of neuronopathic GD, illustrating an important limitation of this therapy. These large molecular weight agents do not cross the blood-brain barrier and therefore are not effective in treating central nervous manifestations of LSDs.[18] Enzyme replacement therapy was subsequently tested in other conditions, including Fabry disease. One ERT trial showed improvements in pain in the group of patients taking agalsidase alfa (Repagal, Shire Human Genetic Therapies [HGT] Pharm) and another form of recombinantly produced α-galactosidase (agalsidase beta, Fabrazyme) was associated with clearance of microvascular endothelial deposits of storage material (globotriaosylceramide, Gb3) from kidney, heart, and skin.[19] Mucopolysaccharidosis is a group of LSDs with substantial clinical heterogeneity resulting in difficulties in the design of clinical studies with relevant endpoints. The recombinant form of α-iduronidase produced in CHO cells, laronidase (Aldurazyme, manufactured by BioMarin Pharmaceutical Inc and commercialized by Genzyme-Sanofi Corp) is available for patients affected with MPS type I (MPS-I) (deficiency of α-iduronidase). The first clinical trial showed reduction of glycosaminoglycan (GAG) excretion and reduction in liver and spleen volumes.[20] A randomized, controlled, double-blind trial showed improvements on percent of predicted forced vital capacity (FVC) and 6-minute walk test. Patients with MPS-VI, Maroteaux-Lamy syndrome, caused by deficiency of arylsulfatase B, have been shown to benefit from recombinant arylsulfatase B infusion in the form of galsulfase (Naglazyme, Biomarin Pharmaceutical Inc). Using the same endpoints, clinical trials showed improvement in walking distance, climbing stairs, and FVC in patients with MPS-6 receiving ERT. In addition, reduction of liver and spleen volumes were observed.[21] Enzyme replacement therapy has been developed for MPS-II, Hunter syndrome with the use of idursulfase (Elaprase, Shire HGT Pharm).[22]

Pompe disease is an LSD caused by deficiency of α-glucosidase and is characterized by an infantile form with hypotonia, weakness, poor ventilatory effort, and hypertrophic cardiomyopathy, in addition to a late-onset form with primarily skeletal muscle involvement and pulmonary compromise that ultimately leads to the need for ventilatory support. The first clinical trials of ERT were performed in patients with the infantile form using recombinant human enzyme produced in CHO cells and from milk of transgenic rabbits. Improvement of survival and motor function was significant along with decrease in the left ventricular mass index.[23,24] In another trial involving the infantile form, patients receiving the recombinant human enzyme from rabbit milk had improvement of cardiac function and all survived beyond 4 years of age. Alglucosidase alfa (Myozyme, Genzyme-Sanofi Corp) has been available for Pompe disease and US Food and Drug Administration (FDA)-approved since 2006. A major limitation has been that nearly half of treated patients have developed antibodies against the recombinant enzyme, and the IgG titers have been correlated with poor or loss of clinical response to treatment. In a trial of alglucosidase alfa, 5 out of 18 infants with Pompe disease had no significant improvement of their motor function, and 6 ended up needing ventilatory assistance.[24] A recent clinical trial with 44 patients with late-onset Pompe disease receiving alglucosidase alfa (Lumizyme, Genzyme-Sanofi Corp), recombinant enzyme for late-onset Pompe patients (>8 years old), had stabilization of neuromuscular deficits over 1 year with mild functional improvement.[25] Although antibody production was not a significant impediment to treatment efficacy with early ERT, the experience in treating Pompe disease has made it clear that development of antibodies can be a significant limitation to effective protein therapy for genetic diseases.[26]

Clinical trials for genetic disorders can be a very difficult undertaking considering the rarity of the diseases and their clinical heterogeneity. Biomarkers or surrogate markers are important tools to monitor treatment of genetic diseases and could prove useful as endpoints in clinical trials. Ideally, surrogate markers need to correlate directly with disease severity and should indicate proper response to therapy. In LSDs, 2 classes of surrogate markers exist: those that directly relate to the lysosomal dysfunction, such as the GAG, and those that indirectly relate to the lysosomal defect (eg, the increased activity of chitotriosidase in GD-1, which is due to dysfunction of reticuloendothelial cells). A table of surrogate markers commonly used in the LSDs for which clinical ERT is available is depicted in Table 16-2.

Substrate Reduction Therapy

Substrate reduction therapy (SRT) is a novel alternative approach for the treatment of LSDs. In contrast to ERT, where enzyme is given to reduce the accumulation of toxic substrates, the principle of SRT is to partially inhibit the biosynthesis of substrates in order to reduce substrate influx into the impaired metabolic pathway. An imino sugar, *N*-butyl deoxynojirimycin (*N*B-DNJ), was identified and characterized as a competitive inhibitor of ceramide glucosyltransferase, a regulatory enzyme in the synthesis of glycosphingolipids.[27] This compound was initially tested in patients with GD-1, with the idea that it could reduce substrate accumulation.[28] After 12 months of treatment exclusively with *N*B-DNJ, known as miglustat (Zavesca, Actelion Pharmaceuticals Inc), mean liver and spleen volumes were significantly reduced.[28] Mild improvement of hematologic parameters was observed.[28] The most common adverse event was diarrhea, which has been inconvenient for some patients under this therapy. Miglustat is currently approved by the FDA for the treatment of GD-1 for those in which

ERT is not an option. The proof of principle set the stage for further clinical studies of SRT.[29] Since glucosylceramide is the common precursor for several glycosphingolipids, such as globosides and gangliosides, miglustat, which reduces glucosylceramide synthesis, is an attractive potential therapy for other LSDs such as GM1 (deficiency of β-galactosidase) and GM2 (deficiency of β-hexosaminidase A) gangliosidosis (Figure 16-1). Clinical trials in patients with the juvenile and adult-onset forms of GM2 gangliosi-

Table 16-2. Enzyme Replacement Therapy in Lysosomal Storage Diseases

Lysosomal Storage Disease	Drug–Enzyme Generic Names (Brand—Manufacturer)	Intravenous Dose	Surrogate Markers
Gaucher disease (GD-1)	Imiglucerase (Cerezyme—Genzyme Sanofi Corp) 200 U/vial and 400 U/vial	7.5–60 U/kg—every 14 days	Chitotriosidase Serum angiotensin converting enzyme Tartrate-resistant acid phosphatase
Fabry disease[a]	Agalsidase beta (Fabrazyme—Genzyme-Sanofi Corp) 5 mg/vial	1 mg/kg every 14 days	Globotriaosylceramide—urine and plasma
MPS-I	Laronidase (Aldurazyme—Genzyme-Sanofi Corp, manufactured by Biomarin Pharm Inc) 2.9 mg/vial	0.58 mg/kg every 7 days	GAGs—urine
MPS-II	Idursulfase (Elaprase—Shire HGT Pharm) 6 mg/vial	0.5 mg/kg every 7 days	GAGs—urine
MPS-VI	Galsulfase (Naglazyme—Biomarin Pharm Inc) 5 mg/vial	1 mg/kg every 7 days	GAGs—urine
Pompe disease (GSD-II)	Alglucosidase alfa (Myozyme—Genzyme-Sanofi Corp) for infantile Pompe disease (Lumizyme—Genzyme-Sanofi Corp) for late-onset forms (≥8 years old) 50 mg/vial	20 mg/kg every 14 days	Tetrasaccharide—urine and serum

Abbreviations: GAGs, glycosaminoglycans; GSD, glycogen storage disease; MPS, mucopolysaccharidosis.

[a]Another electron transport chain drug for Fabry disease is agalsidase alpha (Replagal by Shire HGT Pharm), which is not approved by the US Food and Drug Administration. It is approved by Health Canada, European Medicines Agency, and by drug regulatory agencies in more than 50 countries. It presents as 3.5 mg/vial. Recommended dose: 0.2 mg/kg every 14 days.

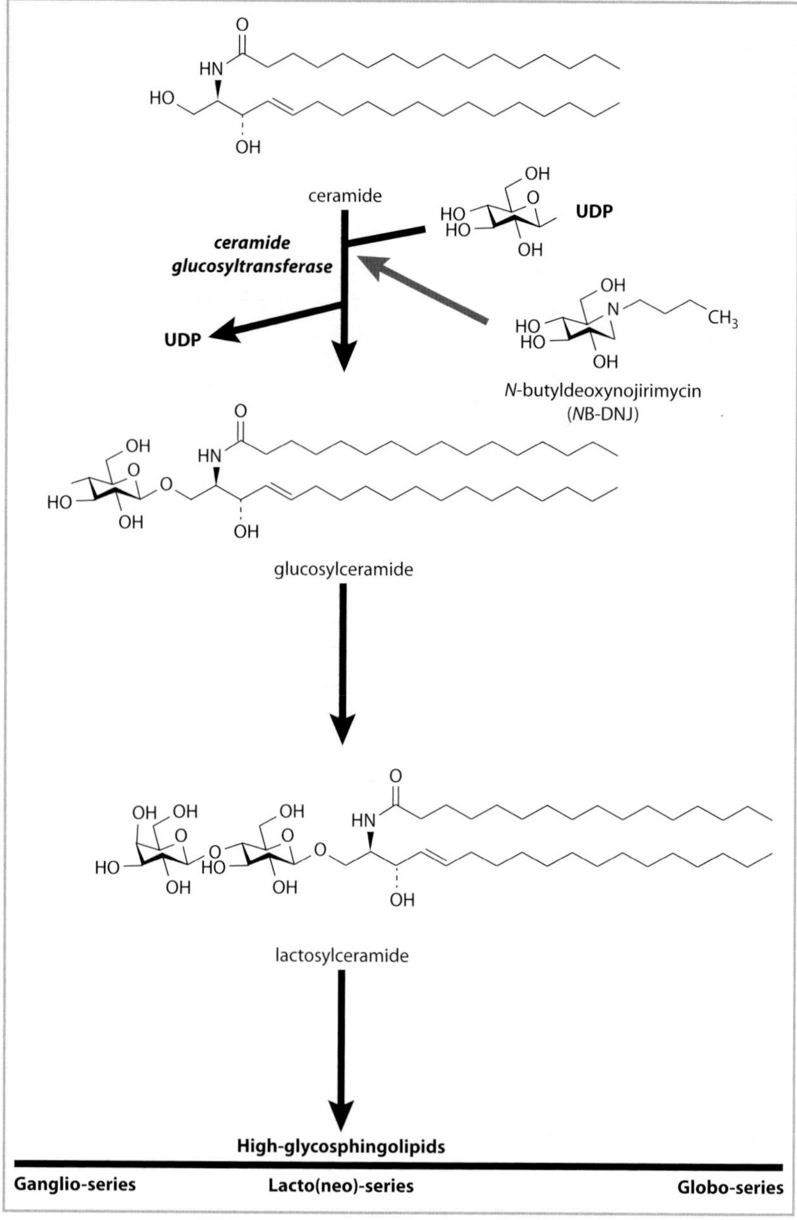

Figure 16-1. The rationale of the substrate reduction therapy in LSDs. The small molecule *N*-butyl deoxyjirimycin (*N*B-DNJ, miglustat) is a competitive inhibitor of ceramide glycosyltransferase and results in reduction of the biosynthesis of glucosylceramide, the substrate accumulated in GD-1 due to the deficiency of glucosylceramidase. *N*B-DNJ also reduces the biosynthesis of other high-glycosphingolipids including ganglio-series, lacto-series, and globo-series.

dosis (Tay-Sachs and Sandhoff diseases) failed to improve or change the natural progression of several neurologic endpoints.[30,31] Miglustat, however, was shown to be a safe drug in children, with similar pharmacokinetic profiles to those observed in adult patients.[32]

Recently SRT with miglustat was tested in juvenile patients with Niemann-Pick C disease, an LSD caused by deficiency of NPC1, a lysosomal protein involved in endosomal-lysosomal transport of lipids. In this study, SRT showed stabilization of clinically relevant outcomes, such as swallowing capacity, stable auditory acuity, and mobility in patients older than 12 years. The study supports SRT as a disease-modifying therapeutic approach for late-onset forms of Niemann-Pick C disease.[33]

Hematopoietic Stem Cell Therapy

In addition to ERT and SRT, hematopoietic stem cell transplantation (HSCT) remains a therapeutic option for some types of LSDs. The rationale for this form of genetic disease treatment is to ameliorate enzyme defects by providing hematopoietic stem cells from an unaffected donor within and outside the blood compartment. Patients with MPS-IH (Hurler syndrome, the early onset form of MPS-I) have shown good outcomes when they receive transplants before 2 years of age or before the onset of psychomotor retardation. Patients with MPS-IH who underwent HSCT, and have a satisfactory engraftment, generally demonstrate reduction of GAG excretion, improvement of respiratory obstructive disease, and decreases in liver and spleen volumes, along with amelioration and stabilization of cardiomyopathy.[34] On the other hand, skeletal abnormalities, such as spine deformities, did not respond to HSCT.[34] Cognitive function has been shown to improve in some patients, while in others the typical intellectual deterioration was noted.[35] Interestingly, 2 HSCT centers demonstrated that umbilical cord blood as the source of HS cells increases the likelihood of sustained engraftment associated with normal enzyme levels and may be considered as a preferential cell source in HSCT for LSDs. In MPS-II and MPS-III, HSCT has not been shown to alter the natural course of the disease. In MPS-IV, in which the skeletal system is predominantly affected, HSCT has little to offer. Hematopoietic stem cell transplantation may also be beneficial in select patients with metachromatic leukodystrophy (deficiency of arylsulfatase A), Krabbe disease (deficiency in β-galactocerebrosidase), and α-mannosidosis (deficiency of α-mannosidase) when performed early. Other genetic diseases not in the LSD category, especially X-linked adrenoleukodystrophy (X-ALD), a peroxisomal disorder caused by defective β-oxidation of very long-chain fatty acids (VLCFAs), have been shown to benefit from

HSCT, and it is the only effective treatment for the symptomatic childhood cerebral form of X-ALD. If HSCT is carefully performed at early stages of the disease in select cases, patients may respond and develop only mild neurologic symptoms.[35,36] For other phenotypes of X-ALD, such as adrenomyeloneuropathy, which is characterized by adrenal insufficiency and peripheral neuropathy presented after the third and fourth decade, HSCT is not recommended.

Cofactor Supplementation

Replacement of a missing enzyme is sometimes impossible and/or unnecessary in the treatment of genetic disorders. Instead, addition of a cofactor may be useful. The use of cofactors is based on the fact that many enzymes require nonprotein elements, such as vitamins and minerals, as cofactors to exert full catalytic activity and prevent disease. Table 16-3 depicts most of the cofactors used therapeutically in managing genetic diseases.

The defects in absorption of minerals or vitamins, and even the nutritional deficiencies, can lead to severe metabolic disturbances. Vitamin B_{12} deficiency due to dietary deficiency or genetic defect in absorption of vitamin B_{12} may be indistinguishable clinically. Parenteral administration of cyanocobalamin, which bypasses intestinal absorption, results in dramatic improvement of symptoms in nutritional vitamin B_{12} deficiency, and in

Table 16-3. Inherited Metabolic Diseases That May Respond to Cofactor Administration

Disease	Cofactor	Dose	Mechanism of Function
Biotinidase deficiency Holocarboxylase synthase deficiency	Biotin	5–20 mg/day (oral)	Carboxylation reactions (eg, pyruvate carboxylase)
PDH deficiency TRMA syndrome	Thiamine hydrochloride (vitamin B_1)	200 mg/day IV initially, followed by 100 mg PO daily (TRMA); 150–300 mg PO daily in MSUD and PDH	Chemical reactions involving acetate groups (eg, transaldolase, transketolase)
MADD	Riboflavin (vitamin B_2)	100–400 mg/day PO	Increase the intramitrochrondrial FAD concentration and promote FAD binding to ETF:QO[a]

Table 16-3. Inherited Metabolic Diseases That May Respond to Cofactor Administration *(cont)*

Disease	Cofactor	Dose	Mechanism of Function
Homocystinuria Pyridoxine-responsive seizures Cystathioninuria Xanthurenic aciduria Hyperornithinemia with gyrate atrophy	Pyridoxine (vitamin B_6)	100–500 mg IV single dose; 10 mg/kg/day—maintenance up to 500 mg/day	Transaminations and decarboxylations
Methylmalonic aciduria (cblA, cblB) Homocystinuria and methylmalonic acidemia (cblC, cblD, cblF)	Cobalamin (vitamin B_{12})	1–5 mg/day (various other regimens are in use also [IM])	Transesterification reactions
Homocystinuria	Folic acid	15 mg/kg/day (oral)	Nucleic acid synthesis and one-carbon-metabolism
Pyridoxal phosphate-responsive seizures	Pyridoxal phosphate	30 mg/kg/day (PO)	Pyrodox(am)ine 5′-phosphate oxidase (*PNPO*)
Hartnup disease	Nicotinamide	50–300 mg/day (PO)	Oxidation and reduction reactions
Carnitine transporter defect; organic acidemias and fatty acid oxidation defects	Carnitine	50–100 mg/kg/day	Restoration of free coenzyme A; scavenger of free organic acids
Mitochondrial electron transport defects Coenzyme Q_{10} deficiency	Coenzyme Q_{10}	30 mg/kg/day (PO)	Improves function of electron transport in mitochondria; free radical scavenger

Abbreviations: ETF:QO, electron transfer flavoprotein-ubiquinone oxidoreductase; FAD, flavin adenine dinucleotide; IM, intramuscular; IV, intravenous; MADD, multiple acyl-CoA dehydrogenase deficiency; MSUD, maple syrup urine disease; PDH, pyruvate dehydrogenase deficiency; PO, oral; TRMA, thiamine-responsive megaloblastic anemia.

[a] Zhang J, Frerman FE, Kim JJ. Structure of electron transfer flavoprotein-ubiquinone oxidoreductase and electron transfer to the mitochondrial ubiquinone pool. *Proc Natl Acad Sci U S A.* 2006;103(44):16212–16217.

some genetic diseases causing vitamin B_{12} deficiency. In methylmalonic acidemia caused by deficiency of mitochondrial cobalamin-dependent enzyme, binding of obligatory cofactor adenosylcobalamin is required for normal enzyme function. Defects in the synthesis of the adenosyl-cobalamin cofactor (cblA and cblB) result in a similar clinical presentation as methylmalonic aciduria. However, patients with cblA respond to treatment with large doses of vitamin B_{12} in the hydroxocobalamin form, whereas patients with cblB may respond variably, and sometimes poorly.

Mutations in the region of enzymes encoding the binding site of the cofactor (vitamin or mineral) can also result in genetic diseases; these defects in particular may respond dramatically to administration of cofactor. Clinical response in patients with these types of mutations can be achieved by administration of cofactor at higher concentrations, which can result in the correction of the metabolic defect. These inherited metabolic diseases depend on the exogenous administration of specific cofactors (Table 16-3). In pyridoxine-responsive homocystinuria, pyridoxine (vitamin B_6) is an obligatory cofactor for cystathionine β-synthase in performing its catalytic function.

Abnormally high, toxic levels of methionine and homocysteine are therapeutically amenable to decrease with the administration of pyridoxine in about one-third of patients with homocystinuria. Mitochondrial disorders consist of another subset of genetic diseases of energy production that are also amenable to cofactor treatment. Mitochondrial electron transport also depends on several nonprotein cofactors, including flavins, nicotinamide, ubiquinone, iron-sulfur clusters, and heme. Some compounds may only be involved in electron transport under special circumstances. This observation has prompted attempts to treat mitochondrial electron transport defects with compounds involved in the transport process. Studies have shown accumulation of free radicals in tissue of patients with mitochondrial transport defects. Based on these studies, administration of free radical scavengers, such as dimethylglycine, is given in an attempt to reduce the damaging effects of the accumulated free radicals secondary to dysfunctional mitochondria.

Dichloroacetate (DCA) has been tested as a treatment for lactic acidosis caused by various genetic diseases of energy metabolism. Dichloroacetate inhibits the pyruvate dehydrogenase (PDH) kinase and, therefore, prevents phosphorylation-mediated inactivation of PDH, which can be beneficial along with thiamine (vitamin B_1) and ketogenic diet in patients with the genetic disorder of energy metabolism PDH deficiency.[37] However, DCA

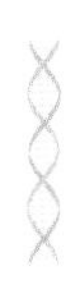

can cause peripheral nerve toxicity when used long term, particularly in the mitochondrial disease MELAS (mitochondrial myopathy, encephalopathy, lactic acidosis, and stroke).[38]

One of the most dramatic examples of cofactor therapy for genetic diseases is in disorders of creatine metabolism. Patients with defects in creatine biosynthesis pathway have shown significant clinical improvement when dietary creatine supplementation is administered in those with arginine:glycine aminotransferase deficiency, or creatine along with ornithine supplementation and arginine restriction in those with guanidine acetate methyltransferase deficiency. Some patients with primary or secondary coenzyme (Co) Q deficiencies may respond to oral supplementation, but others show progression of neurologic symptoms. Coenzyme Q can also serve as a scavenger of free radicals.[38] Carnitine has the same role when used in organic acidemias. It promotes the transesterification of organic acyl-CoA ester with the release of free CoA, and formation of organic acylcarnitines, which per se facilitates excretion of organic acids (renal clearance of conjugated acylcarnitine is larger than free organic acids). In addition, endogenous carnitine depletion is often seen in patients with organic acidemias, fatty acid oxidation effects, and carnitine transport defects. Carnitine treatment of these genetic disorders, although likely efficacious and without serious toxicity, has not been studied in randomized, controlled clinical trials in most of these diseases in which it is routinely used.[37] Indeed, the lack of randomized, controlled studies underscores the importance of evidence-based medicine and clinical trials in rare genetic disorders going forward.[39]

Toxic By-product Management

Toxic by-product management is another approach to treat genetic disorders. In patients with disorders of the urea cycle, for example, management is based on controlling the production of a toxic substance: ammonium. Besides increasing the high-caloric intake orally or parenterally, and reducing protein intake in order to attenuate the breakdown of proteins (which would generate more ammonia), the use of combination sodium benzoate and sodium phenylacetate (Ammonul) can increase the excretion of nitrogen and help to control ammonium levels. If this method fails to diminish the ammonium levels in the acute illness, dialysis in the form of hemodialysis or continuous venous-venous filtration is required. In addition, sodium phenylbutyrate can be useful in maintaining the lower levels in between acute illnesses.[40]

In tyrosinemia type I, caused by deficiency of fumarylacetoacetate hydrolase, the accumulation of fumarylacetoacetate and maleylacetoacetate, intermediates of tyrosine metabolism, may lead to severe hepatorenal dysfunction. The dietary control of tyrosine and phenylalanine levels has failed to prevent these complications, including liver and renal failure, cirrhosis, increased risk of hepatocarcinoma, and acute porphyria attacks. The use of 2-(2-nitro-4-trifluoromethylbenzoyl)-1,3-cyclohexanedione (nitisinone; Orfadin), blocking the production of the toxic tyrosine inter- mediate metabolites, has been shown to significantly alter the course of this disorder, preventing the manifestation of liver and renal complications.[41]

Smith-Lemli-Opitz syndrome (SLOS), caused by the deficiency of microsomal 7-dehydrocholesterol (7-DHC) reductase, which catalyzes the conversion of 7-DHC to cholesterol, is an inborn error of metabolism characterized by multiple malformations and intellectual disability. The metabolic defect results in accumulation of 7-DHC and 8-DHC, and deficiency in cholesterol. Dietary cholesterol supplementation was shown to increase the serum cholesterol levels and reduce the levels of 7-DHC, with some studies showing beneficial effects on growth, behavior, and frequency of infections.[42,43] Since the accumulation of cholesterol precursors was thought to be harmful in several components of SLOS, the use of 3-hydroxy-3-methylglutaryl CoA inhibitors was considered. Treating 2 patients with simvastatin along with cholesterol resulted in reduction of 7-DHC and 8-DHC, along with improvements in cognition and motor and social development.[44] However, in a retrospective study of 39 patients, the same benefits in growth parameters and behavior problems were not observed. Additionally, a reduction of 7-DHC + 8-DHC/total cholesterol ratios were seen in patients with enriched cholesterol diet only and those receiving additional simvastatin.[45]

In the peroxisomal disorder, X-ALD, "Lorenzo's oil," a mixture of oleic and erucic acids, has shown reduction of the levels of VLCFAs in plasma. In this case and as frequently seen in the treatment of many other genetic disorders, the lack of appropriate and necessary clinical studies before the drug is adopted in clinical practice poses difficulties in proving its therapeutic efficacy. Lorenzo's oil has not resulted in major benefits in patients already exhibiting neurologic symptoms, but it may reduce the risk of progression to the childhood cerebral form of X-ALD.[46] Most of the treatments described previously are not curative and must be administered indefinitely.

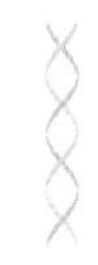

Future Treatments

Gene Therapy

The ideal treatment for genetic diseases is the substitution of the defective (or mutated) gene with a normal gene that has a normally regulated long-term expression in affected tissues. The risk inherent in this form of therapy has precluded many trials in patients. Several studies have now been focused on treating somatic cells. Gene transfer therapy for most genetic diseases is still experimental. The approach has been shown successful in transferring a "normal gene" into hematopoietic stem cells for management of a few genetic defects affecting blood cells. Two examples are adenosine deaminase (ADA) deficiency and X-linked severe combined immunodeficiency (X-SCID; caused by mutations in the *IL2RG* gene encoding the gc-chain of cytokine receptors). Using γ-retrovirus and ex vivo gene transfer, patients with ADA and X-SCID were treated successfully, although this was tempered by the toxic effects seen in one trial of X-SCID.[47] In the latter trial, patients developed T-cell proliferation due to insertional mutagenesis and aberrant expression of a proto-oncogene. This turned out to trigger a fatal leukemia-like disease in one patient, although this complication was effectively reversed by chemotherapy in others. This experience has illustrated both the potential for gene therapy to cure genetic disease while once again demonstrating that gene therapy is highly complex and can lead to untoward events. Much additional research is needed in this area.

Enzyme Enhancement Therapy

Most patients with the late-onset forms of several LSDs have residual enzyme activity.[48] Interestingly, symptoms do not manifest unless genetic mutations lead to more than 90% reduction in the residual activity of the deficient enzyme. Thus the critical threshold of enzyme activity must be achieved, or overcome, to avoid specific substrate storage which, ultimately, may arrest or significantly reverse the disease process. In late-onset forms, the mutations correlating with residual enzyme activity are mostly missense, which encode a mutant enzyme that retains a degree of catalytic activity. Lysosomal enzymes are synthesized in the endoplasmic reticulum (ER) of the cell, where they achieve their proper folding with the assistance of ER resident chaperones, before being released from ER to the Golgi apparatus, and then targeted to the lysosomes. If a mutant protein, after several attempts, persists in the misfolded state, it is directed to ER-associated degradation (ERAD), and subsequently to the ubiquitin proteosomal system (UPS) for degradation. In the case of LSDs, genes with specific missense mutations encode an enzyme that preserves some catalytic function, resulting in the residual enzyme activity often seen in cultured cell lines from patients with late-onset disease. However, most of these mutant enzymes result in a misfolded and unstable protein, which is consequently retained, and ultimately directed to the ERAD. The enzyme enhancement therapy (EET) consists of using small molecules (<500 D) that assist the misfolded mutant lysosomal enzymes to achieve a stable and native-like conformation in the ER, and escape ERAD and subsequently reach the lysosomal compartment, where they are still able to exert some catalytic function. Several pharmacological chaperones (PCs), small molecules used as EET, have been characterized for several LSDs.[49] Some of these molecules have been tested in clinical trials such as pyrimethamine (GM2 gangliosidosis), isofagomine (GD-1), ambroxol (neuronopathic GD-3), and *N*B-DNJ (Fabry disease).[50–52]

Another example of enzyme enhancement therapy is the use of sapropterin dihydrochloride (Kuvan), a synthetic formulation of the active 6R-isomer of tetrahydrobiopterin, a naturally occurring cofactor for the PAH for treatment of PKU. Although originally developed as a cofactor, this compound has been shown to work primarily as a PC by binding to PAH and preventing misfolding. It is FDA-approved to reduce blood Phe levels in patients with hyperphenylalaninemia due to tetrahydrobiopterin-responsive PKU and provides a promising non-dietary treatment option for patients with PKU who are responsive to this form of therapy.

Stem Cell Therapy

Stem cell therapy has been applied as a tool to deliver the correct gene to the specific affected tissues. This approach has been applied to the LSDs group (see page 321). In MPS-IH (Hurler disease), the principle is that the penetration of macrophage-derived microglia cells from the donor cells will engraft and produce and secrete the deficient enzyme that can be uptaken by neighboring cells, leading to amelioration of disease. If performed before the developmental delay or cognition is affected, hematopoietic stem cell therapy will be able to arrest the neurologic effect of the condition in the central nervous system. It was shown to be ineffective in other LSDs with neurologic symptoms. Somatic donor stem cells are also found in brain, muscle, gut, heart, skin, liver, and pancreas of the recipient. These cells have relevant therapeutic application since they can

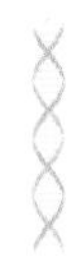

be used to recover the damage of specific tissue caused by progression of a genetic condition.[53] Somatic stem cells isolated from human fetal brain may be used as potential therapy for genetic disorders with major neurologic phenotype, such as neuronal ceroid lipofuscinosis (NCL). In a knockout mice model for palmitoyl-protein thioesterase-1 deficiency (model for infantile form of NCL), human brain fetal cells were transplanted and were shown to differentiate in neuronal cells and reduce significantly lipofuscin and promote neuroprotection.[54] A clinical trial in patients with infantile and late infantile NCL is investigating the safety and potential therapeutic benefits of this approach (personal communication, N. Seldon, February 2013).

Key Points

- Managing genetic diseases involves not only the care of the patient but also seeks detailed family history, relevant information on the patient's family members that can be helpful for diagnostic, management, and counseling perspectives.
- Advances in treating genetic disorders are related to a better understanding of the pathogenesis, the natural history, and the development of different therapeutic strategies.
- Management of genetic diseases can be approached from different levels—from the mutated gene (hematopoietic stem cell transplantation in Hurler syndrome) up to the level of the family of the affected patient (carrier screening for Tay-Sachs disease).
- Treatment for PKU (phenylalanine-restricted diet) and galactosemia (galactose-restricted diet) are classical examples where dietary control treatment is efficacious to prevent severe neurologic and manifestations of these diseases.
- Chemical inducers, such as hydroxyurea and butyrate, to enhance the endogenous levels of fetal hemoglobin have been shown to be of clinical benefit for patients with SCD and β-thalassemia.
- Enzyme replacement therapy, the intravenous administration of recombinant enzyme, for the treatment of LSDs is now considered the standard of care for GD-1 (non-neuronopathic), MPS-I, -II, -VI; Fabry disease; and Pompe disease.
- Enzyme replacement therapy administered systemically is unable to treat neurologic symptoms, as the recombinant enzyme, a large molecular weight molecule, is unable to cross the blood-brain barrier.
- Substrate reduction therapy with miglustat showed some benefit to ameliorate symptoms in specific LSDs.

- Hematopoietic stem cell transplantation remains as a therapeutic option for some LSDs and peroxisomal diseases.
- Supplementation with cofactors can be of clinical benefit in some inherited metabolic disorders.
- Most inborn errors of metabolism result in the accumulation of an intermediate metabolite or by-product that is harmful to the organism, and the elimination of these toxic metabolites is crucial to prevent permanent neurologic debilitation.
- Replacement of the defective gene through gene therapy has shown initial and encouraging results in the treatment of congenital immunodeficiencies, but safety issues are still to be resolved.
- Small molecules can be used to increase the stability and promote folding of mutant proteins that are still partially functional, and small molecules are more likely to cross the blood-brain barrier and treat neurologic manifestations of certain conditions.
- Stem cell therapies have the potential for recovering the damage of specific tissues caused by progression of a genetic condition, especially neurodegenerative conditions.

References

1. Bickel H, Gerrard J, Hickmans EM. Influence of phenylalanine intake on phenylketonuria. *Lancet.* 1953;265(6790):812–813
2. Sarkissian CN, Gamez A, Scriver CR. What we know that could influence future treatment of phenylketonuria. *J Inherit Metab Dis.* 2009;32(1):3–9
3. Scriver CR. The PAH gene, phenylketonuria, and a paradigm shift. *Hum Mutat.* 2007;28(9):831–845
4. Huijbregts SC, de Sonneville L, Mvan Spronsen FJ, et al. The neuropsychological profile of early and continuously treated phenylketonuria: orienting, vigilance, and maintenance versus manipulation-functions of working memory. *Neurosci Biobehav Rev.* 2002;26(6):697–712
5. Levy HL. Historical background for the maternal PKU syndrome. *Pediatrics.* 2003; 112(6 pt 2):1516–1518
6. Walter JH, Collins JE, Leonard JV. Recommendations for the management of galactosaemia UK. Galactosaemia Steering Group. *Arch Dis Child.* 1999;80(1):93–96
7. Waggoner DD, Buist NR, Donnell GN. Long-term prognosis in galactosaemia: results of a survey of 350 cases. *J Inherit Metab Dis.* 1990;13(6):802–818
8. Fratantoni JC, Hall CW, Neufeld EF. Hurler and Hunter syndromes: mutual correction of the defect in cultured fibroblasts. *Science.* 1968;162(853):570–572
9. Watson J. A study of sickling of young erythrocytes in sickle cell anemia. *Blood.* 1948;3(4):465–469
10. Testa U. Fetal hemoglobin chemical inducers for treatment of hemoglobinopathies. *Ann Hematol.* 2009;88(6):505–528
11. Hayes A, Costa T, Scriver CR, et al. The effect of Mendelian disease on human health. II: response to treatment. *Am J Med Genet.* 1985;21(2):243–255

12. Treacy E, Childs B, Scriver CR. Response to treatment in hereditary metabolic disease: 1993 survey and 10-year comparison. *Am J Hum Genet.* 1995;56(2):359–367
13. Meikle PJ, Hopwood JJ, Clague AE, et al. Prevalence of lysosomal storage disorders. *JAMA.* 1999;281(3):249–254
14. Mechtler TP, Stary S, Metz TF, et al. Neonatal screening for lysosomal storage disorders: feasibility and incidence from a nationwide study in Austria. *Lancet.* 2012;379(9813):335–341
15. Barton NW, Brady RO, Dambrosia JM, et al. Replacement therapy for inherited enzyme deficiency—macrophage-targeted glucocerebrosidase for Gaucher's disease. *N Engl J Med.* 1991;324(21):1464–1470
16. Poll LW, Koch J, Avom Dahl S, et al. Magnetic resonance imaging of bone marrow changes in Gaucher disease during enzyme replacement therapy: first German long-term results. *Skeletal Radiol.* 2001;30(9):496–503
17. Poll LW, Maas M, Terk MR, et al. Response of Gaucher bone disease to enzyme replacement therapy. *Br J Radiol.* 2002;75(suppl 1):A25–A36
18. Prows CA, Sanchez N, Daugherty C, et al. Gaucher disease: enzyme therapy in the acute neuronopathic variant. *Am J Med Genet.* 1997;71(1):16–21
19. Eng CM, Banikazemi M, Gordon RE, et al. A phase 1/2 clinical trial of enzyme replacement in Fabry disease: pharmacokinetic, substrate clearance, and safety studies. *Am J Hum Genet.* 2001;68(3):711–722
20. Kakkis ED, Muenzer J, Tiller GE, et al. Enzyme-replacement therapy in mucopolysaccharidosis I. *N Engl J Med.* 2001;344(3):182–188
21. Harmatz P, Ketteridge D, Giugliani R, et al. Direct comparison of measures of endurance, mobility, and joint function during enzyme-replacement therapy of mucopolysaccharidosis VI (Maroteaux-Lamy syndrome): results after 48 weeks in a phase 2 open-label clinical study of recombinant human N-acetylgalactosamine 4-sulfatase. *Pediatrics.* 2005;115(6):e681–e689
22. Muenzer J, Wraith JE, Beck M, et al. A phase II/III clinical study of enzyme replacement therapy with idursulfase in mucopolysaccharidosis II (Hunter syndrome). *Genet Med.* 2006;8(8):465–473
23. Amalfitano A, Bengur AR, Morse RP, et al. Recombinant human acid alpha-glucosidase enzyme therapy for infantile glycogen storage disease type II: results of a phase I/II clinical trial. *Genet Med.* 2001;3(2):132–138
24. Kishnani PS, Corzo D, Nicolino M, et al. Recombinant human acid [alpha]-glucosidase: major clinical benefits in infantile-onset Pompe disease. *Neurology.* 2007;68(2):99–109
25. Strothotte S, Strigl-Pill N, Grunert B, et al. Enzyme replacement therapy with alglucosidase alfa in 44 patients with late-onset glycogen storage disease type 2: 12-month results of an observational clinical trial. *J Neurol.* 2009;257(1):91–97
26. Kishnani PS, Goldenberg PC, DeArmey SL, et al. Cross-reactive immunologic material status affects treatment outcomes in Pompe disease infants. *Mol Genet Metab.* 2010;99(1):26–33
27. Platt FM, Neises GR, Dwek RA, Butters TD. N-butyldeoxynojirimycin is a novel inhibitor of glycolipid biosynthesis. *J Biol Chem.* 1994;269(11):8362–8365
28. Cox T, Lachmann R, Hollak C, et al. Novel oral treatment of Gaucher's disease with N-butyldeoxynojirimycin (OGT 918) to decrease substrate biosynthesis. *Lancet.* 2000;355(9214):1481–1485
29. Elstein D, Hollak C, Aerts J, et al. Sustained therapeutic effects of oral miglustat (Zavesca, N-butyldeoxynojirimycin, OGT 918) in type I Gaucher disease. *J Inherit Metab Dis.* 2004;27(6):757–766

30. Shapiro BE, Pastores GM, Gianutsos J, et al. Miglustat in late-onset Tay-Sachs disease: a 12-month, randomized, controlled clinical study with 24 months of extended treatment. *Genet Med.* 2009;11(6):425–433
31. Maegawa GH, Banwell BL, Blaser S, et al. Substrate reduction therapy in juvenile GM2 gangliosidosis. *Mol Genet Metab.* 2009;98(1–2):215–224
32. Maegawa G, Hvan Giersbergen PL, Yang S, et al. Pharmacokinetics, safety and tolerability of miglustat in the treatment of pediatric patients with GM2 gangliosidosis. *Mol Genet Metab.* 2009;97(4):284–291
33. Patterson MC, Vecchio D, Prady H, et al. Miglustat for treatment of Niemann-Pick C disease: a randomised controlled study. *Lancet Neurol.* 2007;6(9):765–772
34. Aldenhoven M, Boelens J, de Koning TJ. The clinical outcome of Hurler syndrome after stem cell transplantation. *Biol Blood Marrow Transplant.* 2008;14:485–498
35. Peters C, Steward CG. Hematopoietic cell transplantation for inherited metabolic diseases: an overview of outcomes and practice guidelines. *Bone Marrow Transplant.* 2003;31(4):229–239
36. Peters C, Charnas LR, Tan Y, et al. Cerebral X-linked adrenoleukodystrophy: the international hematopoietic cell transplantation experience from 1982 to 1999. *Blood.* 2004;104(3):881–888
37. Stacpoole PW, Gilbert LR, Neiberger RE, et al. Evaluation of long-term treatment of children with congenital lactic acidosis with dichloroacetate. *Pediatrics.* 2008;121(5):e1223–e1228
38. DiMauro S, Mancuso M. Mitochondrial diseases: therapeutic approaches. *Biosci Rep.* 2007;27(1–3):125–137
39. Kruer MC, Steiner RD. The role of evidence-based medicine and clinical trials in rare genetic disorders. *Clin Genet.* 2008;74(3):197–207
40. Enns GM, Berry SA, Berry GT, et al. A survival after treatment with phenylacetate and benzoate for urea-cycle disorders. *N Engl J Med.* 2007;356(22):2282–2292
41. Masurel-Paulet A, Poggi-Bach J, et al. NTBC treatment in tyrosinaemia type I: long-term outcome in French patients. *J Inherit Metab Dis.* 2008;31(1):81–87
42. Elias ER, Irons MB, Hurley AD, et al. Clinical effects of cholesterol supplementation in six patients with the Smith-Lemli-Opitz syndrome (SLOS). *Am J Med Genet.* 1997;68(3):305–310
43. Kelley RI, Hennekam RC. The Smith-Lemli-Opitz syndrome. *J Med Genet.* 2000;37(5):321–335
44. Jira PE, Wevers R, Ade Jong J, et al. Simvastatin. A new therapeutic approach for Smith-Lemli-Opitz syndrome. *J Lipid Res.* 2000;41(8):1339–1346
45. Haas D, Garbade SF, Vohwinkel C, et al. Effects of cholesterol and simvastatin treatment in patients with Smith-Lemli-Opitz syndrome (SLOS). *J Inherit Metab Dis.* 2007;30(3):375–387
46. Moser HW, Raymond GV, Lu SE, et al. Follow-up of 89 asymptomatic patients with adrenoleukodystrophy treated with Lorenzo's oil. *Arch Neurol.* 2005;62(7):1073–1080
47. Cavazzana-Calvo M, Lagresle C, Hacein-Bey-Abina S, et al. Gene therapy for severe combined immunodeficiency. *Annu Rev Med.* 2005;56:585–602
48. Tropak MB, Mahuran D. Lending a helping hand, screening chemical libraries for compounds that enhance beta-hexosaminidase A activity in GM2 gangliosidosis cells. *FEBS J.* 2007;274(19):4951–4961
49. Fan JQ. A counterintuitive approach to treat enzyme deficiencies: use of enzyme inhibitors for restoring mutant enzyme activity. *Biol Chem.* 2008;389(1):1–11

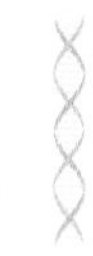

50. Osher E, Fattal-Valevski A, Sagie L, et al. Pyrimethamine increases beta-hexosaminidase A activity in patients with late onset Tay Sachs. *Mol Genet Metab.* 2011;102:356–363
51. Clarke JT, Mahuran DJ, Sathe S, et al. An open-label phase I/II clinical trial of pyrimethamine for the treatment of patients affected with chronic GM2 gangliosidosis (Tay-Sachs or Sandhoff variants). *Mol Genet.* 2011;102:6–12
52. Maegawa GHB, Tropak M, Buttner JD, et al. Identification and characterization of ambroxol as an enzyme-enhancement agent for Gaucher disease. *J Biol Chem.* 2009;284(35):23502–23516
53. O'Connor TP, Crystal RG. Genetic medicines: treatment strategies for hereditary disorders. *Nat Rev Genet.* 2006;7(4):261–276
54. Tamaki SJ, Jacobs Y, Dohse M, et al. Neuroprotection of host cells by human central nervous system stem cells in a mouse model of infantile neuronal ceroid lipofuscinosis. *Cell Stem Cell.* 2009;5(3):310–319

Chapter 17

Newborn Screening in the United States

Michele A. Lloyd-Puryear, MD, PhD
Alex R. Kemper, MD, MPH, MS

Newborn screening, which began in the 1960s with the testing for phenylketonuria (PKU) using dried blood spots collected on filter paper,[1] was the first genetic population-based screening program for the nation's newborns. Newborn screening in most states now includes more than 30 congenital or inherited conditions, and novel technologies likely will continue to expand the number of conditions that can be identified through newborn screening. Despite the challenges in implementation, there is no doubt that newborn screening has improved the health of many individuals.

Overview

Newborn screening is not simply a process of testing, but it is an organized, systematic approach to ensure that every infant identified as screen positive will undergo diagnostic evaluation and, when necessary, treatment and management. The newborn screening system includes both short-term follow-up (ie, ensuring screening was conducted, reviewing the results, and conducting diagnostic testing when necessary) and long-term follow-up (ie, all of the activities that occur after confirmation of a condition), as well as processes for education and quality assurance. In order for the newborn screening system to be successful there must be careful coordination and communication between public health agencies, primary health care providers, specialists, and families.

The American Academy of Pediatrics (AAP), at the request of the Health Resources and Services Administration (HRSA), convened the Newborn Screening Task Force in 1998, in anticipation of expanding newborn screening programs. This effort was cosponsored by federal agencies, professional provider and public health organizations, and family groups. Some of the significant obstacles at the time included the lack of uniformity in conditions screened among states and subsequent disparities for individual infants; poor communication practices from state programs to pediatricians; and the lack of systematic education of parents, pediatricians, and obstetricians about newborn screening. The AAP recommendations that arose from the work of the task force[2] became the blueprint for subsequent federal legislation establishing a federal advisory committee and many state and federal activities.

Significant activity is underway to continue to implement the AAP recommendations, address the expansion of newborn screening, and improve the effectiveness of the process related to newborn screening. Any summary of specific activities would be quickly out of date. Instead, we review the general precepts. For information on specific disorders, refer to the following resources:

- American Academy of Pediatrics newborn screening fact sheets (www.medicalhomeinfo.org/how/clinical_care/newborn_screening.aspx)
- American College of Medical Genetics and Genomics (ACMG) (www.acmg.net)
- National Library of Medicine Genetics Home Reference (ghr.nlm.nih.gov)
- Baby's First Test (www.geneticalliance.org/nbs)

Identifying Conditions for Newborn Screening

Each state determines the conditions included on their newborn screening panel. In the mid-1990s dramatic differences across states began to develop, primarily because of variations in the implementation of tandem mass spectrometry, a technology that can detect a wide array of metabolic conditions.[3] In response, the federal Maternal and Child Health Bureau (MCHB) of HRSA commissioned the ACMG to convene an expert panel to make recommendations about which conditions should be included in screening.[4] This expert panel recommended 29 core conditions based on the availability of an accurate screening test and efficacious treatment with added benefit from early intervention. In addition, the expert panel identified 25 secondary conditions that would be identified in the process of screening for the core conditions but for which the efficacy of treatment or the added benefit of early intervention is unclear. The federal Department of Health and Human Services (DHHS) Secretary's Advisory Committee on Heritable Disorders in Newborns and Children (www.hrsa.gov/heritabledisorderscommittee/default.htm) recommended this panel to the secretary of DHHS in 2006. These conditions are listed in Table 17-1. Since then there has been significant harmonization across states in the conditions included in newborn screening. The National Newborn Screening and Genetics Resource Center (http://genes-r-us.uthsca.edu/) posts the latest information on the conditions included in newborn screening.

Since then, the advisory committee has developed a process for evaluating potential additions or deletions to its recommended uniform panel for screening infants and children. Individuals or organizations can nominate conditions for consideration by the committee. If there is sufficient evidence for the benefit of screening based on an internal evaluation, an external evidence review group will conduct a systematic review and interview experts in the area. This report is then presented to the advisory committee, which then makes recommendations to the secretary of the DHHS. Similar to the secretary's Advisory Committee on Immunization Practices, states may choose to adopt or not adopt the recommendations made by the advisory committee to the secretary. After deliberation by the advisory committee, possible recommendations are as follows: (1) recommend adding the condition to the uniform panel; (2) recommend not adding the condition to the uniform panel; (3) recommend not adding the condition, but instead recommend specific additional studies; and (4) recommend not adding the condition based on current knowledge. Recommendations are made based on the level of certainty of the expected net benefit of screening. The decision process for these 4 criteria is described in Table 17-2.

As of October 2010, the advisory committee has considered nominations for screening newborns for Fabry disease, Krabbe disease, Neimann-Pick disease, Pompe disease, spinal muscular atrophy, α-thalassemia, severe combined immunodeficiency (SCID), and critical cyanotic congenital heart disease. The evidence regarding newborn screening for Fabry and Neimann-Pick disease and spinal muscular atrophy was not considered sufficient for developing a complete evidence review by the external evidence review group. Although Krabbe disease (category 4) and Pompe disease (category 3) were not recommended to be added to the standard newborn screening panel, the committee endorsed screening for SCID and critical cyanotic congenital heart disease.

Table 17-1. Conditions Recommended for Newborn Screening Blood Spot Testing in 2006[4]

Core Conditions	Secondary Target Conditions
Endocrine Disorders	
Thyroid Disorders	
Primary congenital hypothyroidism Disorders of adrenal steroidogenesis Congenital adrenal hyperplasia	
Metabolic Disorders	
Organic Acid Disorders	
Propionic academia Methylmalonic acidemia Isovaleric acidemia 3-Methylcrotonyl-CoA carboxylase deficiency I 3-Hydroxy-3-methyglutaric aciduria Holocarboxylase synthetase deficiency β-Ketothiolase deficiency Glutaric acidemia type I	Methylmalonic acidemia Malonic acidemia Isobutyrylglycinuria 2-Methylbutyrylglycinuria 3-Methylglutaconic aciduria 2-Methyl-3-hydroxybutyric aciduria
Fatty Acid Oxidation Disorders	
Carnitine uptake defect/carnitine transport defect Medium-chain acyl-CoA dehydrogenase deficiency Very long-chain acyl-CoA dehydrogenase deficiency Long-chain L-3-hydroxyacyl-CoA dehydrogenase deficiency Trifunctional protein deficiency	Short-chain acyl-CoA dehydrogenase deficiency Medium-/short-chain L-3-hydroxyacyl-CoA dehydrogenase deficiency Glutaric acidemia type II Medium-chain ketoacyl-CoA thiolase deficiency 2,4-Dienoyl-CoA reductase deficiency Carnitine palmitoyltransferase I deficiency Carnitine palmitoyltransferase II deficiency Carnitine acylcarnitine translocase deficiency
Amino Acid Disorders	
Argininosuccinic aciduria Citrullinemia, type I Maple syrup urine disease Homocystinuria Classic phenylketonuria Tyrosinemia, type I	Argininemia Citrullinemia, type II Hypermethioninemia Benign hyperphenylalaninemia Biopterin defect in cofactor biosynthesis Biopterin defect in cofactor regeneration Tyrosinemia, type II Tyrosinemia, type III

Core Conditions	Secondary Target Conditions
Hemoglobin Disorders	
S,S disease (sickle cell anemia) S, β-0-thalassemia S,C disease (Sickle C disease)	Other hemoglobinopathies
Vitamin Disorders	
Biotinidase deficiency	
Other Disorders	
Galactose disorders Classic galactosemia Galactose epimerase deficiency Galactokinase deficiency	
Pulmonary Disorders	
Cystic fibrosis	

Table 17-2. Decision Matrix for Advisory Committee Recommendations

Category	Recommendation	Level of Certainty	Magnitude of Net Benefit
1	Recommend adding the condition to the uniform panel.	Sufficient	Significant
2	Recommend not adding the condition to the uniform panel.	Sufficient	Zero or net harm
3	Recommend not adding the condition, but instead recommend specific additional studies.	Insufficient, but the potential for net benefit is compelling enough to recommend specific additional studies to evaluate.	Potentially significant, and supported by contextual considerations
4	Recommend not adding the condition based on current knowledge.	Insufficient, and substantial additional evidence is needed to make a conclusion about net benefit.	Potentially significant or unknown

The Question of Benefit

Newborn screening policies have been guided by principles presented in a 1968 World Health Organization monograph by James Wilson and Gunnar Jungner[5] and by the principles set forth in the report *Genetic Screening* from the National Research Council (NRC) of the National Academy of Sciences (NAS) in 1975.[6] In their monograph, Wilson and Jungner identified 10 criteria for including a condition in a population-based screening program. (Also see Chapter 16.) Although designed for the evaluation of screening for adult chronic diseases, the criteria have been applied to newborn screening programs. There are 4 general categories of criteria set forth by Wilson and Jungner: (1) considerations about the condition itself (eg, important health problem, well-described natural history with a recognizable presymptomatic or early symptomatic stage), (2) considerations about screening and diagnosis (eg, suitable and acceptable tests), (3) considerations about treatment (eg, accepted treatment), and (4) considerations about the capacity for providing care (eg, ability to continuously engage in case-finding, availability of diagnosis and treatment, acceptability of cost-effectiveness of the screening program). Generally, newborn screening has adhered to the principle that infants should be screened at birth only for conditions that present in the newborn period for which an effective treatment already exists. Treatment is usually construed as a medical therapy that significantly improves the infant's health. In its 1975 report, the NAS/NRC introduced a broader concept of benefit as part of its decision criteria.[6] The NAS/NRC report noted that genetic screening may be appropriate even when a direct medical treatment is not available if there is benefit to the infant to provide management and support, the family to inform subsequent reproductive decisions, and society to provide knowledge about the condition. Consider the following:

- The Wilson and Jungner criteria do not consider multiplex technology (testing that analyzes for multiple disorders at the same time).[4,7]
- Many of the screening methods can identify a wide range of conditions, not just those that are the focus of screening. Although multiplex technology can decrease the cost of screening, it also can identify conditions that were not necessarily targeted by the screening test. Tandem mass spectrometry is a prime example because of its ability to detect metabolic conditions about which little is known in regard to either natural history or treatment efficacy. However, some other older technology is similar. For example, screening for hemoglobinopathies can not only identify abnormal hemoglobin chains, but also identify those who are carriers.

- The criteria impair the development of innovation.[8]
- The conditions that are identified through newborn screening are rare. Some have argued that without screening and systematic case finding, effective treatments will not be able to be developed and assessed.
- The criteria too narrowly consider treatment benefit.[9]

The criteria focus on the direct benefit of screening to the affected individual. However, families may benefit from knowing that their child has a specific health condition, even if there is no recognized treatment.

The advisory committee considers separately each potentially identifiable condition and weighs the potential net benefit to the affected child. The advisory committee has created a decision framework that builds on the Wilson and Jungner, NAS/NRC, and ACMG Newborn Screening Expert Panel principles and takes into consideration the full array of opinions and interests in regard to the broad concept of benefit. The advisory committee's process aims to balance different perspectives and values of the population.

Testing for Conditions Not Recommended by the Advisory Committee

As indicated previously, states may choose to test for conditions recommended or not recommended by the advisory committee. If a state screens for a condition not currently on the advisory committee's recommended uniform screening panel, states often will collect detailed data on the clinical outcomes resulting from such testing, leading to the collection of much more complete evidence regarding the benefit of screening. Examples include Krabbe disease screening in New York, SCID screening in Wisconsin, and α-thalassemia screening in California. In addition, commercial laboratories also offer newborn screening tests to supplement those available through state newborn screening programs. Unlike state newborn screening programs, these commercial laboratories do not systematically collect data to fill in the evidence gaps, nor do they engage in the necessary follow-up activities, rather they may rely on the state newborn screening program to conduct the follow-up. This often leads to an uncoordinated system of diagnosis, treatment, and management.

Because the number of potential screening tests is expanding and because the cost of these tests is also falling (eg, microarray technology), we anticipate that parents will face bewildering choices. Inevitably it will fall to obstetricians to discuss such testing as a part of prenatal care and pediatricians to discuss such testing in the prenatal visit or in early infancy.[10] Some information about these tests will be available on the previously mentioned Web sites. However, it is likely that there will be many conditions for which very little information is available. Health care providers will need to be able to review the general tenets used for evaluating the benefits and harms of screening to help families make an informed decision. This will be difficult and potentially time consuming. New strategies will be needed to prepare primary care providers for genomic medicine. This manual was developed in part to address this need.

Newborn Screening: More Than a Test

It is essential that any screening program ensure careful follow-up of both the positive and negative screen tests, and also ensure continuity of care for those infants identified with positive screens. This is especially true for newborn genetic and hearing screening; significant mortality and morbidity are associated with those conditions for which screening is done. The program must have protocols that delineate roles and responsibilities as to who is responsible for follow-up and what that follow-up should be.

Short-term Follow-up

State newborn screening programs rely on the submission of samples. Newborn screening programs have no way to identify when a screening sample is not received from a birthing center. All state newborn screening programs make significant efforts to ensure that children with a positive newborn screen have documented follow-up. This can be challenging because the information provided with the sample often does not have correct information regarding the newborn's primary care physician (PCP). Furthermore, names can change after discharge, and families can move. Because of the inability for state newborn screening programs to check whether a sample was received and the difficulty of tracking newborns, the programs rely on PCPs to independently check the results. Some states have developed Web-based systems to monitor newborn screening outcomes. Therefore, as part of the infant's first outpatient visit, the pediatrician should confirm that a newborn screen was performed and received by the state public health laboratories.

In addition, state newborn screening programs generally have infrastructure capacity only for short-term follow-up for those conditions that benefit from early intervention. There is usually no follow-up by the state program when carriers are identified (eg, sickle cell trait). Therefore, it is essential

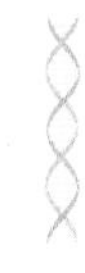

that the pediatrician assume the role of following up on all newborn screen results. The identification of carriers has important implications for integrating the results of newborn screening into lifelong electronic and personal health records.

Following up a positive newborn screen may be stressful for both health care providers and families. Many health care providers have little knowledge about the conditions and may be unsure of the steps that need to be taken after an initial positive result. To help, the MCHB/HRSA funded the ACMG to develop action sheets (ACT sheets) that describe all steps that should be taken (www.acmg.net/resources/policies/ACT/condition-analyte-links.htm) by a PCP. These sheets were endorsed by the AAP. Sample ACT sheets and a full list of available ACT sheets are found in Appendix B. The Web site contains the latest version of the ACT sheets, which are regularly revised based on the availability of new tests and new information received about newborn screening.

The news of a positive newborn screen can be upsetting to families. In our experience, having a well-prepared health care provider (ie, knowledgeable about the ACT sheets) make the initial contact can relieve some of this anxiety. The AAP has recently developed a guideline that defines the steps required for short-term follow-up, including a description of how to incorporate the ACT sheets into practice.[11] The ACT sheets are designed to be practical. These 1- or 2-page sheets provide a brief differential diagnosis for the condition, a short description of the condition, a bulleted list of actions for the primary care provider to take immediately after the positive newborn screen, the process to confirm the diagnosis, and a short paragraph about the expected course of the condition. In addition, the ACT sheets provide links to more information about testing, treatment, and outcomes. Individual newborn screening programs may add additional information about local resources for diagnosis and treatment.

Long-term Follow-up

Most state newborn screening programs do not have the resources to systematically follow and collect outcomes regarding the management of individuals identified through newborn screening. However, systems are now in development to assist public health agencies not only to conduct surveillance but also to help improve the quality of care that individuals receive. Regardless, both primary care providers and specialty care providers are expected by newborn screening programs to be responsible for providing long-term care. Ideally, individuals with conditions identified through newborn screening would receive such care through a patient- and family-centered medical home. The workforce shortage of geneticists and pediatric subspecialists in general highlights the need for carefully constructed care plans to ease the burden on families and the health care system in providing accessible care for rare conditions. These care plans can enable PCPs to manage many problems, thus decreasing the need for families to travel far distances or filling up limited specialty clinic appointment slots.

To be effective, it is critical that an explicit care management document be developed and shared with the family and affected individual to

- Delineate the role of all health care providers.
- Manage the condition, including specific drugs and diet recommendations.
- Provide symptom-specific care, including guidelines for when to seek emergency care.
- Provide care plans for health care providers who may not know the patient or only little about the particular health condition (eg, emergency department physicians).

These care plans should be developed with the input of families and affected individuals and should be regularly reviewed and updated. In addition to having a copy of the care plans in the medical record, families and affected individuals should have up-to-date copies of the care plan. The AAP has developed sample forms for care coordination (www.medicalhomeinfo.org/tools/doc_guide.html).

Transitions to Adult Care

The life expectancy and quality of life for children with conditions identifiable through newborn screening has improved dramatically. We fully expect these improvements to continue. However, this has created challenges as children transition to adult care. For some, health insurance has been an important barrier to care. For example, some have problems getting necessary but expensive medical food or formula. Additionally, few adult care providers are familiar with these conditions because historically these children did not survive into adulthood. We believe that primary care pediatricians should incorporate planning for transition to adult care into care plans. This includes working with adolescents, when possible, to understand their chronic health problems and to engage in their own

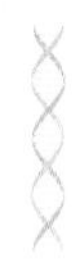

health care and anticipate the challenges of becoming an adult. For example, some families and affected individuals need help with determining how to live independently.

Challenges in Newborn Screening

Case 1

Bobby was born unexpectedly at 31 weeks' gestation in a local emergency department. He had respiratory distress and was transferred immediately to a neonatal intensive care unit, where he stayed for 4 weeks. Later he was transferred to a nursery closer to the family, and eventually discharged home when he was 2 months old. When he was 5 months old he developed a viral illness with poor appetite and some vomiting. Two days later Bobby died. Subsequently it was learned that Bobby had medium-chain acyl CoA dehydrogenase deficiency (MCAD). Unfortunately, Bobby did not receive newborn screening.

It is easy for a child to miss newborn screening when sick or when transferred across health care settings. Newborn screening programs have no way to know when a child has not been tested. We believe that it is incumbent on all primary care providers to ensure that testing has been done and the results have been checked. No news is not necessarily good news. This can be challenging because families may not remember or know that their child was tested. We believe that all newborns should have documentation that testing occurred at the time of their first visit, and the results should be recorded in a standardized place within the medical record by 1 month of age or at the first well-child visit if that is after 1 month of age. Ensuring completion of newborn screening is critical because it identifies conditions that require early intervention. Many, like MCAD, can be lethal if appropriate management is not begun. Also, like MCAD, the treatment for some is well-defined and straightforward.

Case 2

Jessica is a 3-year-old with galactosemia diagnosed through newborn screening who is coming in for a routine preventive maintenance visit. Jessica's family lives in a rural community. They are happy that they only travel to see their geneticist and metabolic dietitian every 4 months and that they are able to get her health taken care of by her general pediatrician. Jessica's parents also feel comfortable letting her travel out of town with her grandparents for holiday trips because of the care plan that has been developed.

There is a workforce shortage of pediatric specialists. Children with conditions identified through newborn screening often have to travel long distances for care. Some of these conditions can be managed by primary care providers if there is clear communication between the specialist and the primary care health provider about the roles that each will play in care management and the indications for seeking emergent care from the specialist. Sharing this information through a carefully documented care plan can be tremendously empowering to families and, in our experience, can lead to improved health outcomes.

Case 3

David is a 16-year-old star of his high school's track and field team. David usually feels bad because his brother, who has sickle cell disease, cannot participate in sports like he can. David knows that he doesn't have sickle cell disease because he had a negative newborn screen. During practice one afternoon David developed significant pain in his legs while running and then collapsed on the field.

For some conditions like sickle cell disease or cystic fibrosis, newborn screening can identify newborns who are carriers. Sharing this information with families is critical. Parents should consider that they may both be carriers, which would have implications for future child planning issues. Similarly, children should have information that they are carriers. Communicating this information in a way that it can be used is challenging but important. Finally, being a carrier is not always benign. For example, children with sickle cell trait (sickle cell carriers) are at increased risk for exertional rhabdomyolysis. As newborn screening expands, it is likely that more will be learned about the association between being a carrier and the development of specific conditions. Primary care providers should ensure that any identified carrier state is well marked in the child's medical record and that a review be made on an annual basis of new information regarding the relationship between that carrier state and health outcomes.

Case 4

Sarah is a 23-year-old recently married graduate student with PKU. Although Sarah earned excellent grades in college, she has had trouble completing her graduate school assignments, and her overall concentra-

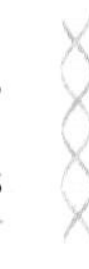

tion has been poor. After finishing college, she was no longer able to be on her parent's health insurance plan. Her current plan does not cover medical foods. Sarah is now planning to start a family of her own.

Appropriate dietary management leads to dramatic improvements for children with metabolic conditions such as PKU. Unfortunately, medical foods and formula are expensive, and coverage by health insurance is highly variable. This can lead to poor metabolic control. Women with PKU who have poor metabolic control may have severely developmentally delayed children, even if the children do not have PKU (ie, maternal PKU syndrome). Primary care providers should be aware of these financial challenges and work with families and state health agencies to develop a plan at times of health insurance transition. Primary care providers can also be strong advocates for policy reform to ensure that medical foods and formulas are available to those with metabolic conditions identified through newborn screening.

Key Points

Newborn screening is a great example of a modern success of the public health system. Pediatricians play a central role in ensuring that their patients benefit from newborn screening. The expansion of state newborn screening panels and the availability of tests outside of state newborn screening panels present challenges to already busy pediatricians. However, there is tremendous opportunity to improve the lives of affected individuals and their families.

- Be aware of the conditions included in newborn screening within your state.
- Understand the implications of ordering additional testing.
- Be able to talk about newborn screening and additional optional available screening with parents.
- Ensure that all newborns are tested and that results are documented in the medical record.
- Be aware of the ACT sheets and how to conduct newborn screening.
- Be able to talk with families about the meaning of a positive newborn screen.
- Be able to talk about the carrier status.
- Know local resources for specialty referral.
- Develop and monitor care plans.

- Ensure that families are engaged in the development and revision of care plans.
- Develop plans for transition to adult care.
- Be able to work with public health agencies in monitoring the impact of newborn screening and subsequent treatment.

The views expressed in this chapter are those of the authors and do not necessarily reflect those of the authors' respective institution or agencies within the US Department of Health and Human Services or the US Department of Health and Human Services as a whole.

References

1. Guthrie R. The introduction of newborn screening for phenylketonuria: a personal history. *Eur J Pediatr.* 1996;155:S4–S5
2. American Academy of Pediatrics Newborn Screening Task Force. Serving the family from birth to the medical home: newborn screening: a blueprint for the future. Executive summary: Newborn Screening Task Force report. *Pediatrics.* 2000;106:386–388
3. Wilcken B, Wiley V, Hammond J, et al. Screening newborns for inborn errors of metabolism by tandem mass spectrometry. *N Engl J Med.* 2003;348:2304–2312
4. Watson MS, Mann MY, Lloyd-Puryear MA, et al. Newborn screening: toward a uniform screening panel and system—executive summary. *Genet Med.* 2006;8:1S–11S
5. Wilson JMG, Jungner G. *Principles and Practice of Screening for Disease.* World Health Organization public health papers, No. 34, 1968
6. National Academy of Sciences/National Research Council. *Genetic Screening: Programs, Principles, and Research.* Washington, DC: National Academy of Sciences; 1975
7. Botkin JR, Clayton EW, Fost NC, et al. Newborn screening technology: proceed with caution. *Pediatrics.* 2006;117:1793–1799
8. Alexander D, Van Dyck PC. A vision of the future of newborn screening. *Pediatrics.* 2006;117:S350–S354
9. Bailey DB, Skinner D, Warren SF. Newborn screening for developmental disabilities: reframing presumptive benefit. *Am J Pub Health.* 2005;95:1889–1893
10. American College of Obstetricians and Gynecologists. Ethical issues in genetic testing. ACOG Committee Opinion No 410. *Obstet Gynecol.* 2008;111:1495–1502
11. American Academy of Pediatrics Newborn Screening Authoring Committee. Newborn screening expands: recommendations for pediatricians and medical homes—implications for the system. *Pediatrics.* 2008;121:197–217

Chapter 18

Preventable Disabilities: The Road Ahead

Tiina K. Urv, PhD
R. Rodney Howell, MD

Introduction

Preventing disabilities is a long-standing challenge facing the medical community. Identifying the optimal time to screen and treat individuals with life-altering disorders is imperative to prevention. Currently newborn screening is the most widespread means of identifying infants who are presymptomatic and could benefit from treatment of disease, while prenatal diagnosis of fetal chromosomal abnormalities is the most common indication for prenatal testing. Both approaches have played an important role in the early identification of infants with disabilities.

Newborn Screening

Newborn screening (Chapter 17) has expanded from its early groundbreaking days of detecting and treating a single disorder to prevent intellectual disability in the 1960s into a vital national public health program. The voices of family and advocacy groups, long a driving force behind newborn screening, have been heard, as is evidenced by state mandates for newborn screening and the federal Newborn Screening Saves Lives Act of 2008.[1] This rapid expansion of newborn screening in recent years was driven by multiple factors, including

- Development of new, sophisticated technologies to identify an ever-growing number of disorders
- Improvement in the understanding and treatment of existing disorders
- Discovery of new disorders that may benefit from newborn screening

- Enhanced technologies that allow for increased communication and collaboration between the key players in the field

The further evolution of newborn screening requires an alliance of stakeholders, including

- Policy (state and federal)
- Research (federally and privately funded)
- Clinical care
- Advocacy groups
- Families
- Industry

Prenatal Testing

For the last 30 years research efforts have focused on developing a better understanding of a woman's risk of having a child with a disability or serious illness, including the creation of noninvasive screening methods to identify these children prenatally. Ultrasound and serum screening may be performed on mothers and fetuses to monitor pregnancy outcomes. Prenatal screening tests may decrease the need for more invasive diagnostic testing and may reduce the risk of procedure-related miscarriage. The American College of Obstetricians and Gynecologists has indicated that prenatal testing, including amniocentesis and chorionic villus sampling, should be available to all women,[2] and the American College of Medical Genetics and Genomics (ACMG)[3] recommends that this diagnostic testing should be made available if requested, and after appropriate counseling of the risks and benefits of the testing.

Coordination of Policies in Newborn Screening

Historically there have been inconsistencies in access to newborn screening due to differences in state law, although in the last 10 years a concerted effort has been made to reduce variability. The Advisory Committee on Heritable Disorders in Newborns and Children (ACHDNC) authorized by the Children's Health Act of 2000 received the central charge to advise the secretary of the Department of Health and Human Services (DHHS) regarding the most appropriate application of universal newborn screening tests, technologies, policies, guidelines, and standards for effectively reducing morbidity and mortality in newborns and children with, or at risk for, heritable disorders. In 2006 the ACMG was commissioned by the Maternal and Child Health Bureau (MCHB) of the Health Resources and

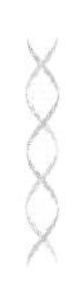

Services Administration (HRSA) to develop newborn screening guidelines. They recommend that newborns be screened for 29 "core conditions" and that 25 secondary conditions that can also be identified during the "core conditions" evaluations be reported.[4] In 2008 the ACHDNC recommended to the secretary that the ACMG report be accepted. These guidelines are endorsed by the ACHDNC, the American Academy of Pediatrics, and the March of Dimes. Most state newborn screening laboratories have also accepted these screening guidelines. In 2011 the DHHS accepted this recommendation as national policy.

Criteria for Including Conditions in Newborn Screening Panels

Newborn screening (Chapter 17) is more than a process for testing a spot of blood. It is an organized, systematic approach to ensure that every infant identified as screen positive undergoes a diagnostic evaluation and, when necessary, treatment and management (Figure 18-1). Screening also includes hearing screening and the use of pulse oximetry to detect critical congenital cyanotic heart disease. Serum bilirubin testing may soon be included. The guidelines developed by the ACMG have provided an initial framework for

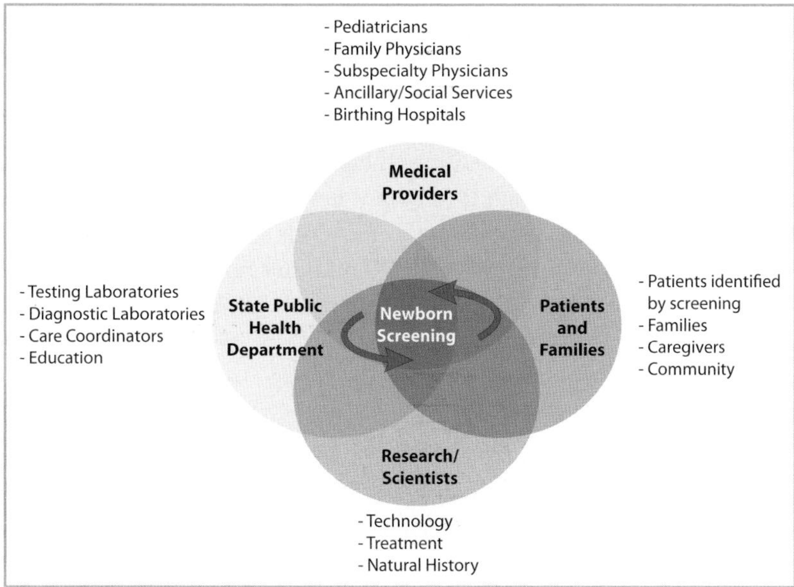

Figure 18-1. Coordination of resources.

determining which conditions to recommend for screening. The guidelines[4] propose that policies related to newborn screening be determined through

- Analysis of the severity and incidence of each condition under consideration
- The specificity and sensitivity of the screening test
- The natural history of the disorder
- The efficacy, safety, and effectiveness of treatments available for the disorder

Currently there are numerous candidate conditions being considered for newborn screening panels; however, for many conditions there is a lack of evidenced-based research to support the inclusion of these conditions. There is a dire need to

- Develop and evaluate the capabilities of screening technology.
- Understand the natural history of these candidate conditions.
- Develop therapeutic interventions for these conditions.

Dozens of new conditions may be added to the core newborn screening panel in coming decades.

Expanded Evidence Base

Novel Technologies in Newborn Screening

New technologies are being explored and modified for use in newborn screening, including microchips, microbeads, nanotechnologies, micro-fluidics, DNA assays, biophysical assays, and technologies based on RNA or protein analysis. Equally important is the ability of the technology to function efficiently and effectively in the appropriate environment, be it in a high throughput newborn screening laboratory or at the point of care. Despite the tremendous strides made in developing new technologies in recent years, limitations remain in the type of conditions that can be screened for clearly indicating that more research is needed.

Treatment Interventions

Early detection and treatment can have a profound impact on the clinical severity of numerous conditions. One of the primary objectives of newborn screening is to detect potentially fatal or disabling conditions in newborns providing physicians with a window of opportunity to treat an asymptom-

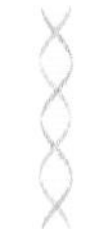

atic child before irreversible neurologic damage; intellectual, developmental, and physical disabilities; and even death occur.

Severe combined immune deficiency, a primary immune deficiency, usually results in the onset of one or more serious infections within the first few months of life. A bone marrow or stem cell transplant within the first 3 months of life is life-saving and prevents infection, disability, and premature death.[5] Early treatment is very cost-effective. Without newborn screening most children are diagnosed after this critical period and experience severe infections before diagnosis. If the child survives these infections, transplantation is much less effective than if diagnosed before 3 months of age. Severe combined immune deficiency has recently been added to the newborn screening core panel on the recommendation of ACHDNC.

The Natural History of Screenable Disorders

Understanding the natural history of a disorder is a necessary element in providing appropriate treatment for infants identified by newborn screening. In recent years research has concentrated on the development of screening tools and treatments for disorders, placing less emphasis on identifying the natural history of a disorder. This gap in knowledge weakens the ability to develop and measure the most effective treatments and interventions for infants and children identified via newborn screening, particularly as they age. To address this imbalance, California (a state with ~560,000 births annually, or one-eighth of all children born in the United States) has established a database designed to track positive cases to learn more about the natural history of these diseases. This is especially important for disorders that have demonstrated a great deal of genetic and clinical heterogeneity, resulting in difficulty in identifying individuals most suitable for specific interventions and the proper ages at which to initiate treatment. Knowledge of specific genotype-phenotype correlations may allow prediction of the clinical course of a disorder, and it may also provide an opportunity of modifying genetic, epigenetic, or environmental factors that will enhance our understanding of the clinical outcome for a condition. For example, Krabbe disease has varying manifestations. Not all who test positive in the newborn screen develop the full-blown phenotype. Stem cell transplantation has limited effectiveness with significant potential morbidity and mortality. Aggressive intervention in such disorders must be carefully considered, since a full understanding of such issues is critical in the decision-making process.[6]

The development of comprehensive data on the natural history of conditions suitable for newborn screening will benefit our ability to

- Accurately diagnose the disorder.
- Understand the genetic and clinical heterogeneity and phenotypic expression of the disorder.
- Identify underlying mechanisms related to basic defects.
- Potentially prevent, manage, and treat symptoms and complications of the disorder.
- Provide children and their families with needed support and predictive information about the disorder.

Comparative Effectiveness Research

As new technologies for screening and treatment are developed and the breadth of knowledge related to the natural history of disorders is expanded, the need to compare existing and newly developed methods and technologies becomes increasingly evident. Comparative effectiveness research is defined as research that compares the benefits and harms of different interventions and strategies used to prevent, diagnose, treat, and/or monitor health conditions in "real world" settings.[7] This type of research is valuable as the results generated from such studies can be shared with stakeholders (policy makers, researchers, clinicians, advocacy groups, families, and commercial enterprises), allowing them to make informed decisions regarding policy, treatment, and research.

Examples of comparative effectiveness studies might include the comparison of existing treatments for phenylketonuria (PKU) and Pompe disease to newly discovered interventions. The gold standard and very effective treatment for PKU is dietary treatment. However, an exciting new drug, a biopterin compound, is proving very effective in certain patients. Myozyme is the standard treatment for Pompe disease; however, the possibility of using chaperone therapy (small molecules that can bind to misfolded protein [due to a mutation]) to stabilize the defective enzyme is on the horizon.[8,9] While research evaluating specific treatment is important, the knowledge of which treatment is most effective for which patients depending on the stages of disease progression is invaluable.

New Directions in Prenatal Screening

Noninvasive prenatal diagnosis is the study of fetal genetic material circulation in maternal peripheral blood. The separation of fetal cells in maternal blood was first described in the late 1970s, and researchers have

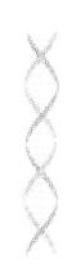

been refining the process since then. Circulating cell-free fetal DNA testing in maternal plasma was originally limited to the study of paternal DNA sequences; however, new techniques and technology have broadened its use to include molecular studies in high-risk families, general screening, and pregnancy management.[10]

Pregnancy-associated plasma protein-A has proven to be a highly efficient serum marker in the first-trimester screening for chromosomal abnormalities. This marker is associated with adverse pregnancy outcomes, such as preterm delivery, intrauterine growth retardation, preeclampsia, and still birth.[11]

Other minimally invasive techniques that have been identified include cervical mucus aspiration, cervical swabbing, and cervical or intrauterine lavage. These techniques have been used to retrieve trophoblast cells during the first trimester for diagnostic purposes, including for prenatal genetic analysis.[12]

Coordination of Resources

In recent years federal agencies, along with partners, have developed resources targeted at meeting the needs of specific stakeholder groups (eg, newborn screening service providers, researchers, clinicians, and families). Although each resource is individually beneficial, the field of newborn screening as a whole would reap greater benefits from a collaborative and cooperative approach between the resource providers.

National Coordinating Center for the Regional Genetic and Newborn Screening Service Collaboratives

In 2004 the MCHB/HRSA Genetic Services Branch (GSB) established 7 genetics and newborn screening regional collaborative groups (RCs) and a National Coordinating Center (NCC) (Table 18-1). The RCs work regionally to strengthen and support the genetics and newborn screening capacity of states. The NCC provides the needed infrastructure, including coordination, technical assistance, and needed resources for local and pilot projects.

The Newborn Screening Translational Research Network

In 2008 The Hunter Kelly Newborn Screening Research Program, at The Eunice Kennedy Shriver National Institute of Child Health and Human Development in a collaborative effort with ACMG established

Table 18-1. Regional Genetics and Newborn Screening Collaborative Groups[a]

Region	States Served
New England Genetics Collaborative	Connecticut, Massachusetts, Maine, New Hampshire, Rhode Island, and Vermont
New York-Mid-Atlantic Consortium for Genetics and Newborn Screening Services	Delaware, District of Columbia, Maryland, New Jersey, New York, Pennsylvania, Virginia, and West Virginia
Southeast NBS & Genetics Collaborative	Alabama, Florida, Georgia, Louisiana, Mississippi, North Carolina, Puerto Rico, South Carolina, Tennessee, and the Virgin Islands
The Region 4 Genetics Collaborative	Illinois, Indiana, Kentucky, Michigan, Minnesota, Ohio, and Wisconsin
Heartland Genetics and Newborn Screening Collaborative	Arkansas, Iowa, Kansas, Missouri, Nebraska, North Dakota, Oklahoma, and South Dakota
Mountain States Genetics Regional Collaborative Center	Arizona, Colorado, Montana, Nevada, New Mexico, Texas, Utah, and Wyoming
Western States Genetic Services Collaborative	Alaska, California, Guam, Hawaii, Idaho, Oregon, and Washington

[a] There are 7 regional genetics and newborn screening collaborative groups in the United States, supported by the Department of Health and Human Services/Health Resources and Services Administration/Maternal and Child Health Bureau/Genetic Services Branch.

the Newborn Screening Translational Research Network Coordinating Center (NBSTRN-CC). The purpose of the NBSTRN-CC is to facilitate research that develops new screening methods, or conducts clinical trials for new therapeutic interventions, and that explores the natural histories of disorders identified through newborn screening.

The primary goals of the NBSTRN-CC are to

- Facilitate an organized network of state newborn screening programs and clinical centers.
- Develop, implement, and refine a national *research* informatics system for investigators and policy makers that dovetails with established national clinical networks.
- Establish and administer an efficient and reliable repository of residual dried blood spots.
- Provide expertise and support related to regulatory requirements associated with informed consent, institutional review boards, and state and local research policies associated with newborn screening.

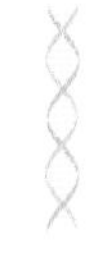

- Facilitate research on the development of new methods and technologies by maintaining close contact with the scientific and biomedical research community.
- Facilitate research on screened and treated patients to define effectiveness of treatments and long-term outcomes.
- Provide statistical leadership and clinical trial design expertise for the individualized needs of researchers through the NBSTRN-CC, and facilitate the timely dissemination of research findings.

Newborn Screening Clearinghouse

To provide information and resources to parents and health care providers in a centralized and coordinated manner, the HRSA GSB established the Newborn Screening Clearinghouse in 2009. This center is being coordinated by the Genetic Alliance and the National Newborn Screening and Genetics Resource Center at the University of Texas Health Science Center at San Antonio (http://genes-r-us.uthscsa.edu). These groups are collaborating with the RCs, the March of Dimes, the Association of Public Health Laboratories, and many other partners.

Newborn Screening Coding and Terminology Guide

To facilitate communication between the various members of the newborn screening team (the laboratories, the primary care and specialty physicians, the state laboratories, and others) a detailed coding and terminology guide suitable for electronic records must be available. The National Library of Medicine (NLM) has developed a Newborn Screening Coding and Terminology Guide (http://newbornscreeningcodes.nlm.nih.gov/). The use of standard terminology

- Speeds the delivery of newborn screening reports
- Facilitates the care and follow-up of infants with positive test results
- Enables the use (and comparison) of data from different laboratories
- Supports the development of strategies for improving the newborn screening process

Key Points

- New technology and discovery of new disorders have led to a rapid expansion in newborn screening.
- Focus on screening has superseded an emphasis on understanding the natural history of genetic disorders for which there are screens. With

primary care physicians and specialists systematically gathering information on disease manifestation, particularly for those conditions that have variable phenotypes, treatment options should improve over time.

- Genetics and newborn screening regional collaborative groups support physicians and families in diagnosing and treating genetic disorders, and in advising states on their newborn screening policies.
- Standard terminology developed by the NLM helps in gathering and comparing data, reporting newborn screen results, and supporting improvement of newborn screening processes.
- Primary care physicians should anticipate continued advances in the prevention of disabilities as newborn screening programs continue to evolve.

References

1. Newborn Screening Saves Lives Act of 2007 (Pub L No. 110-204)
2. American College of Obstetricians and Gynecologists. ACOG Practice Bulletin No. 88, December 2007. Invasive prenatal testing for aneuploidy. *Obstet Gynecol.* 2007;110(6):1459–1467
3. Driscoll DA, Gross SJ. Fetal aneuploidy and neural tube defects. *Genet Med.* 2009;11(11):818–821
4. Watson MS, Mann MY, Lloyd-Puryear MA, Rinaldo P, Howell RR. Newborn screening: toward a uniform screening panel and system—executive summary. *Genet Med.* 2006;8:1S
5. Grunebaum E, Mazzolari E, Porta F, et al. Bone marrow transplantation for severe combined immune deficiency. *JAMA.* 2006;295(5):508–518
6. Steiner RD. Commentary on: "Newborn screening for Krabbe Disease: the New York state model" and "the long-term outcomes of presymptomatic infants transplanted for Krabbe disease. A report of the workshop held on July 11 and 12, 2008, Holiday Valley, New York". *Genet Med.* 2009;11(6):411–413
7. Federal Coordinating Council for Comparative Effectiveness Research. Report to the President and the Congress. June 30, 2009
8. Parenti G. Treating lysosomal storage diseases with pharmacological chaperones: from concept to clinics. *EMBO Mol Med.* 2009;1(5):268–279
9. Beck M. New therapeutic options for lysosomal storage disorders; enzyme replacement, small molecules and gene therapy. *Hum Genet.* 2007;121(1):1–22
10. Bustamante-Aragones A, Gonzalez-Gonzalez C, Rodriquez de Alba M, Ainse E, Ramos C. Noninvasive prenatal diagnosis using ccffDNA in maternal blood: state of the art. *Expert Rev Mol Diagn.* 2010;10(2):197–205
11. Kirkegaard I, Uldbjerg N, Oxvig C. Biology of pregnancy-associated plasma protein-A in relation to prenatal diagnostics: an overview. *Acta Obst Gynecol Scand.* 2010;89(9):1118–1125
12. Imudia AN, Kumar S, Diamond MP, DeCherney AH, Armant DR. Transcervical retrieval of fetal cells in the practice of modern medicine: a review of the current literature and future direction. *Fertil Steril.* 2010;93(6):1725–1730

Chapter 19

Personalized Medicine

Emily Chen, MD, PhD

Introduction

Personalized medicine is a rapidly advancing field that promises greater precision and effectiveness than disease-based traditional medicine because it is targeted to an individual's unique clinical, genomic, and environmental information. Personalized medicine uses tools that make use of the molecular profile (DNA sequence and variations, RNA and protein data) to better understand the genetic makeup of the patient. Treatment is based on the individual genomic profile that will differ from person to person. Care of the patient is optimized when molecular data, individual risk assessments, and family history can be individualized and combined to predict responsiveness to therapy or drugs. Whereas disease-based traditional medicine as we know it is based on only clinical criteria or genotypic information (DNA mutation of specific genes), personalized care integrates a person's individualized history with the most precise science.[1] Personalized medicine has the most promise if all known concurrent therapies and diseases for one individual are included in the assessment.

Goal of Personalized Medicine

The goal of personalized medicine is to customize the best possible treatment, medications and dosages, and prevention strategies for an individual.[2] The focus is wellness and disease prevention, uniquely tailored and optimized for each patient. Understanding which environmental factors may affect the patient and should be altered is central to personalized medicine. See Box 19-1 for advantages of personalized medicine.

Box 19-1. Rewards of Personalized (Individualized) Medicine[a]

1. Ability to make more informed and precise medical decisions
2. Higher probability to achieve desired outcomes due to better targeted therapies (ie, choosing the right drugs, interventions, surveillance and monitoring, surgical options, and other testing for the right person at the right time)
3. Reduced probability of negative side effects by determining sensitivity of a drug
4. Ability to focus on prevention and prediction of disease before it occurs
5. Reduced health care costs because of the promise of prevention
6. Using a whole genome approach, more data can be obtained all at once to help make decisions
7. Ability to suggest lifestyle changes, including diet and nutritional supplements
8. Opportunity to offer presymptomatic genetic testing to at-risk family members or to offer genetic counseling and recommendations for the entire family
9. A statistical approach to estimation of risk
10. More motivation to comply with recommendations and make changes that are based on lifetime risks of having certain medical disorders
11. Reduce the time and cost of clinical trials
12. Revive drugs that are failing in clinical trials or were withdrawn from the market, and use them in other beneficial ways

[a] From Abrahams E. Personalized medicine realizing its promise. *Genet Eng Biotechnol News.* 2009;29:70–73; Personalized Medicine Coalition. *The Case for Personalized Medicine.* 3rd ed. Washington, DC: Personalized Medicine Coalition; 2011

Types of Genetic Testing

Genetic testing can either be diagnostic (offered to those who have presumed medical conditions) or predictive (offered to individuals with no specific symptoms or health concerns). Predictive testing can be offered for childhood-onset disorders, or for adult-onset disorders to show increased susceptibility for a genetic condition. However, before genetic testing is initiated, much forethought, planning, and possibly even consultation with other providers is prudent, weighing the pros and cons of offering a genetic test, taking into account the additional testing that could follow, the value of testing for the patient, ambiguities of potential results, the implications of potential results, ethical factors (especially for children), and emotional impact for the patient and family. Discussions with the family should occur before genetic testing so that the family can make an informed decision (consent) and to ensure that the family will not be surprised about the results and implications once the genetic testing has been done. Genetic testing should only be done if beneficial for the patient. (See Chapter 15.)

Interpreting genetic test results can pose many challenges. The following genetic results may be obtained:

- Finding a pathogenic mutation or variant that alters the product of the gene (protein) in such a way that the function of the protein is either altered or absent. The most clear-cut mutations that are pathogenic are those that produce protein truncation (stop codons or premature truncation). Some variants have been previously reported as deleterious or pathogenic while others are novel and predicted to be associated with the genetic condition.
- No mutation or variant is detected. This could mean that the individual does not have that genetic condition, the gene was not completely sequenced, or the wrong gene was sequenced.
- Finding a variant of unknown clinical significance based on genetic databases or published medical literature. In this instance, the results can be ambiguous or indeterminate. Testing other affected family members to see if they have the same variant may be helpful in the interpretation of the results.
- An association or linkage is made, with specific numerical interpretations that address risk.
- A quantitative gene copy number is obtained.

Direct Single Gene Mutation Testing

Direct single gene mutation testing is the DNA test that pediatricians are the most familiar with. Reasons to perform single gene mutation testing can be to (1) confirm a suspected clinical diagnosis, thereby giving the opportunity to test at-risk family members (either to confirm a diagnosis or to provide presymptomatic testing); (2) help give less credence to a diagnosis if the genetic testing does not show any mutation; and (3) help to make some genotype-phenotype correlation, which can dictate management and treatment to some extent.

Example 1: Single Gene Testing to Confirm a Diagnosis

Single gene mutation can be provided to a child suspected to have cystic fibrosis who has failure to thrive and pancreatic insufficiency and an abnormal sweat chloride test (>60 mmol/L). Genetic testing can be done to look for either 2 known pathogenic mutations (2 compound heterozygous mutations) or 2 homozygous mutations in the *CFTR* gene. Each of the parents would be expected to be a carrier of cystic fibrosis. What is exciting is that recently there has been some focus on mutation-specific therapy for cystic fibrosis. Ivacaftor (Kalydeco) (a CFTR potentiator designed to increase the time that activated CFTR chloride channels remain open) is now an approved drug for the treatment of cystic fibrosis patients who had at least one copy of the G551D CFTR mutation. Results of a phase III randomized, double-blind, placebo-controlled trial (VX-770) showed that those treated with the drug showed weight gain, improved pulmonary function, and decreased hospitalizations due to pulmonary exacerbations with no adverse events.[3] An extension of this study would be to investigate this drug, and others like it, to tweak additional activity out of the chloride channels with reduced function in patients with at least one delta F508 mutation, which would be potentially much more widely beneficial.

Example 2: Single Gene Presymptomatic Testing

Confirmatory testing or linkage analysis (*RYR1, MHS4, MHS3, MHS2* genes) for malignant hyperthermia susceptibility can be helpful and potentially life-saving if there is any doubt of this diagnosis in a proband or if presymptomatic testing can be offered. Testing could be helpful even though up to 50% of individuals with malignant hyperthermia susceptibility have undergone anesthesia uneventfully. Those patients who test positive for a mutation all require anesthesia precautions (no use of potent inhalation agents and succinylcholine); treatment with dantrolene sodium for the treatment of malignant hyperthermia; avoidance of azumolene, a congener of dantrolene sodium; and avoidance of overheating in general. Genotype-phenotype correlations exist and may be helpful in management.

Example 3: Genotype-Phenotype Correlation

Mutation testing for maturity-onset diabetes of the young (MODY) is an example of looking for genotype-phenotype correlations. MODY is an autosomal dominant form of type 2 diabetes that usually develops in childhood, adolescence, or young adulthood.[4] MODY1, MODY3, and MODY4 are characterized by mild hyperglycemia and pronounced glucose intolerance, which respond well to oral sulfonylurea drugs. Insulin therapy over time may be required for these forms of MODY. MODY2 is characterized by mild hyperglycemia and glucose intolerance; in contrast this form is generally nonprogressive and usually can be managed with diet and exercise alone. Therefore, knowing which form of MODY a child may have can help with the management plan.

Example 4: Classic Genetic Testing for Preventive Care

When the daughter was 2 years old, a family updated their pediatrician that the father was diagnosed with a pheochromocytoma. The pediatrician further pursued the family history. The father's hypertension started at 16 years of age. At age 18 years he was deferred from the military due to hypertension. His own father had been diagnosed years ago to have hyperparathyroidism.

Subsequent workup for the father revealed he also had medullary thyroid cancer, and he had his thyroid gland removed. He was diagnosed to have Sipple syndrome, or multiple endocrine neoplasia type 2A (MEN2A). The father's sister was known to have abnormal serum calcitonin levels.

The pediatrician recommended screening for pheochromocytoma and hyperparathyroidism for all at-risk individuals in the family, even for the children. The risk of thyroid carcinoma was discussed for individuals affected with MEN2A, and screening was recommended by the end of the first decade for the daughter. Before the wife conceived again, the family sought genetic counseling concerning the probabilities of a child inheriting the gene for MEN2A. At the time, prenatal genetic testing for MEN2A was not available as the gene for MEN2A had not yet been discovered. They were counseled by a geneticist and genetic counselor about the 50% recurrence risk for the pregnancy. After the son was born, he was monitored for his 50% risk to have MEN2A. The father and his 2 children (daughter and son) were monitored by blood pressure checks, serum calcitonin, calcium, and parathyroid hormone levels, and 24-hour urine catecholamine studies biannually.

Gene testing for MEN2A became clinically available when the son was 10 years old, at which time the father was tested. The father had a codon 618 mutation in the RET proto-oncogene on chromosome 10, associated with MEN2A. Mutations are classified based on risk for aggressive medullary cancer. The classification is used in predicting phenotype and in recommendations regarding the ages at which to perform prophylactic thyroidectomy and to begin biochemical testing for phenochromocytoma and hyperparathyroidism.[5]

The 2 children had presymptomatic testing for the same mutation as the father; the son had the same mutation, and the daughter did not. Because the son inherited the mutation, he had a preventive total thyroidectomy at age 10 years, and histopathology revealed there was no evidence of medullary thyroid carcinoma. The right lower parathyroid was also removed. He continued to be under surveillance for hyperparathyroidism and pheochromocytoma.

When the son turned 18 years old, he developed severe headaches, disorientation, and nausea associated with heavy exercise. He was found to have elevated vanillylmandelic acid and elevated urinary metanephrines. Magnetic resonance imaging of the abdomen revealed a small adrenal mass and 123I-MIBG scanning showed uptake in the left adrenal. A 1.5-cm pheochromocytoma was removed from the left adrenal gland. His symptoms of flushing during exercise remitted, and all the labs normalized. He continues to be monitored because of the possibility of bilateral pheochromocytoma.

This family illustrates the role of genotyping for an autosomal dominant genetic disorder, and the benefits of testing at-risk members, even children, presymptomatically. The son, with the same mutation as the father, had prophylactic thyroidectomy at age 10 years. Most (95%) individuals with MEN2A eventually develop medullary thyroid cancer with a risk of metastases if the thyroid gland is not removed. The son was also monitored for a potential pheochromocytoma (50% risk), which he did develop at age 18 years. Genotyping was also helpful for the daughter, because she no longer needed further monitoring, and she does not have an increased risk for her future children to have MEN2A. The paternal aunt elected not to have genetic testing because she assumed she had the same MEN2A mutation. She had her thyroid gland removed after abnormal calcitonin tests; she was found to have medullary thyroid cancer and she was also given the clinical diagnosis of MEN2A. Monitoring guidelines for MEN2A can be found at www.genetests.org.

Example 5: Classic Genetic Prenatal Testing

While pregnant, a woman found out that her father tested positive for a well-described mutation of the *KCNH2* gene for long QT syndrome. He had a history of a cardiac arrest, which occurred several years prior while he was asleep and had a nightmare. Fortunately, he was able to get emergency care right away and he survived. He began taking β-blocker medication, and a pacemaker was placed.

Because of the risks of arrhythmia during delivery associated with long QT syndrome, the pregnant woman asked to also have genetic testing for the same mutation since she was at a 50% risk. She was found to also have the same mutation, despite several previous electrocardiograms that were normal and no history of syncopal episodes. She was started on a β-blocker

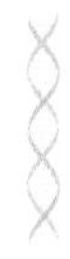

medication during her pregnancy and monitored closely during the delivery of her baby. After her son was born, he was also tested, and he had the same mutation. He too was placed on a β-blocker at about 1 year of age.

This example illustrates an autosomal dominant condition with variable expression/incomplete penetrance and the importance of genetic testing in a condition with preventive, potentially life-saving therapies.

Example 6: Genotyping to Prevent Side Effects Prior to Starting Therapy

Tegretol (carbamazapine) is a drug used to treat epilepsy, bipolar disorder, and neuropathic pain. In 2007 the US Food and Drug Administration (FDA) issued the recommendation to all physicians to test patients of Asian ancestry, including South Asian Indians, for HLA-B*1502 before administering Tegretol therapy. Therefore, prior to deciding to start Tegretol in a patient of Asian background, the pediatrician sent for genotyping for the HLA allele, HLA-B*1502. This genotype was present in the patient, and the pediatrician decided to choose another drug because of the patient's increased risk to develop Stevens-Johnson syndrome. Keep in mind that HLA testing for carbamazepine therapy is population-specific and not 100% specific; most patients who actually have the HLA-B*1502 genotype do not necessarily develop Stevens-Johnson syndrome. A resource for similar drug interactions is www.pharmgkb.org/.

Example 7: Genotyping to Determine Recurrence Risk

A 35-year-old woman is interested in knowing if there is a genetic basis to her moderate to severe nonprogressive bilateral sensorineural hearing loss (SNHL) as she prepares for her first pregnancy. As a newborn infant she had a urinary tract infection and was treated with gentamicin for 5 days. She says that her mother noticed that her hearing may not have been normal as early as 16 months; her mother had told the doctor that she did not turn her head when she was called in kindergarten. She was formally diagnosed to have SNHL at the age of 5 years. She started wearing a left hearing aid at age 5 years and bilateral hearing aids at 18 years. She has a "cookie-cutter" pattern to her audiograms, indicating loss at mid-frequencies. She denies any other health problems. Interestingly, when a family history was obtained, she has only one sister, and she also has bilateral hearing aids for SNHL diagnosed in childhood. This sister has one son with normal hearing. Her mother has adult-onset mild hearing loss and her father has normal hearing. Her husband does not have hearing loss. Options for genetic testing were explored.

Nonsyndromic mitochondrial hearing loss and deafness is characterized by moderate-to-profound hearing loss and a mutation in either *MT-RNR1* or *MT-TS1*. Mutations in *MT-RNR1* can be associated with predisposition to aminoglycoside ototoxicity and/or late-onset SNHL. Mutations in *MT-TS1* are usually associated with childhood onset of SNHL. Hearing loss associated with aminoglycoside ototoxicity is bilateral and severe to profound, occurring within a few days to weeks after administration of any amount (even a single dose) of an aminoglycoside antibiotic such as gentamycin, tobramycin, amikacin, kanamycin, or streptomycin.[6] Results of this testing were negative; therefore, she is less likely to have a maternally inherited aminoglycoside susceptibility as an etiology for her hearing loss.

Since she also has a sister with SNHL, the most common autosomal recessive form of hearing loss was next pursued. She was offered *GJB2* and *GJB6* (connexin 26 and 30 genes or gap junction beta 2 and 6) testing for the *DFNB1* locus-specific hearing loss. She was found to have 2 mutations of the *GJB2* gene: c.299-300delAT and c.235delC. This is useful information for her and her sister to know, as she now knows she has a generally prelingual, stable mild to severe-to-profound autosomal recessive form of hearing loss. Her recurrence risk would be low if her husband is not a carrier of a mutation in the same gene. Based on this information, she feels she would be unlikely to be interested in future prenatal genetic testing for her future children.

Example 8: Genotyping in Celiac Disease and HLA-DQ Typing (Not Usually Recommended)

A mother has the clinical diagnosis of celiac disease. She asks whether her newborn son can have any genetic testing to see if he will develop celiac disease. After much discussion with her pediatrician, who does not recommend presymptomatic testing, she agreed to have her son followed clinically.

The diagnosis of celiac disease relies on characteristic histologic findings on small-bowel biopsy and clinical and/or histologic improvement on a gluten-free diet. Most individuals with celiac disease have celiac disease–associated antibodies and specific pairs of allelic variants in 2 HLA genes: *HLA-DQA1* and *HLA-DQB1*. Because 30% of the general population has one of the celiac disease–associated HLA alleles and only 3% of individuals with one or both of these alleles develop celiac disease, presence of celiac disease–associated HLA alleles is not diagnostic of celiac disease; however, their absence essentially excludes a diagnosis of celiac disease.

Pharmacogenomics

Application of pharmacogenomics to the personalized medicine model is one area that shows great promise.[7–9] With time, targeting specific drugs to specific genotypes will be more widely applied and relevant, particularly in the treatments for cancer and neurologic and psychiatric disorders. The FDA has revised drug labels to reflect relevant pharmacogenetic information and recommendations for consideration of genotyping for certain drugs. See Table 19-1 (and Chapter 20) for some of the associations that have been investigated for children.

Table 19-1. Genotyping and Responses to Specific Drugs[a]

Test for Genotyping	Indication	Uses
Thiopurine S-methyltransferase for thiopurine metabolism	Immunosuppressant for inflammatory bowel disease, rheumatoid arthritis, and other immune disorders; ALL	Adjust starting dose
Valproic acid	Epilepsy, bipolar disorder, migraines	Prevent hepatotoxicity
Methotrexate pathway	Juvenile idiopathic arthritis	Predict response or toxicity
Vincristine/CYP3A5	ALL	Neurotoxicity

[a] From Egbelakin A, Ferguson MJ, MacGill EA, et al. Increased risk of vincristine neurotoxicity associated with low CYP3A5 expression genotype in children with acute lymphoblastic leukemia. *Pediatr Blood Cancer.* 2011;56:361–367; Relling MV, Gardner EE, Sandborn WJ, et al. Clinical pharmacogenetics implementation consortium guidelines for thiopurine methyltransferase genotype and thiopurine dosing. *Clin Pharmacol Ther.* 2011;89:387–391.

Genome-Wide Association Study

A genome-wide association study (GWAS) is a widely used approach to look for specific genetic variations associated with particular common diseases. This method involves scanning the entire genome from hundreds to thousands of different individuals, seeking genetic markers that can be used to predict the presence of a disease. To carry out a GWAS, researchers use 2 groups of participants: people with the disease and similar people without the disease. Researchers obtain DNA from each participant, usually from a blood, saliva, or buccal sample. Each person's complete set of DNA, or genome, is then purified and placed on tiny chips and scanned on automated laboratory machines. The machines quickly survey each participant's genome for strategically selected markers of genetic variation, which are called single nucleotide polymorphisms (SNPs).

If certain genetic variations are found to be significantly more frequent in people with the disease compared with people without disease, the variations are said to be associated with the disease. The associated genetic variations can serve as powerful pointers to the region of the human genome where the disease-causing problem resides. Therefore, GWASs are case-control studies in which genetic variation, often measured as SNPs that form haplotypes (set of closely linked markers on one chromosome that tend to be inherited together) across the entire genome, are compared between people with a particular condition and unaffected individuals.

One must keep in mind that the associated variants themselves may not directly cause the disease. They may just be tagging along with the actual causal variants and are indirectly involved with the disease. For this reason, researchers often need to take additional steps, such as sequencing DNA base pairs in that particular region of the genome, to identify the exact genetic change involved in the disease.

The GWASs have contributed to our understanding of associations for Kawasaki disease.[10] In one study, 2 loci have been associated with Kawasaki disease. The *FCGR2A* gene may not be directly responsible for Kawasaki disease, but its sequence (or polymorphisms) may somehow be associated with susceptibility for Kawasaki disease.

SNP Genotyping and Arrays

Single nucleotide polymorphism genotyping involves scanning the entire genome, searching for patterns of variation that are linked to disease susceptibility or drug response. Single nucleotide polymorphisms are usually single nucleotides that are a product of copy errors. Single nucleotide polymorphisms can be a measure of genetic similarity or diversity, and can give predictions about appearance, disease susceptibility, or response to drugs. While some SNPs lead to differences in health or physical appearance, most SNPs seem to lead to no observable differences between people at all.

The human genome is thought to contain more than 10 million SNPs, about one in every 300 bases. Single nucleotide polymorphisms are by far the most common source of genetic variation. It is now possible to analyze patient samples by using whole genome scans to look at 1 million or more SNPs across the genome (often using array platforms). Results are given to patients in terms of odds ratios, relative risks, adjusted lifetime risk, and a comparison risk, matched for ethnic group and sex. A personalized medical genomic profile looking at SNP associations can be obtained for a large number of conditions such as celiac disease *(HLA-DQA1),* Crohn disease, type 1 diabetes, and altered drug metabolism for genes/enzymes (CYP2C19, CYP2C9, VKORC1, TPMT, DPYD, UGT1A1, CYP3A5, NAT2, ABCB1). At this time, there are no profiles or panels specifically designed for children. No recommendations or regulation about SNP genotyping for children presently exist. Caution must be exercised regarding the ethical and social implications of such highly complex genetic testing for children, although statements and policies about genetic testing in minors in general are available for reference.[11–14] See Chapters 11 and 15.

A massive study, the 1,000 Genomes Project, is underway to sequence and delineate SNPs from 1,000 genomes to provide a catalog of human genetic variation.[15] Studies like these enable us to better understand the 1% of the variations in our genomes, which make each person unique and provide the basis for personalized medicine.

Chromosome (Karyotype) Analysis and Array Comparative Genomic Hybridization

Array comparative genomic hybridization (CGH) is a genetic test that is based on looking at chromosome rearrangements on a larger scale. A routine chromosome analysis can detect large deletions, duplications, marker chromosomes, and balanced and unbalanced rearrangements. Array CGH, a more precise test, will only pick up deletions and duplications and imbalances (not balanced translocations), and determine the size of the imbalances and which genes are involved in the imbalances.

Quantitative Time-Dependent Measurements

Quantitative methods have been studied in the pediatric population for diagnosing acute respiratory infections.[16] A very precise and quantitative measurement is performed, calculating the number of infectious particles accumulated in a set amount of time, and is expressed as copy number, or the logarithm of change from a baseline amount. Real time polymerase chain reaction is the method of choice when the copy number of a gene can be measured quantitatively, particularly when measuring pre- and post-treatments, such as cancer treatments.

Linkage Analysis

Linkage analysis is occasionally used to track genetic variation in multiple family members in different generations. The more members of the family there are to study, the more powerful the linkage analysis is.

Gene Expression Assays

Gene expression assays are measurements of RNA levels and function (transcription) that have started to elucidate the role of the "transcriptome." In the cancer field, gene expression arrays have been useful clinically, primarily in the adult population, but will likely be more widely used in the pediatric age group in the future.

Functional Protein Assays

Functional protein analysis looks at the structure or function of a particular gene product. There is currently limited clinical testing available to look at protein structure and function for a few genetic conditions, such as fragile X syndrome. Affected individuals with deletions in *FMR1* have been shown to have low or no levels of FMR protein, which causes fragile X syndrome.

Whole Exome Sequencing

Whole exome sequencing involves sequencing the coding regions and exon-intron junctions of genes. New genes for certain disorders can be discovered by this method. An example of this technique would be the identification of truncating mutations in human gene *SERPINF1* in an autosomal recessive form of osteogenesis imperfecta.[17] This technique is most useful when multiple genes are sequenced simultaneously, and all the exons are sequenced, generating a lot of data in a short time.

Whole Genome Sequencing

Individuals can have most of their genome completely sequenced, but this is not standard of care yet. Whole genome scanning, while potentially generating a lot of data, poses many medical, ethical, legal, and social challenges when testing adults[18] and even more so for children. The cost to sequence 3 billion bases as a routine clinical test is prohibitively high despite the fact that sequencing costs have decreased by 100,000-fold. A $10 million prize, the Archon X Prize for Genomics, will be awarded to the first team that can build a device and use it to sequence 100 human genomes for $10,000 within 10 days.[19] And there is a race for companies or laboratories to be able to offer the "$1,000 genome," which also will give us more ethnicity-specific information.[20]

No doubt, the cost of sequencing will decrease even further. Up to now, sequencing an adult human genome has been restricted to prominent genetic researchers at biopharmaceutical companies and academic research centers, famous leaders, individuals participating in research, and those who can afford to pay out of pocket. The time will come when whole genome sequencing will be more affordable and accessible.

Specialized Genetic Tests

Specialized genetic tests include epigenetic tests, such as methylation analysis, uniparental studies using SNP arrays or DNA variable number of trinucleotide repeat markers,[21] and telomere length testing. Shorter telomere length is reported to be a marker of biological aging and can increase susceptibility to age-related diseases.[22] Shorter telomeres have been implicated with some cardiovascular disorders and an increased risk of melanoma.[23]

Role and Use of Family History Information for Individualized Care

Family history may still be the determining factor as to which families or individuals are at highest risk for whom testing or intervention would be helpful. Appropriate screening, targeted education, preventive efforts, and genetic counseling can be personalized once family history is obtained. Even with current sophisticated technology, a family history remains the critical element and crucial starting point of a pediatric visit to identify individuals at risk for genetic disorders and should be used in combination with any genotypic data. For some conditions and situations, family history may be the absolute best predictor of the disease or risks. Use of the family history allows clinicians to classify individuals into different risk categories: average, moderate, and high (Figure 19-1). Family history ideally should be obtained from an adult contemplating starting a family prior to a pregnancy (sometimes with the help of a geneticist or genetic counselor), again at a prenatal visit, again at a child's first pediatric visit,[24] and then updated at all subsequent pediatric visits, perhaps annually. Much of the family history can be obtained by the patient or parents in advance of the visit if the right questions are asked ahead of time. Genetic counselors and geneticists should be used as resources. See Chapter 5 for more on the role of family history.

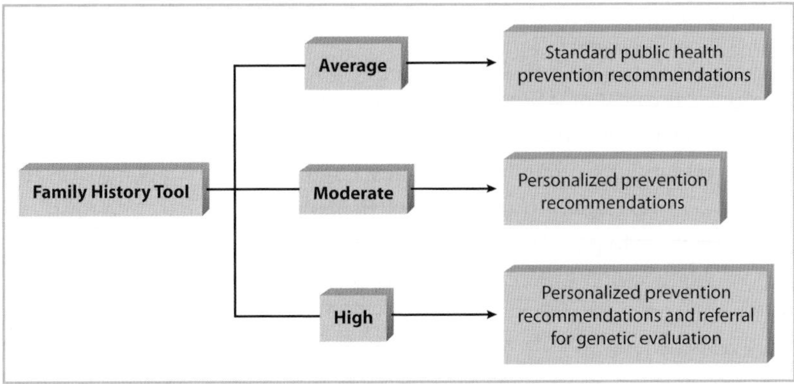

Figure 19-1. Risk classification. From www.nchpeg.org (Family History slide set).

Limitations of Genetic Testing and Caution

Limitations of genetic testing should be well understood before embarking on the testing. Ethical considerations need to be well thought out.[25] Knowing which laboratories to use and why certain methods are used (and in which order to do the testing) takes some knowledge and planning. If a diagnosis is certain based on clinical grounds and molecular confirmation does not change management, there may be no need to offer mutation testing, unless future prenatal testing for parents becomes important. Mutation testing has some important roles, but it is not always necessary. It is important to know that no genetic testing will identify 100% of the mutations for a genetic condition. If a negative or uninformative result is obtained, there needs to be a good understanding of what this means. Fortunately, geneticists, laboratory directors, and genetic counselors can be used as resources.

Interpretation of the results of genetic testing can be complex and may not be black and white. The results of genetic testing, whether it is a specific known pathogenic mutation, a risk calculation, an association, or a variant of unknown clinical significance, can pose dilemmas regarding whether or not the results are a direct cause of a medical condition. Sometimes this cannot be sorted out, even after testing multiple family members or performing additional testing. Sometimes a genetic result may become more interpretable with time. And it is important not to overestimate the predictive power of a certain result. One of the biggest hurdles is that the clinical utility may not have been established. Until large-scale studies are done, results may remain unclear, especially if results are based on only certain ethnic groups. One must be cautioned against overinterpreting genetic results; genetic heterogeneity or variation may play a larger role than we can predict. One must always remember that an individual can coincidentally have more than one genetic condition, or presumed modifier genes can play a role, causing symptoms to be either more or less severe than what is predicted by genotyping. Also, nonpenetrance of a genetic condition in an individual in a family should always be considered. Misattributed paternity (also known as non-paternity) could potentially be uncovered and should be addressed in the most sensitive and appropriate way.

Interpretation of a result, whether a pathogenic mutation, negative, or variant of unknown clinical significance, could change with time as more information becomes available. There have been instances in which a result is interpreted as pathogenic only to be reclassified later as a polymorphism (not clinically significant) once more individuals have been sequenced for that gene, and discovery that the sequence change is more common than originally thought.

Surveillance guidelines for certain medical conditions should be well understood by the patient in the context of the existing medical literature. Understanding the genetic contributions to traits or conditions allows a family to realize what cannot be changed (genes inherited) and what can be changed (environmental factors; diet; lifestyle; medical surveillance for conditions; deciding which genetic tests to do; treatments; medications; other therapies; attitude; choice of job, careers, or schools; whether or not to have more children) and ultimately leads to better acceptance. Identifying at-risk family members for a genetic condition may clarify misunderstandings and potentially be life-saving or at least life-prolonging; on the other hand, identifying family members who did not inherit a particular gene will provide much relief and save time and money on unnecessary monitoring and doctor visits.

Products are being offered to those individuals identified as at-risk to help lower certain health risks with supplements, vitamins, or medications. It can be difficult to sort out which recommendations are backed by solid medical evidence in well-controlled studies and which ones are not. Clinical geneticists and genetic counselors can be consulted.

Direct to Consumer (DTC) Testing

These are genetic tests that are marketed directly to consumers via television, print advertisements, or the Internet. This form of testing, which is also known as at-home genetic testing, provides access to a person's genetic information without necessarily involving a doctor or insurance company in the process. For a list of companies offering DTC testing, go to www.dnapolicy.org/resources/DTCcompanieslist.pdf. For more information on the definition of DTC testing and additional references, go to www.ghr.nlm.nih.gov/handbook/testing/directtoconsumer.

Single nucleotide polymorphism genotyping can scan 500,000 to 1 million DNA variant markers from a blood sample, a saliva sample, or cheek (buccal) swab that is mailed in a test kit. A calculation of a set of disease risks based on the patient's or customer's specific combination of markers can be given online, or in the privacy of an individual's own home. Face-to-face meetings may not be necessary as long as there is adequate education and communication before and after testing and ongoing into the future. Some companies offer monthly updates about new tests or interpretations once testing has been done. The larger question is whether shotgun testing is necessary or cost-effective, or helps to improve quality of life. More information does not always translate into better clinical management and potentially can cause anxiety.[26,27]

A genetic test at a minimum needs to be accurate, replicable, and precise.[28] Pros and cons of DTC testing are listed in Box 19-2. Also see the fact sheet, At-Home Genetic Tests: A Healthy Dose of Skepticism May Be the Best Prescription, from the Federal Trade Commission at www.ftc.gov/bcp/edu/pubs/consumer/health/hea02.pdf. Transparency, provider education, and test and laboratory quality have been addressed in an American Society of Human Genetics statement on DTC testing in the United States.[29]

The 2008 American College of Medical Genetics and Genomics policy statement on DTC testing[30] recommends (1) a knowledgeable professional should be involved in the process of ordering and interpreting a genetic test; (2) the consumer should be fully informed regarding what the test can and cannot say about his or her health; (3) the scientific evidence on which a test is based should be clearly stated; (4) the clinical testing laboratory must be accredited by Clinical Laboratory Improvement Amendments, the state, and/or other applicable accrediting agencies; and (5) privacy concerns must be addressed. These statements recommend involving trained clinical genetics professionals in the genetic testing process, and for consumers to have accurate information both pre- and post-testing (Box 19-3).

There are claims from DTC companies that genetic testing can uncover your ancestry. Certainly this is an area of increasing public interest, and we need more recommendations for facilitating the development of scientifically based, ethically sound, and socially attentive guidelines

Box 19-2. Advantages and Disadvantages of Direct-to-Consumer Testing

Advantages

- Tests are accessible to consumers directly and there is some choice as to the particular test or "package" desired.
- Promotes proactive health care.
- Significant health risks may be identified that would not have been identified otherwise, allowing for some interventions.
- Public education and awareness of the role genes can play in the development of common diseases.
- Some companies provide detailed patient education materials on many common conditions and updated communication for further testing.
- Allows for privacy of genetic information to the consumer.

Disadvantages or Limitations

- Test results may come from a non–Clinical Laboratory Improvement Amendments–certified laboratory and therefore are not well standardized.
- Test interpretation may not be based on peer-reviewed results that have been replicated.
- False sense of security for conditions with environmental risk factors.
- Lack of government regulation.
- No physician or genetic counselor involvement required and more chance for misinterpretation of results.
- Patients may be misled about the significance of the results or about the possible proactive treatments and thus harm could potentially occur.
- Privacy may still be an issue as research involvement is often required.
- Patients may be told they are at risk for conditions with no interventions available.
- Testing may cause more anxiety.
- Different sets of markers or single nucleotide polymorphisms are used in different laboratories.
- Testing of children is sometimes available. Some companies even accept cord blood for testing.

Box 19-3. Questions to Ask About Direct-to-Consumer (DTC) Testing

- How are risks defined? Absolute risk, or the probability that an individual will develop a disease, is reported by some DTC companies. Absolute risk is derived from "relative risk" and "average population risk." Population risk can be gender-, age-, or ancestry-dependent. In one study for 7 diseases, 50% or less of the predictions of 2 companies agreed across 5 individuals. Genetic composite index, relative lifetime risk, relative risk, and odds ratios, or risk relative to a reference population, are reported in some results.
- What set of markers are chosen for a particular condition in the calculation of relative risks? Or, for mutation-based scans, which particular mutations are looked for, and if negative, what are the residual risks? And with the use of markers that have been discovered by genome-wide association studies, how do they explain the genetic heritability of the disease?
- How meaningful are results that show a 0.5 to 2.0 times relative risk?
- How can parents and the general public become more educated about the interpretation of genetic tests?
- Are results confirmed in a Clinical Laboratory Improvement Amendments–certified laboratory and what regulatory standards need to be followed to ensure excellence in the quality and service of the laboratory conducting the testing?

concerning the use of continually evolving technologies to address ancestry testing and its implications.[31,32]

Promises and Hopes: Directions for the Future of Personalized Medicine

It is estimated that before long there will be 30,000 whole human genome sequences available in the databases that can be accessed and used for clinical and research purposes. Future studies include carrying out more prospective studies, replicating associated markers in other ethnicities, establishing clinical utility, and more whole genome sequencing rather than genotyping individual genes. It is too soon to interpret and come up with completely personalized and clear-cut guidelines about monitoring or treatment for many genetic disorders without more data from larger studies. It would be dangerous to draw major conclusions about clinical utility and health impact at this juncture; in the future there may very well be a role for these types of genome scans and associations as more knowledge is available. Evaluation of Genomic Applications in Practice and Prevention (EGAPP) is an initiative launched in 2004 to support a coordinated, systematic process for evaluating genetic tests and other genomic applications that are in transition from research to clinical and

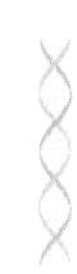

public health practice in the United States. An independent, non-federal EGAPP Working Group, a multidisciplinary expert panel, selects topics, oversees the systematic review of evidence, and makes recommendations based on that evidence.[33] Additional information is also given in recommendations from a multidisciplinary workshop convened by the National Institutes of Health and Centers for Disease Control and Prevention.[34]

Particularly for children, personalized genomic testing is not yet appropriate for clinical application except perhaps in the arena of pediatric oncology. Parents will have to make more and more decisions about how much information they want to know about the genetic risks of their children and, as pediatricians, we have to know how to respond.[35,36]

Key Points

- Personalized medicine is an emerging and rapidly evolving practice of medicine that uses an individual's genetic profile and unique genomic variations to guide decisions made in regard to the prevention, diagnosis, and treatment of disease. Personalized medicine is being advanced through data from the Human Genome Project (www.genome.gov).
- The hope of personalized medicine is that knowledge of a patient's genetic profile can help doctors select the proper medication therapy, administer treatment using the proper dose or regimen, motivate the patient to change his or her lifestyle, and make targeted recommendations based on the genomic testing. The goal is to give the right patient the right dose and treatment at the right time and to minimize trial and error treatments.
- Pediatricians should be well informed about the resources, tests, and tools available to practice personalized medicine. Preventive measures, early treatment, and lifestyle changes ideally should start during childhood.
- The rationale for genotyping is to improve clinical management, prevent adverse drug reactions, and optimize those factors that can be changed or controlled.
- Obtaining an accurate family history and combining it with useful genomic information about a patient is ultimately the best way to interpret genetic risks.

References

1. Ashley EA, Butte AJ, Wheeler MT, et al. Clinical assessment incorporating a personal genome. *Lancet.* 2010;375:1525–1535

2. Grosse SD, McBride CM, Evans JP, Khoury MJ. Personal utility and genomic information: look before you leap. *Genet Med.* 2009;11(8):575–576
3. Ramsey BW, Davies J, McElvaney NG, et al. A CFTR potentiator in patients with cystic fibrosis and the G551D mutation. *N Engl J Med.* 2011;365:1663–1672
4. National Center for Biotechnology Information. Online Mendelian Inheritance of Man. http://www.ncbi.nlm.nih.gov/omim
5. Moline J, Eng C. Multiple endocrine neoplasia type 2. In: Pagon RA, Bird TD, Dolan CR, Stephens K, Adam MP, eds. *GeneReviews* [Internet]. Seattle, WA: University of Washington, Seattle. www.ncbi.nlm.nih.gov/books/NBK1257. Published September 27, 1999. Updated January 10, 2013. Accessed March 22, 2013
6. GeneTests. www.genetests.org
7. Scott SA. Personalizing medicine with clinical pharmacogenetics. *Genet Med.* 2011;13:987–995
8. Conti R, Veenstra DL, Armstrong K, Lesko LJ, Grosse SD. Personalized medicine and genomics: challenges and opportunities in assessing effectiveness, cost-effectiveness, and future research priorities. *Med Decis Making.* 2010;30:328–340
9. Manolopoulos VG, Dechairo B, Huriez A, et al. Pharmacogenomics and personalized medicine in clinical practice. *Pharmacogenomics.* 2010;12:597–510
10. Khor CC, Davila S, Breunis WB, et al. Genome-wide association study identifies FCGR2A as a susceptibility locus for Kawasaki disease. *Nat Genet.* 2011;43(12): 1241–1246
11. American College of Medical Genetics. Points to consider in preventing unfair discrimination based on genetic disease risk: a position statement of the American College of Medical Genetics. 2001. http://www.acmg.net/StaticContent/StaticPages/Discrimination.pdf
12. American College of Medical Genetics, American Society of Human Genetics. Report: points to consider: ethical legal and psychosocial implications of genetic testing in children and adolescents. *Am J Hum Genet.* 1995;57:1233–1241
13. American College of Obstetricians and Gynecologists Committee on Ethics, Committee on Genetics. Ethical issues in genetic testing. *ACOG Comm Opin.* 2008;410. http://www.acog.org/Resources_And_Publications/Committee_Opinions/Committee_on_Ethics/Ethical_Issues_in_Genetic_Testing
14. Genetic Information Nondiscrimination Act (GINA), 2008. www.genome.gov/10002328
15. 1000 Genomes: A Deep Catalog of Human Genetic Variation. Web site. www.1000genomes.org
16. Wishaupt JO, Russcher A, Smeets LC, Versteegh FG, Hartwig NG. Clinical impact of RT-PCR for pediatric acute respiratory infections: a controlled clinical trial. *Pediatrics.* 2011;128:e1113–1120
17. Becker J, Semler O, Gilissen C, et al. Exome sequencing identifies truncating mutations in human SERPINF1 in autosomal recessive osteogenesis imperfecta. *Am J Hum Genet.* 2011;88:362–371
18. Ali-Khan SE, Daar AS, Shuman C, Ray PN, Scherer SW. Whole genome scanning: resolving clinical diagnosis and management amidst complex data. *Pediatr Res.* 2009;66:357–363
19. Archon Genomics. X Prize Web site. http://genomics.xprize.org
20. Davies K. *The $1000 Genome: The Revolution in DNA Sequencing and the New Era of Personalized Medicine.* New York, NY: Free Press; 2010

21. Shaffer LG, Agan N, Goldberg JD, Ledbetter DH, Longshore JW, Cassidy SB. American College of Medical Genetics statement on diagnostic testing for uniparental disomy. *Genet Med.* 2001;3:206–211
22. Aubert G, Lansdorp PJ. Telomeres and aging. *Physiol Res.* 2008;88:557–579
23. Nan H, Qureshi AA, Prescott J, De Vivo I, Han J. Genetic variants in telomere-maintaining genes and skin cancer risk. *Hum Genet.* 2011;129:247–253
24. Trotter TL, Martin HM. Family history in pediatric primary care. *Pediatrics.* 2007;120(suppl 2):560–565
25. American College of Obstetricians and Gynecologists. Ethical issues in genetic testing. ACOG Committee Opinion No. 410. *Obstet Gynecol.* 2008;111:1495–1502
26. Hunter DJ, Khoury MJ, Drazen JM. Letting the genome out of the bottle–will we get our wish? *N Engl J Med.* 2008;358:105–107
27. Evans JP, Green RC. Direct to consumer genetic testing: avoiding a culture war. *Genet Med.* 2009;11:568–569
28. Ng PC, Murray SS, Levy S, Venter JC. An agenda for personalized medicine. *Nature.* 2009;461:724–726
29. Hudson K, Javitt G, Burke W, Byers P; ASHG Social Issues Committee. ASHG statement on direct-to-consumer genetic testing in the United States. *Am J Hum Genet.* 2007;81:635–637
30. American College of Medical Genetics. ACMG statement on direct-to-consumer genetic testing. April 2008. American College of Medical Genetics Web site. www.acmg.net/StaticContent/StaticPages/DTC-statement.pdf. Published April 7, 2008. Accessed March 13, 2013
31. Royal CD, Novembre J, Fullerton SM, Goldstein DB, Bamshad MJ, Clark AG. Inferring genetic ancestry: opportunities, challenges, and implications. *Am J Hum Genet.* 2010;86:661–673
32. American Society of Human Genetics Ancestry Testing Statement 2008. www.ashg.org/pdf/ASHGAncestryTestingStatement_FINAL.pdf
33. Teutsch SM. The Evaluation of Genomic Applications in Practice and Prevention (EGAPP) initiative: methods of the EGAPP Working Group. *Genet Med.* 2009;11:3–14
34. Khoury MJ, McBride CM, Schully SD, et al. The scientific foundation for personal genomics: recommendations from a National Institutes of Health-Centers for disease control and prevention multidisciplinary workshop *Genet Med.* 2009;11:559–567
35. Collins F. Has the revolution arrived? *Nature* 2010;464:674–675
36. Personalized Medicine Coalition. PMC Web site. www.personalizedmedicinecoalition.org

Chapter 20

Pharmacogenomics

Brad T. Tinkle, MD, PhD

Introduction

Pharmacogenomics is the general study of the interindividual differences in reactions to medications, both positive and negative, that are influenced by genes.[1] Sometimes used interchangeably, pharmacogenetics is the use of such information to predict a person's response to a drug, including but not limited to absorption, metabolism, clearance, and excretion of said drug. Such predictive testing based on pharmacogenetic analysis may aid the practitioner in determining the effective dosage and possible likely side effects.

An individual's reaction to a specific drug is a complex trait that is influenced by age, body weight, other medications, and many different genes. The metabolism of certain medications has a stronger genetic influence than others (Table 20-1). Cytochrome P450 (CYP) is a very large family of heme-containing enzymes responsible for the breakdown of various medications and the conversion of pro-drugs. Cytochrome P450 is only one family of drug-metabolizing enzymes (DMEs), although it accounts overall for a large portion of the body's drug metabolism.

Variations in the DNA of the CYP genes can greatly influence an individual's ability to metabolize certain drugs. Wide variations include gene deletion, gene duplication, or small changes in genes called single nucleotide polymorphisms, many of which affect drug metabolism in incremental changes (Figure 20-1). Single nucleotide polymorphisms are sequence variations that occur when a single nucleotide (A, C, G, or T) in the gene sequence is altered. Missing or duplicated genes significantly affect a drug's metabolism. Individuals with predicted reduced DME activity may be referred to as poor metabolizers (PM) and those with increased activity as ultra-rapid metabolizers (UM). This wide range of enzymatic variation can account for an up to 1,000-fold difference in the plasma levels of certain drugs.

This wide variation of drug levels will affect therapeutic effectiveness and may result in adverse drug reactions (ADRs). Drugs whose metabolism is affected greatly by only a few genetic variations are more likely to have wider range of activity, including no therapeutic response to toxicity (Table 20-1). Therefore, the use of such genetic variations for such drugs may aid in the prediction of therapeutic response as well as ADRs. The predictive value in turn may be used to guide dosing or use of alternative therapies.

Table 20-1. Drug Metabolizing Enzymes and Clinically Relevant Drugs Significantly Impacted by Genetic Alterations

DME	Overall Drug Metabolizing Activity	Phenotypes	Drug Classes
CYP1A2	–	Whites: 12% PMs	• Antiarrhythmics (eg, mexiletine) • Antiemetics (eg, ondansetron) • Antipsychotics (eg, clozapine) • CCBs (eg, verapamil) • Muscle relaxants (eg, cyclobenzaprine, tizanidine) • SNRIs (eg, duloxetine) • SSRIs (eg, fluvoxamine) • TCAs (eg, clomipramine)
CYP2C9	~15%	Whites: 2%–6% PMs	• Anticoagulants (eg, warfarin) • Anticonvulsants (eg, mephenytoin, phenytoin) • Angiotensin II receptor blockers (eg, losartan) • β-blockers (eg, carvedilol) • Oncologics (eg, tamoxifen) • Oral hypoglycemic agents (eg, glimepiride, glipizide, tolbutamide) • SSRIs (eg, fluoxetine)

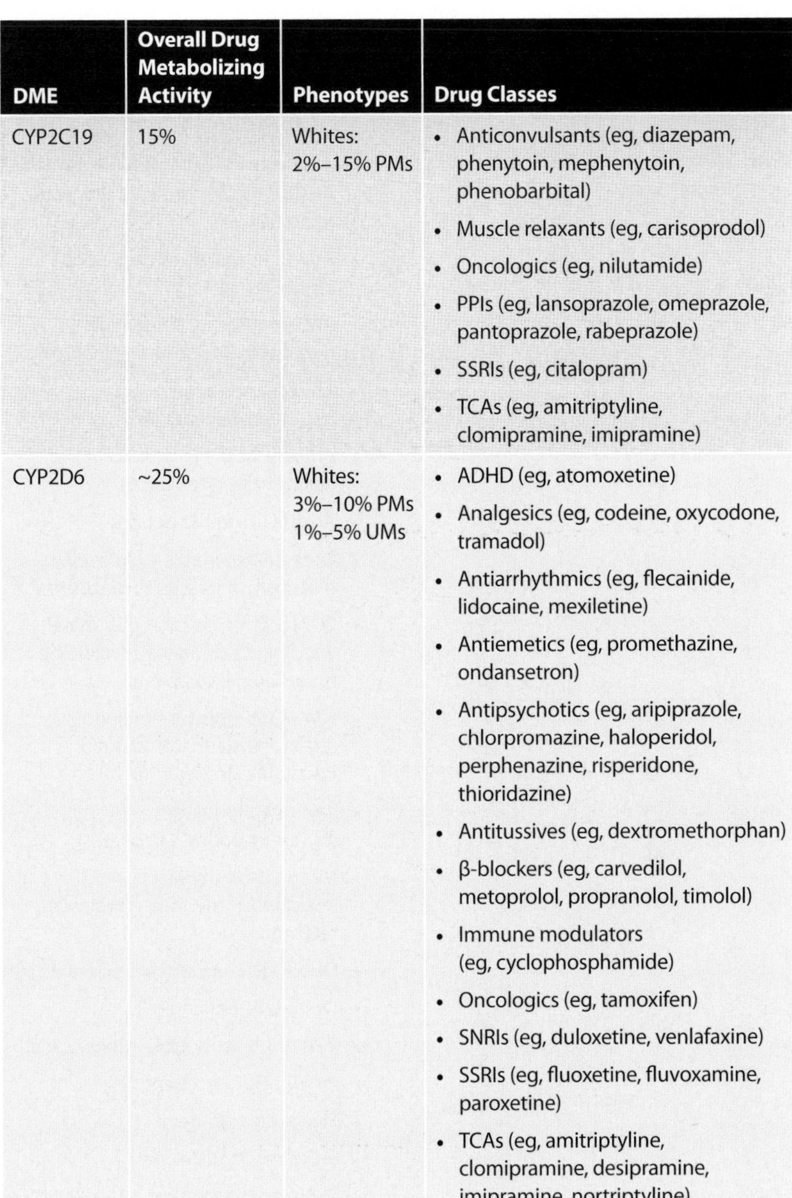

DME	Overall Drug Metabolizing Activity	Phenotypes	Drug Classes
CYP2C19	15%	Whites: 2%–15% PMs	• Anticonvulsants (eg, diazepam, phenytoin, mephenytoin, phenobarbital) • Muscle relaxants (eg, carisoprodol) • Oncologics (eg, nilutamide) • PPIs (eg, lansoprazole, omeprazole, pantoprazole, rabeprazole) • SSRIs (eg, citalopram) • TCAs (eg, amitriptyline, clomipramine, imipramine)
CYP2D6	~25%	Whites: 3%–10% PMs 1%–5% UMs	• ADHD (eg, atomoxetine) • Analgesics (eg, codeine, oxycodone, tramadol) • Antiarrhythmics (eg, flecainide, lidocaine, mexiletine) • Antiemetics (eg, promethazine, ondansetron) • Antipsychotics (eg, aripiprazole, chlorpromazine, haloperidol, perphenazine, risperidone, thioridazine) • Antitussives (eg, dextromethorphan) • β-blockers (eg, carvedilol, metoprolol, propranolol, timolol) • Immune modulators (eg, cyclophosphamide) • Oncologics (eg, tamoxifen) • SNRIs (eg, duloxetine, venlafaxine) • SSRIs (eg, fluoxetine, fluvoxamine, paroxetine) • TCAs (eg, amitriptyline, clomipramine, desipramine, imipramine, nortriptyline)

Table 20-1. Drug Metabolizing Enzymes and Clinically Relevant Drugs Significantly Impacted by Genetic Alterations *(cont)*

DME	Overall Drug Metabolizing Activity	Phenotypes	Drug Classes
CYP3A4/A5	~50%		• Analgesics (eg, fentanyl, lidocaine, methadone) • Angiotensin II receptor blockers (eg, losartan) • Antiemetics (eg, aprepitant, ondansetron) • Antihistamines (eg, chlorpheniramine) • Antipsychotics (eg, aripiprazole, haloperidol, quetiapine) • Anxiolytics (eg, buspirone) • Benzodiazepines (eg, alprazolam, diazepam, midazolam, triazolam) • CCBs (eg, amlodipine, diltiazem, felodipine, nifedipine, nisoldipine, nitrendipine, verapamil) • HMG CoA reductase inhibitors (eg, atorvastatin, cerivastatin, lovastatin, simvastatin) • Immune modulators (eg, cyclosporine, tacrolimus) • Macrolide antibiotics (eg, clarithromycin, erythromycin, telithromycin) • Oncologics (eg, tamoxifen, vincristine) • Opioids (eg, alfentanil) • PPIs (eg, lansoprazole, rabeprazole) • Prokinetics (eg, cisapride) • Sleep (eg, zolpidem) • SNRIs (eg, venlafaxine) • SSRIs (eg, citalopram)
TPMT	–	Whites: 1% PMs	• 6-mercaptopurine • 6-thioguanine • Azathioprine

Abbreviations: ADHD, attention-deficit/hyperactivity disorder; CCB, calcium channel blocker; DME, drug-metabolizing enzyme; HMG-CoA, 3-hydroxy-3-methylglutaryl-coenzyme A; PM, poor metabolizer; PPI, proton pump inhibitor; SNRI, serotonin/norepinephrine reuptake inhibitor; SSRI, selective serotonin reuptake inhibitor; TCA, tricyclic antidepressant; TPMT, thiopurine S-methyltransferase; UM, ultra-rapid metabolizer.

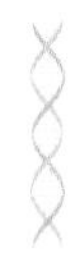

GCGCTAATTCGA CGCGATTAAGCT	GCGCAAATTCGA CGCGTTTAAGCT
The normal nucleotide sequence for gene *A*.	The nucleotide sequence showing a single nucleotide polymorphism (SNP) for gene *A*.

FIGURE 20-1. Nucleotide sequence alteration substituting an "A" in place of a "T" resulting in a single nucleotide polymorphism. Such an alteration can greatly affect drug metabolism.

Importance of Pharmacogenomics

In 1994 ADRs resulted in over 100,000 deaths and 2.2 million cases of serious adverse events as one of the leading causes of hospitalizations and deaths in the United States.[2] Therefore, iatrogenic disease has become one of the leading causes of morbidity and death. There is no easy method to determine how a particular person reacts to medications. Most will react as expected with good treatment effect with minimal side effects, which is sometimes referred to as the "one-size-fits-all" approach in drug development.[3] However, some individuals will experience little or no treatment effect while others will have major adverse reactions. Ideally, treatment is best individualized to maximize effectiveness while avoiding ADRs.

Specific Examples

Warfarin

Warfarin (Coumadin) is used for the prophylactic treatment of venous thrombosis, pulmonary embolism, and other thromboembolic events. It specifically interferes with the vitamin K–dependent metabolic pathways that are important in the synthesis of the clotting factors II, VII, IX, and X (Figure 20-2). In the United States, more than 2 million people receive warfarin. Unfortunately, side effects are common and severe side effects are experienced by approximately 1% of those taking warfarin. Dosing of warfarin is complicated by its nonlinear dose response and narrow therapeutic index. Factors affecting warfarin dosing include comorbid conditions (eg, liver disease), concurrent medications, dietary intake of vitamin K, age, body mass, and genetics. Inappropriate dosing can cause

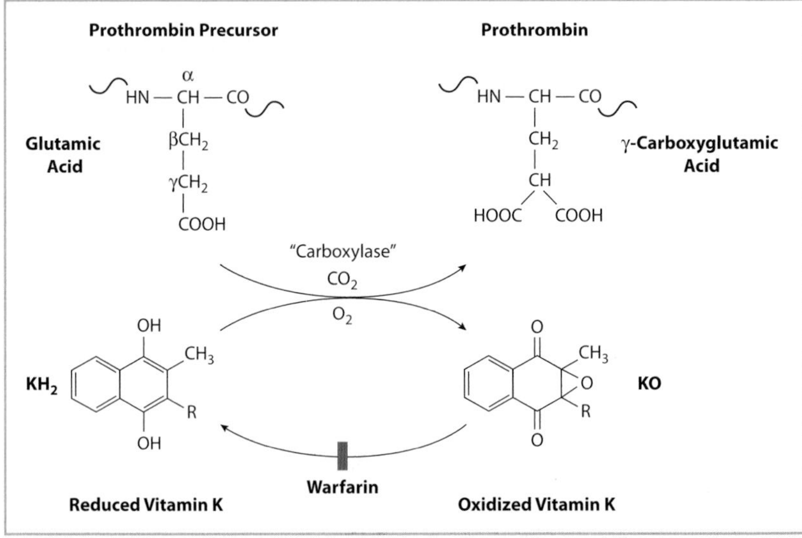

Figure 20-2. Vitamin K use in the making of a clotting factor and its inhibition by warfarin.

a fatal thrombosis when underdosed, and bleeding when overdosed. In 2010 the US Food and Drug Administration (FDA) updated the labeling of Coumadin to include pharmacogenomically guided dosing instructions.[4] Cytochrome P450 is the key enzyme that metabolizes and inactivates warfarin. Of the 3 common genetic (ie, allelic) variants, *CYP2C9*1* is the usual variant with normal activity, while *CYP2C9*2* has only 12% enzyme activity and *CYP2C9*3* has only 5% activity. Approximately 80% of the white population has the normal variant, but 20% has 1 of the 2 variants with decreased enzyme activity. To avoid improper dosing and the subsequent risk of bleeding, those with decreased enzyme activity ("poor metabolizers") require lower doses of warfarin (Table 20-2).

In a systematic review and a meta-analysis, Lindh et al[5] calculated the warfarin dose reduction prescribed for individual with the common variants of *CYP2C9*. Thirty-nine studies (7,907 patients) were included. Compared to the normal genotype (*CYP2C9*1/*1)* those persons with the *CYP2C9*1/*2, CYP2C9*1/*3, CYP2C9*2/*2, CYP2C9*2/*3*, and *CYP2C9*3/*3* genotypes required warfarin doses that were 19.6%, 33.7%, 36.0%, 56.7%, and 78.1% lower, respectively. Individuals with allelic variations resulting in reduced ability to metabolize warfarin are at significantly elevated risk of bleeding due to excessive anticoagulation.

Table 20-2. Warfarin Clearance by CYP2C9 Genotype[a]

CYP2C9 Genotype	Mean Warfarin Clearance (mL/min/kg) Mean (SD)
*1/*1	0.065 (0.025)
*1/*2 or *1/*3	0.041 (0.021)
*2/*2, *2/*3, or *3/*3	0.020 (0.011)

[a]Modified from Bristol-Meyers Squibb package insert for Coumadin.

Warfarin exerts its anticoagulant properties by interrupting the vitamin K regeneration cycle mediated by the enzyme vitamin K 2,3-epoxide reductase (VKOR). One of the subunits of the VKOR complex, VKORC1, has been associated with both warfarin sensitivity and resistance. The *VKORC1* gene has within it a common set of variations that affect the enzymatic activity level. The effects of these variations appear to be linear. Individuals homozygous for 2 variant *VKOR* genes are twice as sensitive as heterozygotes (one variant gene) when compared to the drug sensitivity of those homozygous for a normal *VKOR* gene.

Limdi et al[6] studied 521 patients (250 African Americans and 271 European Americans) who required warfarin treatment. Dose response in the rate of international normalized ratio (INR) change, number of dosage adjustments, and anticoagulation maintenance were correlated to *VKORC1* and *CYP2C9* variant status. Differences between the various variant groupings in the rate to attain target INR, number of dosage changes, and maintenance dosing were recorded (Figure 20-3).

Together, individuals with *VKORC1* and *CYP2C9* genetic variants have been reported to account for nearly half of the variability in warfarin dosing in whites. These variants both contribute independent information to help establish an appropriate warfarin dose. A slightly higher proportion of overall variability in warfarin dose is due to the presence of the *VKORC1* variant (20%–30%) than *CYP2C9* variant (~10%). This effect occurs mainly because the *VKORC1* variant associated with reduced dosage is more common in the white population. Other important factors needed to accurately predict an effective warfarin dose are body weight (9% of variability) and age (7% of variability). Altogether, genotyping data and physical attributes account for nearly 60% of the drug variability,[7] which can be used in an algorithm to predict warfarin dosage in adults.[8] Genotype-based dosing algorithms including variants of both *CYP2C9* and

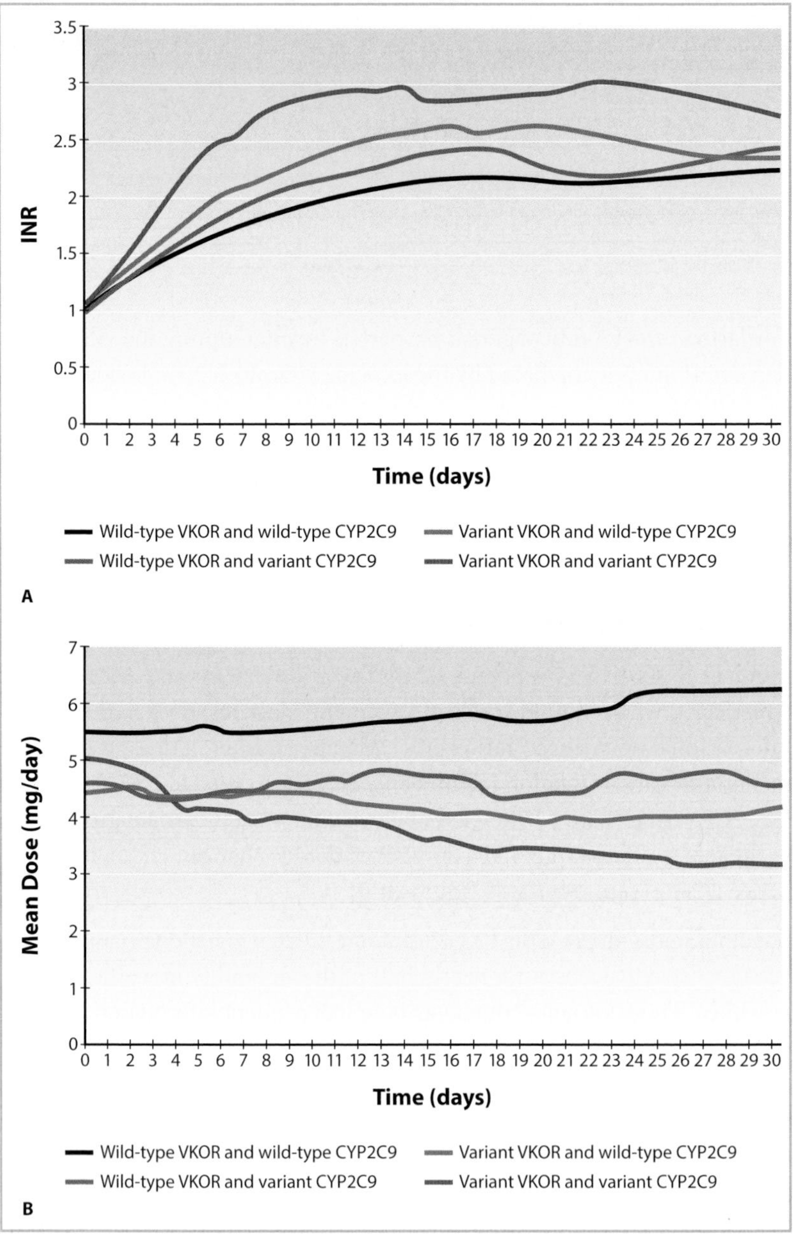

Figure 20-3. The combined effect of VKOR and CYP2C9 variants in the time to attain international normalized ratio and the mean dosage necessary. From Limdi et al. Influence of CYP2C9 and VKORC1 on warfarin response during initiation of therapy. *Blood Cell Mol Dis.* 2009;43:119–128, with permission from Elsevier.

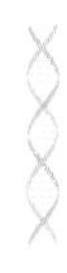

VKORC1 have been proposed and are being considered by the FDA with regard to recommendations for labeling changes to warfarin and for design and commercialization of associated diagnostic tests.[9]

Thiopurines

Most anticancer agents are enzymatically transformed into active, inactive, or toxic metabolites. Efficacy and adverse reactions are therefore related to the activity of enzymes that metabolize these drugs. A better understanding of the genetic and nongenetic factors that govern enzymatic activity is important to improve treatment outcome and safety.

An effective treatment for childhood leukemia includes the class of medications called thiopurines, and includes 6-mercaptopurine (6-MP), 6-thioguanine, and azathioprine. Thiopurines are pro-drugs that become active once processed to thioguanine nucleotides. Individuals with a poor ability to metabolize thiopurines run the risk of toxic doses of 6-MP and even death. The enzyme thiopurine S-methyltransferase plays an important part in the metabolism of these thiopurines. Unfortunately, about 1 in 300 whites has a genetic variation that prevents them from metabolizing these drugs, which causes accumulation of the thiopurines in the body in toxic levels. Currently, the FDA suggests that physicians be aware that pharmacogenetic testing is clinically available. Some clinicians currently use these tests in clinical practice.

Analgesics

The psychopharmacological treatment of pain is often unsatisfactory. The metabolism of multiple drugs from many different classes is significantly affected by genetic alterations in DMEs. These include nonsteroidals, cyclooxygenase-2 inhibitors, opioids, anticonvulsants, anxiolytics, antidepressants, neuroleptics, local anesthetics, and anti-migraine medications.

Codeine, for example, is a commonly prescribed opioid either alone or in combination. Some patients respond well to codeine while others may have little to no analgesic effect (PM), and some have increased sedation, respiratory depression, and even death (UM). Codeine is metabolized to morphine. Poor metabolizers with reduced *CYP2D6* activity may be at risk for little or no analgesia. Ultra-rapid metabolizers can have an equivalent to an overdosage of morphine.

Of particular relevance to pediatricians, the UM genotype in a mother given codeine postpartum for obstetrical pain has been associated with at least one neonatal death from central nervous system depression.[10] Moreover, severe neonatal toxicity in breastfeeding infants has been associated with the *CYP2D6* UM genotype in combination with *UGT2B7*2/*2*.[11] The latter is a variant in the enzyme uridyl glucuronyltransferase 2B7, which catalyzes the conversion of morphine to its active metabolite, morphine-6-glucuronide (M6G). The variant results in higher levels of M6G.

Serotonin Norepinephrine Reuptake Inhibitors (SNRIs)

Atomoxetine (Strattera) is an effective drug for attention-deficit/hyperactivity disorder. The precise mechanism by which atomoxetine produces its therapeutic effects is largely unknown, but is thought to be related to selective inhibition of the presynaptic norepinephrine transporter. It is extensively eliminated by oxidative metabolism through the *CYP2D6* pathway. A small fraction of whites (about 7%) and African Americans (2%) are poor metabolizers, resulting in a 5-fold higher peak plasma concentration and slower elimination phase of atomoxetine compared with people with normal enzymatic activity. Coadministration of atomoxetine with any potent inhibitor of *CYP2D6* (eg, fluoxetine or paroxetine) can also result in a substantial increase in atomoxetine plasma concentration. Therefore, the product's labeling includes a description from the FDA that pre-therapeutic pharmacogenetic testing be considered prior to initiating treatment with Strattera.

Antiepileptic Drugs (AEDs)

Genetic variation is known to play a role in both the clinical efficacy of AEDs as well as their tolerability and safety. Polymorphisms in the gene *ABCB1* (multidrug resistance 1) are known to impact the function of drug efflux transporters that are expressed in the gut, facilitating or inhibiting drug absorption. Bioavailability of phenytoin, carbamazepine, and valproate may be influenced by these variants. Moreover, these polymorphisms may play a role with respect to drug penetration of the blood-brain barrier and AED resistance.[12]

Antiepileptic drugs are one of the most common causes of cutaneous ADRs, ranging from mild maculopapular eruptions to Stevens-Johnson syndrome. Variants in inflammatory mediators, such as HLA and tumor necrosis factor, appear to play an important role in mediating cutaneous and systemic adverse reactions to this category of agent. For example HLA-B*1502 has shown strong association with carbamazepine-induced Stevens-Johnson syndrome in Asian individuals.[12–16]

Box 20-1. The Promise of Pharmacogenomics

- Facilitate drug discovery.
- Improve the development of better and safer drugs.
- Provide more accurate methods to determine the appropriate drug dosing.
- Aid in the advanced screening for disease potential.
- Aid in the development of better vaccines.
- Improve the safety and speed of drug trials.
- Decrease health care costs.

The Future of Pharmacogenomics

Pharmacogenomics holds promise for many aspects of medicine (Box 20-1).[1] Drug discovery and development takes approximately 8 to 10 years and costs several hundred million dollars on average.[17] Genetic screening can benefit drug development and testing by allowing the exclusion of those study participants who may react poorly to a given medication. Therefore, one of the promises of pharmacogenomics is safer, faster, and cheaper drug trials, yet comprehensive studies will still need to be done to ensure analysis of the individual variations.[18] Additionally, avoiding serious ADRs that result in hospitalization or even death, as well as reducing office visits for ineffective drug treatments, will improve medical care and reduce medical costs.

Drugs with a narrow therapeutic index (eg, warfarin, 6-MP) require close and frequent dosage adjustments to maintain efficacy while avoiding toxic side effects. Pharmacogenetic testing can be used to predict those individuals with a higher risk of ADRs and potentially guide dosing. Knowledge that an individual possesses a genotype that is associated with a high risk of ADR allows selection of alternative modes of treatment. Ultimately this saves lives and reduces the costs of medical care.

Effect of Pharmacogenomics on Prescription Writing

Pharmacogenomics has the potential to provide information ensuring that initial treatment will have less guesswork as far as the selection of the medication and its dosage. To achieve this potential, pharmacogenetic information needs to be readily available, ideally as point-of-care testing. While it is not the case currently, rapid technological advancements could mean receiving pharmacogenetic information as quickly as one would obtain a liver or renal profile before initiating specific medications. Alternatively, this DNA information could be obtained once in a lifetime as part of a newborn or childhood screen and be readily available as part of the future of the electronic medical record (EMR) for every patient.

Ideally, computerized algorithms using the DME genotype information from the EMR would be used and incorporate other medications, comorbidities, age, weight, and pharmacogenetic information to aid the practitioner in selecting the most correct medication and its dosing for that particular patient.

Key Points

- Pharmacogenomics is the study of interindividual differences in the reactions to medications.
- Adverse drug reactions are a leading cause of morbidity and mortality, and also escalating health care costs.
- The metabolism of certain medications is greatly influenced by individual genetic differences.
- Genetic differences, particularly in certain enzymes, can result in decreased effectiveness or increased toxicity.
- Pharmacogenetics can be used to select the appropriate drug and/or dose for an individual patient, increasing safety and effectiveness while decreasing costs.
- Individual genetic variations are only a part of the overall factors effecting drug metabolism and reduce their effectiveness of tailoring medications to any single patient.

References

1. Pharmacogenomics, Human Genome Project Information. http://www.ornl.gov/sci/techresources/Human_Genome/medicine/pharma.shtml. Accessed June 11, 2012
2. Lazarou J, Pomeranz BH, Corey PN. Incidence of adverse drug reactions in hospitalized patients: a meta-analysis of prospective studies. *JAMA*. 1998;279:1200–1205
3. National Center for Biotechnology Information. One Size Does Not Fit All: The Promise of Pharmacogenomics. http://www.ncbi.nlm.nih.gov/About/primer/pharm.html. Accessed June 11, 2012
4. Coumadin prescribing information. http://www.accessdata.fda.gov/drugsatfda_docs/label/2010/009218s108lbl.pdf. Accessed June 11, 2012
5. Lindh JD, Holm L, Andersson ML, Rane A. Influence of *CYP2C9* genotype of warfarin dose requirements—systemic review and meta-analysis. *Eur J Clin Pharmacol.* 65:365–375

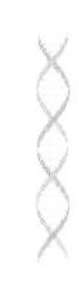

6. Limdi NA, Wiener H, Goldstein JA, Acton RT, Beasley TM. Influence of *CYP2C9* and *VKORC1* on warfarin response during initiation of therapy. *Blood Cell Mol Dis.* 2009;43:119–128
7. Miao L, Yang J, Huang C, Shen Z. Contribution of age, body weight, and *CYP2C9* and *VKORC1* genotype to the anticoagulant response to warfarin: proposal for a new dosing regimen in Chinese patients. *Pharmacogenet.* 2007;63:1135–1141
8. The Warfarin Dose Refinement Collaboration. Warfarin dosing (calculator). http://www.warfarindosing.org. Accessed June 11, 2012
9. McClain MR, Palomaki GE, Piper M, Haddow JE. A rapid ACCE review of *CYP2C9* and *VKORC1* allele testing to inform warfarin dosing in adults at elevated risk for thrombotic events to avoid serious bleeding. *Genet Med.* 2008;10:89–98
10. Koren G, Cairns J, Chitayat D, Gaedigk A, Leeder SJ. Pharmacogenetics of morphine poisoning in a breastfed neonate of a codeine-prescribed mother. *Lancet.* 2006;368:704
11. Madadi P, Ross CJD, Hayden MR, et al. Pharmacogenetics of neonatal opioid toxicity following maternal use of codeine during breastfeeding: a case-control study. *Clin Pharmacol Ther.* 2009;85:31–35
12. Löscher W, Klotz U, Aimprich F, Schmidt D. The clinical impact of pharmacogenetics on the treatment of epilepsy. *Epilepsia.* 2009;50:1
13. Kim WJ, Lee JH, Yi J, et al. A nonsynonymous variation in MRP2/ABCC2 is associated with neurological adverse drug reactions of carbamazepine in patients with epilepsy. *Pharmacogenet Genomics.* 2010;(4):249–256
14. McCormack M, Alfirevic A, Bourgeois S, et al. HLA-A*3101 and carbamazepine-induced hypersensitivity reactions in Europeans. *N Engl J Med.* 2011;24;364(12):1134–1143
15. Depondt C, Godard P, Espel RS, et al. A candidate gene study of antiepileptic drug tolerability and efficacy identifies an association of *CYP2C9* variants with phenytoin toxicity. *Eur J Neurol.* 2011;(9):1159–1164
16. Chen P, Lin JJ, Lu CS, et al. Carbamazepine-induced toxic effects and HLA-B*1502 screening in Taiwan. *N Engl J Med.* 2011;364(12):1126–1133
17. Rawlins MD. Cutting the cost of drug development? *Nat Rev Drug Discov.* 2004;3:360–364
18. Froehlich TE, Epstein JN, Nick TG, et al. Pharmacogenetic predictors of methylphenidate dose-response in attention-deficit/hyperactivity disorder. *J Am Acad Child Adolesc Psych.* 2011;50(11):1129–1139

Chapter 21

Information Technology and Primary Care Genetics

Marc S. Williams, MD

Introduction

The problem of information overload is well recognized in pediatrics and medicine in general. In 1980 the doubling time of medical knowledge was estimated to be 30 years, and now is estimated to be 7 years. The sheer volume of information quickly outstrips the brain's ability to retain all but a fraction (and it may not retain the pertinent fraction). Information regarding genomics magnifies this problem. With the increasing emphasis on delivery of evidence-based medicine, the importance of incorporating current and relevant knowledge into practice cannot be overstated.

Criticism of medical education in an environment of rapid change and knowledge expansion can be generally characterized in 2 ways. (1) Classroom knowledge is acquired (and subsequently forgotten) years before the opportunity to apply the knowledge arises. An example of this in pediatric practice is a brief discussion of a genetic condition (such as Angelman syndrome) in the genetics coursework in the first or second year of medical school. It is likely that most general pediatricians will encounter a patient either with Angelman syndrome or with Angelman syndrome in the differential diagnosis at some point in their clinical practice. However, this encounter could be years or even decades after the brief lecture on this condition, making it unlikely that the pertinent information is retained or accurate. (2) Situations arise that require an informed response before the knowledge is acquired. Expanded newborn screening is an excellent example of this. Although lectures on inborn errors of metabolism are standard in most medical schools, unless a physician is a recent graduate, the lectures were likely limited to a handful of disorders (phenylketonuria, galactosemia, etc) for which screening existed. So when the first positive screen for long-chain 3-hydroxyacyl coenzyme A dehydrogenase deficiency arrives, how does the pediatrician find accurate and clinically actionable information quickly to respond to the patient situation?

One proposed solution is to condense important information into clinical guidelines. Unfortunately, simply providing evidence-based best practice resources even in the form of relatively clear-cut guidelines does not automatically result in changes in practice. One study in adults[1] showed that only 50% of Americans receive recommended preventive care. Of patients with acute illness, 70% received recommended treatments and 30% received contraindicated treatments. Of patients with chronic illnesses, 60% received recommended treatments and 20% received contraindicated treatments.

It does not appear that pediatricians fare better in this area. Fewer than 50% of pediatricians studied provided recommended anticipatory guidance.[2,3] Barriers to incorporating clinical knowledge into practice fall into 2 general categories

- Physician-related obstacles
  - Failure to recognize an information need
  - Answers are not thought to exist
- Resource-related obstacles
  - Excessive time required to find answers
  - Lack of seamless access
  - Inability of literature search technology to directly answer clinical questions
  - Lack of evidence (and guidelines for all situations)

Formal studies of physician information needs by Ely and colleagues[4–6] were able to distill all clinical questions into 64 generic question types, of which the 3 most frequent were What is the drug of choice for condition X? (11%), What is the cause of symptom X? (8%), and What test is indicated in situation X? (8%)

Perhaps even more surprising is where physicians seek clinical information. Approximately 64% consult a textbook or go down the hall to ask a colleague. Only 16% used electronic resources and, of those, no single electronic resource was used more than 7% of the time.

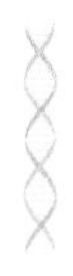

One proposed solution to quickly accessing accurate information has been to promote change in the delivery of health care through the use of informatics. It is clear that simply converting paper records and processes into an electronic format will not substantially alleviate the problem. However, incorporating electronic health records (EHRs) with advanced capabilities into the workflow of care delivery has the potential to dramatically improve the quality and consistency of care. Sophisticated EHRs that can represent information about family history, newborn screening, or other genetic or genomic test results in a coded fashion such that the information can be computed (ie, analyzed, stored, combined with other information, etc) will be essential if personalized medicine is to be a reality.

The remainder of this chapter will provide a series of case studies that demonstrate how informatics can facilitate practical incorporation of genetics and genomics into pediatric practice.

Lowering the Barriers in the Office: Point of Care "Just-in-Time" Education

Just-in-time education is the acquisition of knowledge or skills as they are needed. The ultimate example of this occurs in the movie *The Matrix* when the character Trinity needs to pilot a helicopter. A quick call to the command center and the knowledge (and presumably experience) to fly the chopper is immediately uploaded just in time for a daring rescue. The increasing availability of content that can be accessed in the course of the clinical workflow in a timely manner has the potential to remove some resource-related obstacles. While just-in-time education is typically focused on electronically available resources, it is important to note that print resources can serve this role as well. A premier example of this is the American Academy of Pediatrics (AAP) *Red Book: Report of the Committee on Infectious Diseases*. When faced with an unusual infectious disease process, a physician can find needed information from the print *Red Book* within a couple of minutes.

Increasingly there is a move to incorporate multifunctional EHRs into the clinic. These systems can dramatically enhance the quality and efficiency of practice if the systems are well-designed with an appropriately customized interface—something that is not incorporated into many off-the-shelf systems. In systems where an interface fully integrated within the office is not readily available, the use of handheld devices that either contain or are able to access electronic resources has also expanded. A number of systems are now completely paperless.

Electronic Resources in the EHR

Example 1: Enabled EHRs

Figure 21-1 depicts a screen shot from Intermountain Healthcare's homegrown EHR system. The arrow points to the E-Resources link on the left-hand navigation bar. Clicking on this link takes the user to the E-Resources home page (Figure 21-2). There is an extensive collection of external resources (both free and subscription) available to the user, as well as links to system medical libraries, patient education resources, and a variety of internal resources, including internally developed care guidelines, protocols, clinical programs, and laboratory and formulary information. To provide access to genetic resources, links were added to several external genetics resources (circled) as well as a link to an internal program, the Clinical Genetics Institute (arrow). Clicking any one of the links takes the user to the home page of the resource. The user must then enter search terms to identify the information required. While the E-Resources link lowers the barrier to accessing information during a patient encounter because it can be accessed directly from a patient's EHR, it still requires the user to search the targeted resource for information. If relevant information is not identified, then the user needs to move to

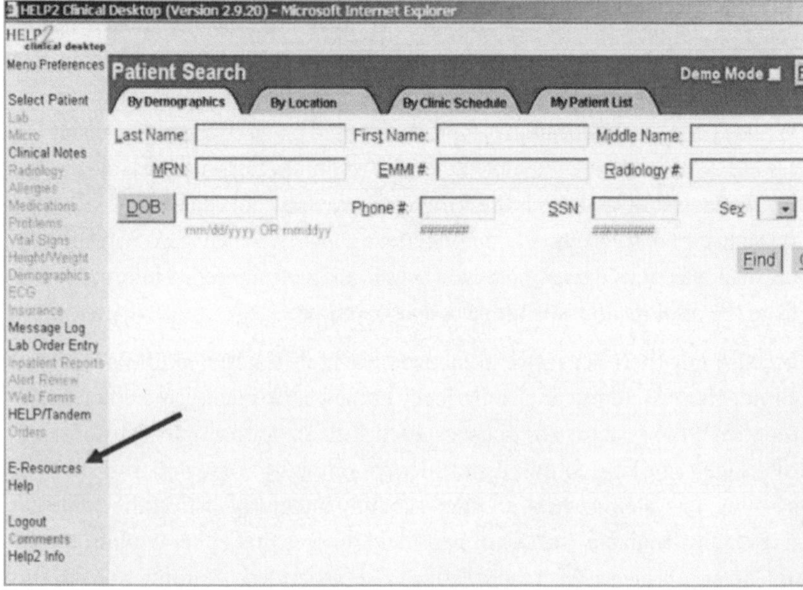

Figure 21-1. Screen shot highlighting E-Resources link on navigation bar. Copyright Intermountain Healthcare 2009. All rights reserved.

another resource and repeat the process until the information is found, or the user ends the search from lack of time or frustration.

Example 2: Marfan Syndrome

Consider a pediatrician seeing a new patient with the diagnosis of rule out Marfan syndrome. The parent asks, "How do we know if she has it? How should we be treating her? Are there tests that should be done or medications she should take?" Because the physician is not familiar with the condition, there are several options: refer to a geneticist, consult a text (eg, *Management of Genetic Syndromes,*[7] *Harriet Lane,* or the AAP text *Medical Genetics in Pediatric Practice*), search personal files of journal articles, search PubMed, or try to find information online.

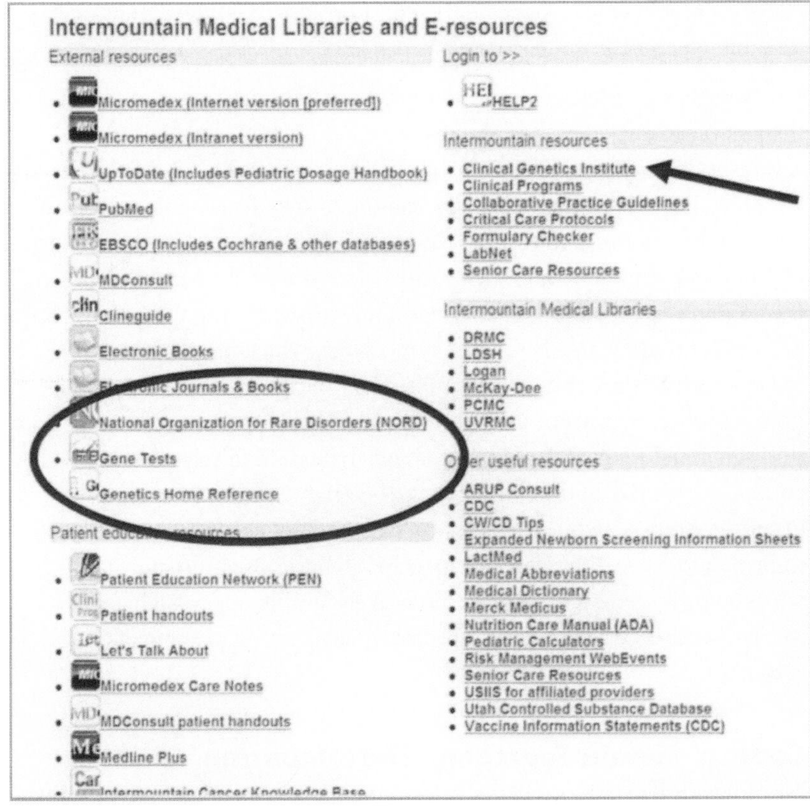

Figure 21-2. The E-Resources page. The circled external resources are specific to genetic and rare diseases. The arrow is a link to the internal genetics resource. Clicking any of the links takes the user to the resource's home page where searching can begin.

A geneticist is not available locally and the pediatrician does not have ready access to a book or articles that discuss Marfan syndrome. Fortunately, there is access to electronic resources. Initially the pediatrician accesses UptoDate, logs in, and types in the search term "Marfan syndrome." A list of 74 hits appears (>2 pages). The navigation bar at the top allows prioritizing by pediatric topics, so this is selected and the reordered list is presented. The first topic is "The Marfan Syndrome" and this is chosen. When the cursor rolls over the topic an outline appears to the right that contains, in order, Introduction, Genetics, Histopathology, Pathogenesis, The Marfan Phenotype, Management, Pregnancy, Prognosis, etc. The parent's first question was about diagnosis, but there isn't a subject heading for diagnosis. Careful reading identifies the subheading Diagnostic Criteria under Marfan Phenotype. Clicking on this reveals a text-dense page with 15 bulleted items, and more. While a diligent pediatrician could with many clicks eventually find answers to the questions posed by the parent, it is difficult to accomplish this in a busy practice.

On average, a physician spends no more than 2 minutes trying to locate the answer to a specific question. A recent study by Levy et al[8] tested several commonly used electronic resources available through EHRs or handheld devices for their usability relating to specific genetic questions. None of the resources were able to consistently provide the given answer within this 2-minute window. Of more concern were numerous errors in the content, particularly in the general resources, raising the potential problem of finding an answer that is incorrect, which has the potential to negatively impact patient care. (One site indicated that the autosomal dominant breast/ovarian susceptibility genes could not be inherited through a male—an incorrect statement that could falsely reassure a patient at high risk of developing breast/ovarian cancer). In contrast, the genetics resources, while much more likely to have accurate and complete information, were difficult to navigate for all but those intimately familiar with them (ie, geneticists). Even a relatively simple query such as the Marfan syndrome search is extraordinarily frustrating in some of these resources.

Context-Specific Searching: The Infobutton

To address the search problems, informaticists have explored the idea that the location from which the physician navigated in the patient EHR may provide context for the search. This allows the opportunity to "pre-search" content libraries, enabling the physician to access a filtered set of resources that could facilitate receiving applicable answers while minimizing search time. Infobuttons build and run queries against electronic resources based on patient data and clinical context to take the user to the most appropriate section(s) within a content collection with a minimum number of clicks. In EHRs with this capability, infobuttons appear in locations relevant to the most commonly asked questions—usually the problem list, laboratory results, and medication list (including medication ordering).

Example 1: Marfan Syndrome

Returning to the Marfan syndrome example, in this case the pediatrician goes to the problem list and enters Marfan syndrome. This is added to the problem list and a blue button with an "*i*" in it appears (Figure 21-3). This is the infobutton. The infobutton is a hyperlink and, when clicked, it takes the user directly to content relevant to the context—in this case the clinical problem Marfan syndrome. Figure 21-4 depicts the result of this one click. By choosing the infobutton the pediatrician is taken directly to an external content resource's article on Marfan syndrome. This resource is preselected based on input from users and content experts (in this case geneticists and

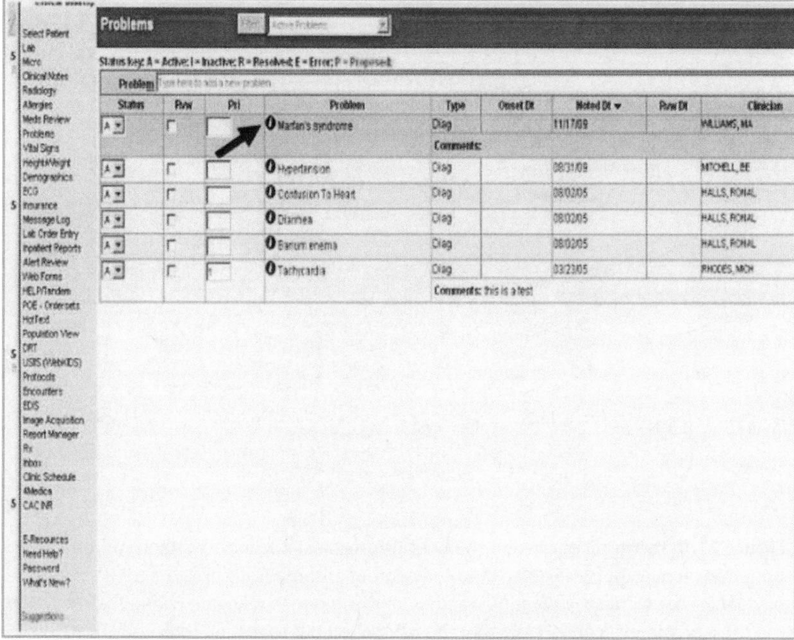

Figure 21-3. A screen shot of a test patient problem list from an electronic health record. The arrow indicates the infobutton associated with the disorder of interest.

genetic counselors) based on the ease of use and likelihood that answers may be found quickly. In addition the external resource's navigation index is active (circle), allowing this to be used to rapidly move within the topic's content. Assuming that the answer isn't found (or the pediatrician is more familiar with an alternative resource), the EHR's content navigation bar is active (bracket), allowing the pediatrician to change to a different external resource with a single click. As before, the content appears in the window. It should also be noted that if there were a practice guideline for Marfan syndrome (either an internal guideline developed by content experts within the system or one by a specialty society such as the AAP), links to these could be provided and, where appropriate, could be the preselected resource. Finally, this system has the ability to capture user feedback on 2 items: Did you find the answer? How did the content impact your patient care decision? The submission of this information and information that is automatically captured by the system (time within each resource, navigation, etc) can be used in an iterative fashion to improve the infobutton's ability to rapidly present the best content for the user, thus constantly improving the functionality and efficiency.

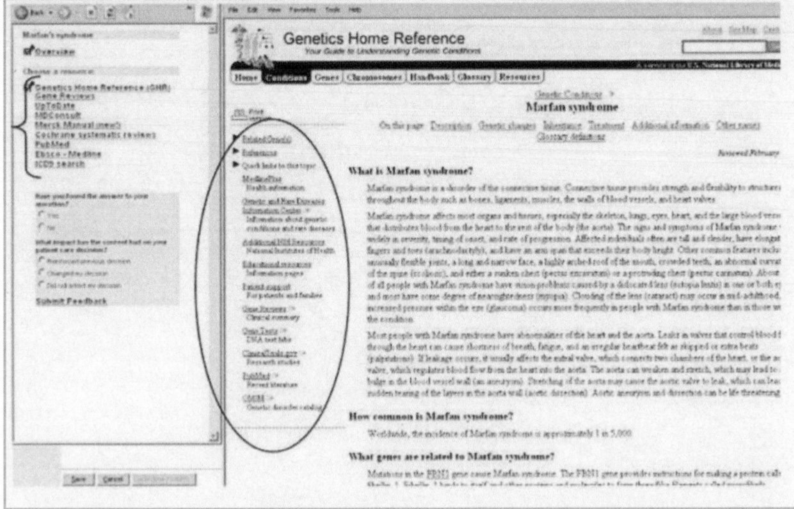

Figure 21-4. The result of clicking the infobutton associated with Marfan syndrome. The preferred resource is preselected, and the content automatically appears to the right. The navigation bar within the content is active, allowing one to navigate within the content to the topic of interest (circle). Note that the navigation bar to the left (bracket) allows the user to move to different resources with a single click, at which time the new content resource would appear in the right-hand window. Finally, the user can quickly submit feedback (gray box), which can be used by the infobutton manager to alter resource presentation based on immediate user feedback. Copyright Intermountain Healthcare 2009. All rights reserved.

Example 2: Newborn Screening

Upon arriving in the office in the morning the pediatrician logs into her clinical workstation. Immediately an alert appears on the screen "Critical Laboratory Result." Clicking on the alert takes the pediatrician to the electronic newborn screening result of Baby Smith, a patient under her care from the newborn nursery. The report indicates "Biotinidase ABNORMAL." Next to this is an infobutton. Clicking this immediately takes the pediatrician to the confirmatory algorithm from the American College of Medical Genetics and Genomics (ACMG) (Figure 21-5) or perhaps to the ACMG ACT sheet or to locality-specific resources, such as are available in California and other states. The decision on which resource to link to resides with the users and content experts. In addition to rapidly linking to critically needed information, because the physician is working in the EHR environment the physician has immediate access to contact information for the

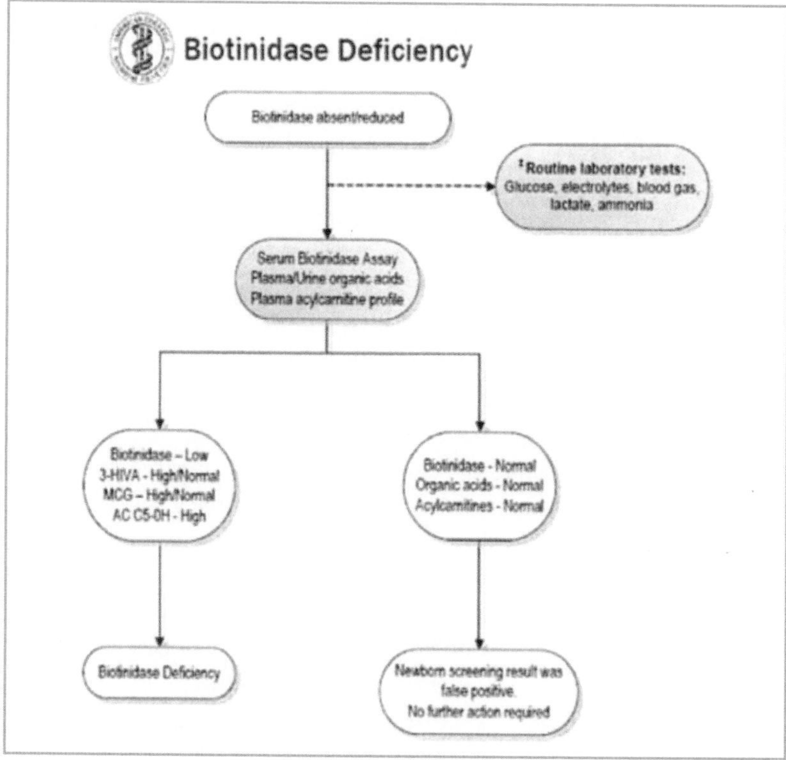

Figure 21-5. Treatment algorithm for biotinidase deficiency from American College of Medical Genetics and Genomics. The algorithm provides instructions for routine tests to assess the infant's current metabolic state as well as listing the confirmatory tests needed. The algorithm also provides information regarding interpretation of the confirmatory tests, allowing the physician to decide if this is a true- or false-positive screening result. © American College of Medical Genetics, 2006

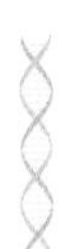

family and access to laboratory order entry. This example requires that the pediatrician's EHR have the ability to receive newborn screening results from the laboratory in a coded electronic format (not just an electronic image like a pdf or text document). The results can be analyzed by the EHR system and, in this case, trigger an automated alert to the treating physician (also available as coded information in the report) and automatically enable the infobutton. (Further functionality is discussed in Clinical Decision Support.)

Interestingly, in systems that have both electronic resources and infobuttons, more than 90% of physicians use the electronic resources function rather than infobuttons, despite the decreased efficiency.

Clinical Decision Support

The previous examples address issues related to resource-related obstacles. Provider-related obstacles include the failure to recognize an information need.

Clinical decision support (CDS) systems, according to Dr Robert Hayward of the Centre for Health Evidence, "…link health observations with health knowledge to influence health choices by clinicians for improved health care."[9] The implications of this definition are the existence of an active system to perform the desired linkages more or less automatically, as opposed to relying on providers to input data into a system or rely on their intrinsic knowledge. The active surveillance and linkage by the system then presents actionable information to the provider *at the appropriate time in the workflow,* assisting the provider's decision-making to increase the likelihood of doing the right thing for the patient. Lack of attention to any of these components can result in frustration and failure. An alternative definition by Osheroff and colleagues more explicitly articulates aspects of the process of CDS: "Clinical decision support refers broadly to providing clinicians and patients with clinical knowledge and patient-related information, intelligently filtered, or presented at appropriate times, to enhance patient care."[10] This definition also acknowledges the important role of the patient (or the parent) in using this information to independently manage their child's care in concert with the provider. Examples of provider and patient CDS follow.

Clinical decision support can be passive or active. Passive decision support occurs when a system facilitates access to relevant patient data or clinical knowledge for interpretation by the physician, while active decision support implies some higher level of information processing, or inference. In the traditional laboratory setting, the normal value ranges that accompany a laboratory report can be considered passive decision support, while calling the physician with a critical value on a result is active decision support (at its most simplistic). To illustrate the difference, consider a patient presenting with an acute asthmatic attack. The patient is experiencing air hunger, has a respiratory rate of 50 breaths per minute with retractions, decreased air movement, and tight wheezing. A blood gas is obtained and the partial pressure of carbon dioxide, arterial ($PaCO_2$) is 40 mm Hg. Passive decision support provides a reference range for $PaCO_2$ of 35 to 45 mm Hg. The passive information tells the physician that the result is in the normal range. An experienced physician knows that even though the result is in the normal range, it is not normal *in the context of the clinical presentation*. This patient is experiencing incipient respiratory failure. If this result was assumed to be normal by the physician, the gravity of the situation could be missed and the patient could suffer injury and death. In contrast, were an active decision support system built for this scenario, it would use rules to capture relevant data about the diagnosis and patient parameters (such as respiratory rate) so that when the result returned it would generate an urgent message to the care team indicating that the patient was at risk for respiratory failure and, depending on its sophistication, could suggest possible interventions. The remainder of this section will discuss different types of CDS using genetic examples.

Alerts and Reminders

Alerts and reminders are the most basic types of CDS and are enabled in many proprietary and home-built EHRs. While the alert itself is passive, the algorithms used to generate the alert can actively seek information from a variety of sources, analyze them for patterns and, when a critical pattern is identified, trigger the alert. Many offices have automated reminder systems that can automatically generate a letter or phone call to a parent about the need to schedule an appointment (patient-facing CDS reminder), or to the provider to prompt administration of a lapsed vaccine (provider-facing CDS reminder). The former is triggered simply by a predefined elapsed time and comparison of age to well-child schedule or by a reminder inserted by the pediatrician or staff to facilitate follow-up of a clinical issue, such as a weight check. The immunization reminder is somewhat more sophisticated in that the system must "know" which immunizations have been administered as well as the patient's age to compare that against the recommended immunization schedule. If a gap is identified, the alert is triggered when the patient is scheduled for an appointment of any kind (ie, the reminder system scans the schedule to see which patients are coming in and runs the immunization algorithm on all scheduled patients).

The newborn screening just-in-time example represents an alert triggered by a laboratory result and a facilitated retrieval of information necessary to appropriately treat the patient. The alert automatically connects the specific abnormal result (in this case biotinidase) with the clinical resources (the ACT sheet and algorithm for biotinidase deficiency) and presents those to the clinician.

Alerts of this nature are quite simple to construct and implement. While the previous examples clearly demonstrate the utility of this type of CDS, if too many alerts are enabled in the EHR the physician can suffer the effects of alert fatigue, as often happens with computerized drug order systems with an interaction alert function that can cause nearly every medication order to trigger an alert, 99% of which are clinically insignificant. The consequence is that many providers will find a way to disable the interaction alerts, which are annoying and waste time. The potential problem with this approach is that significant interactions with the potential for negative patient outcomes could be missed. Finding the right balance between alert significance and frequency is an ongoing challenge.

Diagnostic Decision Support

To make accurate diagnoses, physicians must integrate information from a variety of sources (history, family history, physical examination, laboratory reports, imaging studies, etc) and generate a differential diagnosis. This differential diagnosis drives prioritization of subsequent diagnostic and treatment interventions, the results of which further refine the differential diagnosis in a series of iterations until (hopefully) the patient is successfully treated. If the correct diagnosis is not part of the differential, it is extremely unlikely that the diagnosis will be made expeditiously. This is a major dilemma in diagnosing genetic conditions given the rarity of many, if not most, genetic conditions.

Clinical decision support can assist in diagnosing, although for the purposes of illustration we'll use a common pediatric condition with a strong genetic component: asthma. It is well known that asthma is underdiagnosed, particularly in younger children. While some of this relates to a reluctance to label, in many cases not all of the information is available to the treating physician to allow proper construction of the differential diagnosis with asthma at the top. The increasing rate of asthma mortality is a reminder of the serious consequences of underdiagnosis and undertreatment of this common disease.

Imagine a scenario in which an asthma CDS system has been implemented within the EHR. The pediatrician goes in the room to see a 5-year-old patient with the chief complaint of "cough for 2 weeks." When the patient record opens in the EHR an alert appears, "Patient meets criteria for consideration of asthma diagnosis. Peak flow pre- and post-bronchodilator administration recommended." This is a new alert that the pediatrician has not encountered before, and it is not clear why the alert appeared for this patient. Fortunately there is an infobutton, so the pediatrician clicks this and a new screen appears (Figure 21-6). The information contained behind the infobutton lets the pediatrician know that the alert was generated against criteria developed by the medical center to flag patients with potential asthma. This implies that the clinical content experts (ie, pediatric allergists

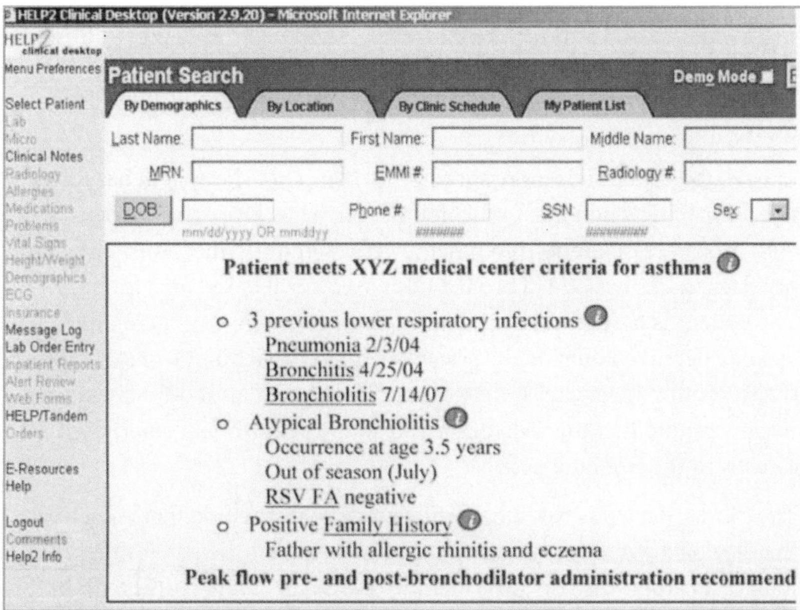

Figure 21-6. Mock asthma diagnosis alert within patient electronic health record (EHR) screen. All underlined text is hyperlinked to content within the patient's EHR. Infobuttons access information about the specifics of the criteria.

or pulmonologists) reviewed the pertinent evidence and guidelines; defined presenting complaints that would inform the algorithm to run (in this case the chief complaint of cough exceeding a given duration); and synthesized clinical criteria such that when defined combinations of criteria were present, a threshold would be exceeded and the alert would trigger. The information provided in this screen allows one to "reverse engineer" the logic model that underlies the alert. In this example, 3 criteria are presented.

The first criterion is a numerical count of lower respiratory tract infections. The system has a list of pertinent diagnostic codes (*International Classification of Diseases, Ninth Revision;* SNOMED; etc) that represent the lower respiratory infections of interest. The electronic data warehouse (EDW) is queried, and the number of hits are counted. The diagnoses could be from the clinic, emergency department, inpatient, or other encounters that contribute data to the EDW. There are likely date limits that aggregate multiple hits into an episode of care (eg, all lower respiratory infection codes that occur within 1 month of the first date are aggregated as one hit). This is necessary, as a single episode of lower respiratory tract infection will be represented in multiple places in the EDW. If all of these were counted, the number of insignificant alerts would multiply and the utility of the system would be lost. Note that each of the episodes is a hyperlink, so that clicking on the link would take the pediatrician directly to the relevant clinic notes for review.

The second criterion is more specific and complex. The system has identified a specific diagnosis, bronchiolitis, which has properties associated with it that are different from other lower respiratory infections. The alert has flagged this episode of bronchiolitis as atypical based on 3 findings: The patient is older than a predetermined age cutoff (say age 2), the episode occurred outside the system-defined bronchiolitis season, and the respiratory syncytial virus immunofluorescent antibody screen was negative (note that this is hyperlinked so the pediatrician could click directly to the laboratory report).

The third criterion is based on family history information that recognizes that having a parent with an atopic disease increases the risk for the child to have an atopic disease (40% lifetime risk if one parent is affected). In this case the system identified that a family history had been obtained at some point and it queried the coded family history information for first-degree relatives (parents or siblings), with a diagnosis of one of the atopic diseases (again a predefined set of codes). A positive hit was returned when the father was identified to have one or more of the codes and the alert provided the specific information. A hyperlink is available to view the family history information.

One could imagine a number of other criteria of interest, including prior use of a bronchodilator (query against the medication list); text searching for terms such as wheezy, wheezing, retraction, rhonchi, etc; exposure to secondhand smoke or pets (coded social history); and many others. As long as the information is coded and represented somewhere in the EDW, queries can be built to retrieve, evaluate, and combine any combination of desired data elements to assist clinical decision-making.

There are infobuttons associated with each of the criteria, which allow the pediatrician to drill down to understand why a certain criterion was flagged. These could link to brief explanatory notes created by the content experts, with links here to relevant sections of clinical guidelines, such as the National Heart, Lung, and Blood Institute Guidelines for the Diagnosis and Treatment of Asthma and, ultimately, to electronically available primary medical literature relevant to the criterion. This allows the pediatrician to expeditiously access as much information as needed to confirm that the alert is appropriate for the patient. The screen also reiterates the recommended diagnostic investigation: peak flow before and after bronchodilator. It is likely that there is a relevant age cutoff, given that 2-year-old children are not able to operate a peak flow meter. The infobutton associated with the peak flow recommendation could provide information about why this is appropriate, normal range (which could automatically be calculated for this specific patient based on age, gender, weight, and height data in the EDW), or how to order this test in the system.

The advantages of this type of system include higher likelihood of making an appropriate diagnosis in a timely fashion, applying best care practices, more rapid initiation of disease-specific treatment, identification of contributing factors (such as secondhand smoke), and others. This type of system, however, will never supplant the importance of collecting the appropriate information by history taking and physical examination.

Laboratory Decision Support

There are 2 opportunities within the laboratory testing workflow where CDS can aid the clinician—pre-analytic (ordering the test) and post-analytic (the test result). The previous newborn screening example illustrates the potential value of CDS in the post-analytic setting, even if limited to providing information. Even now, work is taking place to develop genetic test reports that would be interactive within the EHR. The envisioned report would contain a glossary for unfamiliar terms; links to relevant literature; links to genetic professionals in the area; links to knowledge repositories curated by the laboratory or national databases that contain information about the specific mutation identified; and, in the case of pharmacogenomic testing, links to dosing algorithms that would use the information to determine the specific dose for the patient that will maximize efficacy and minimize adverse events.

To illustrate the role of CDS in the pre-analytic process consider the following situation: A 12-year-old boy is brought in by his mother for genetic testing for familial adenomatous polyposis (FAP), an inherited cancer syndrome due to mutations in the *APC* gene. The boy's father was diagnosed with colorectal cancer at age 35. At the time of surgery hundreds of polyps were present in the colon. The father had testing of the *APC* gene, and a deleterious mutation was identified. The gastroenterologist informed the parents that polyps in gene carriers develop in the second decade, and it is recommended that colonoscopy begin around the age of 10. The parents also met with a genetic counselor who explained that this is an autosomal dominant condition, so their children are at a 50% risk of inheriting this mutation. The counselor also told them that their doctor could order a genetic test that would determine whether or not their son had inherited the mutation from his father. If he did not, then colonoscopy would not be indicated. They are asking you to order the test. The process of ordering the test involves determining which laboratory performs the test, what specimen is needed, which test to order, and whether insurance will cover the testing.

The chief issue at hand is which test to order. When the pediatrician accesses the laboratory's *APC* gene testing information, there are 3 tests that could be ordered: complete *APC* gene sequencing, Ashkenazi founder mutations, and family-specific mutation analysis. Which test is appropriate for the patient? At present the decision would cause the pediatrician to read materials on the laboratory Web site to determine the appropriate test, and potentially contact the laboratory (or the genetic counselor) for assistance with test ordering. In a situation where the laboratory ordering is done through a computerized system, this support can be built into the order entry. In this scenario the pediatrician accesses the computerized laboratory order system and either picks *APC* gene testing from a pick list or enters *APC* or FAP into a search box. When selected, a question appears: Is there another family member with FAP (Figure 21-7)? The pediatrician clicks yes and the second question about the mutation status of a family member appears. Yes is clicked, and the third statement appears requesting that the specific mutation be entered. The pediatrician then enters the mutation identified in the father. An infobutton is present to assist the pediatrician to enter the mutation properly (eg, 2144 delG or A4467G). An algorithm checks to make sure the mutation was entered appropriately. After the mutation is correctly entered, the order test button appears. When clicked, a laboratory test request for the appropriate test (familial mutation analysis) and required information about the patient, insurance, etc, is automatically pulled into the form from the registration information, and this pre-populated form is printed in the pediatrician's office or at the drawing station.

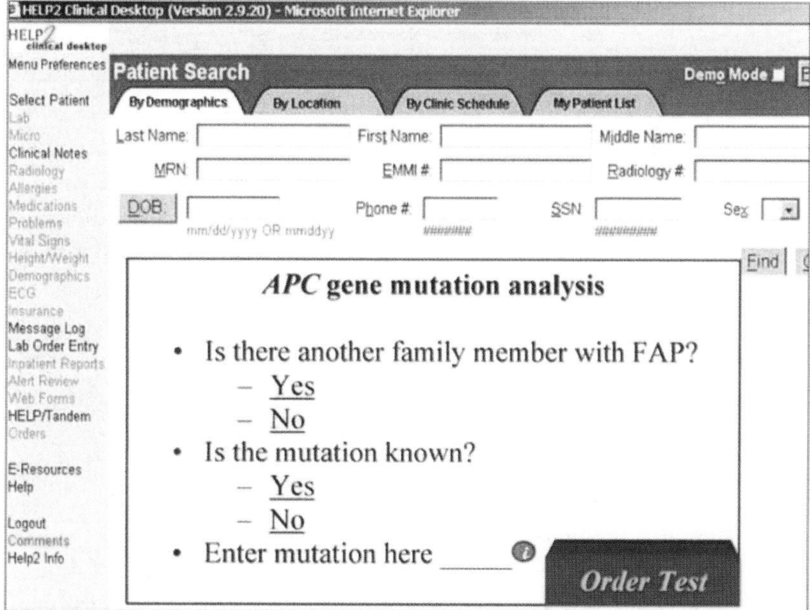

Figure 21-7. Mock laboratory order entry for *APC* genetic testing. Subsequent questions would only appear if "Yes" is selected from the preceding question.

For an adult who presents with multiple adenomatous polyps with no previous testing in the family, the physician would click no to the first question. At that point a second question would appear: "Is the patient Jewish?" If the patient is Jewish the physician checks yes. A third statement would then appear: "The preferred testing strategy is to test for the common Ashkenazi mutations first, for if one is present the cost of testing is significantly reduced. If testing for the Ashkenazi mutations is negative, full *APC* gene sequencing would be appropriate. Would you like to order the testing in this order?" An infobutton would be available for the physician who wanted more information. If yes is chosen, the test order would be for *APC* gene testing for the Ashkenazi mutations *automatically reflexing* to full gene sequencing if none of the Ashkenazi mutations are present. Alternatively, if the physician clicked no, he would be asked to select between *APC* Ashkenazi mutations only or *APC* full gene sequencing. As before, the request would be automatically generated. When the test report is received, the interpretation will be specific for the information that was provided in the request, making it much more likely that the interpretation is correct for this specific patient.

Pharmacogenomic Decision Support

In Chapter 20, the emerging importance of pharmacogenomics in medicine is discussed. While this has been predominantly in adult medicine at present, *TPMT* gene analysis prior to the use of 6-mercaptopurine as well as preliminary information about genes that influence the response of asthmatic patients to β_2-agonists or anti-inflammatory agents, such as inhaled corticosteroids or leukotriene antagonists (being assessed by the PACMAN study), shows that these tests will also be important in pediatric practice in the future. Computerized order entry for medications has been shown to dramatically improve patient safety by catching dosing errors, medically significant interactions (with the caveats about alert fatigue dis- cussed previously), and allergies. This process has the potential to allow pharmacogenomic tests that have proven clinical utility to be rapidly translated to practice.

Example

A 16-year-old boy presents with new onset psychomotor seizures. The pediatrician has followed him for some time because of unstable mood that has only partially improved on previous medications prescribed by the patient's psychiatrist. Given the combination of the psychomotor seizures and the mood disorder, the pediatrician believes that carbamazepine would be the preferred medicine to use given its effectiveness in psychomotor seizures as well as its use as a mood stabilizer. The pediatrician opens the computerized medication order system and chooses carbamazepine. When this medication is chosen an algorithm is run represented by the logic model in Figure 21-8. The information in the left-hand box is automatically collected by the program from various parts of the EDW. In this case the computer determines that the indication is psychomotor epilepsy (this may require the pediatrician to enter this at the time of medication order). The weight is needed to determine the dose; sex is needed to determine if there is a risk of fetal exposure (in this case since the sex is male, this ends the inquiry; if the patient is a female older than a predetermined age and the drug presents a risk to a fetus, the pediatrician would be prompted to order a pregnancy test), allergy to carbamazepine or cross-reacting compounds is determined, and medications with potential interactions are queried. The program also asks about ethnicity because of the knowledge about increased risk for Stevens-Johnson syndrome or toxic epidermal necrolysis in patients of Asian ethnicity. Recently this has been determined to be due to the presence of a specific

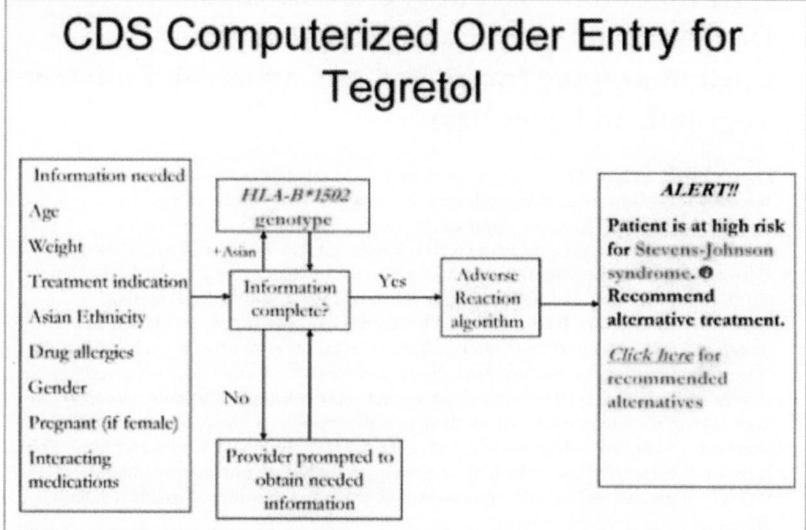

Figure 21-8. Logic model for Tegretol order entry. The left-hand box lists the required information, which is assessed in the next step. The patient is Asian, so the HLA-B*1502 genotype result is sought. Once the information is complete, the next step is analysis by the adverse reaction algorithm, which generates the alert at the right.

HLA marker *HLA-B*1502*, which has a significantly higher prevalence in many Asian populations. It is now recommended that individuals of Asian ethnicity should be tested for this HLA type before initiating therapy with carbamazepine. In this scenario the patient is of Asian ethnicity, so the program automatically queries the laboratory result section looking for the specific HLA test. The psychiatrist had ordered the test when considering carbamazepine for the mood disorder. The patient carries the *HLA-B*1502* allele. Because of this the pediatrician sees the alert represented in the right-hand box of Figure 21-8. If the infobutton is clicked, the pediatrician is taken to the US Food and Drug Administration (FDA) alert abstract (Figure 21-9) where the entire report could be accessed with one more click. In addition, the pediatrician can click in this box for alternative medications. If this is clicked, the system will look at the indication for treatment as well as other factors built into the program and would propose clonazepam as the recommended alternative, given its equivalence to carbamazepine in the treatment of psychomotor seizures (with an infobutton that would link to references that confirm this). Alternatively, if the

Information for Healthcare Professionals: Dangerous or Even Fatal Skin Reactions - Carbamazepine (marketed as Carbatrol, Equetro, Tegretol, and generics)

FDA ALERT [12/12/2007]: Dangerous or even fatal skin reactions (Stevens Johnson syndrome and toxic epidermal necrolysis), that can be caused by carbamazepine therapy, are significantly more common in patients with a particular human leukocyte antigen (HLA) allele, HLA-B*1502. This allele occurs almost exclusively in patients with ancestry across broad areas of Asia, including South Asian Indians. Genetic tests for HLA-B*1502 are already available. Patients with ancestry from areas in which HLA-B*1502 is present should be screened for the HLA-B*1502 allele before starting treatment with carbamazepine. If they test positive, carbamazepine should not be started unless the expected benefit clearly outweighs the increased risk of serious skin reactions. Patients who have been taking carbamazepine for more than a few months without developing skin reactions are at low risk of these events ever developing from carbamazepine. This is true for patients of any ethnicity or genotype, including patients positive for HLA-B*1502. This new safety information will be reflected in updated product labeling.
More...

Figure 21-9. US Food and Drug Administration alert below the infobutton in Figure 21-8. Clicking on "more" will take the user to the full alert and references.

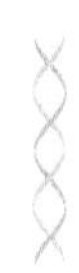

*HLA-B*1502* test had not been done previously, the pediatrician would be alerted to order this test before prescribing carbamazepine, and an infobutton would direct to the FDA information. If the patient weren't of Asian ethnicity, the query about the *HLA-B*1502* would not have triggered and the prescribing would have proceeded with consideration of the other factors.

Not only does a system such as this improve patient safety by minimizing the risk for an unanticipated adverse event, the user is able to rapidly prescribe an alternative within the clinical workflow (or order laboratory tests) with a minimum number of clicks while never leaving the patient's medical record. While technically more challenging, it is possible, at least in theory, to push this information to handheld devices that are used in some settings for prescription ordering.

Example: Dysmorphology

Searching for dysmorphology diagnoses has changed in the Internet era. Multiple medical students recently demonstrated nontraditional ways to use Internet search engines. In one session the students took a history and physical examination about a hypothetical genetics patient. They were to return with a prioritized differential diagnosis and prepared to discuss and defend their choices. Some of the features of the female patient included mental retardation, ataxia, microcephaly, inability to speak, pleasant disposition with frequent spontaneous laughter, and seizures. Many physicians would likely have already made the diagnosis of Angelman syndrome given that set of features. However, many third-year students consistently generated a comprehensive differential diagnosis that was appropriately prioritized. Using search engines (such as Google or Online Mendelian Inheritance in Man [OMIM]), they were able to generate a suitable list of differential diagnoses not easily imaginable in the pre-Internet era. Figure 21-10 demonstrates the first 6 hits if the search phrase "microcephaly ataxia seizures laughter" is entered into the Google search box. Through some trial and error the students had determined the key discriminating terms (or handles) for the diagnoses in the differential. (See Chapter 8 for a more in-depth discussion of dysmorphic features.) This strategy also works very well in the OMIM, another publicly available free resource[11] (Figure 21-11). Online Mendelian Inheritance in Man has much less to search than the entire World Wide Web, so using too many search terms significantly limits the number of hits returned, as demonstrated in Figure 21-11. In either case, playing around with different combinations of search terms allows one to generate a good differential diagnosis in a relatively short time. If used in combination with an illustrated text, such as *Smith's Recognizable Patterns of Human Malformation* (Chapter 8), this approach can facilitate the diagnosis of many genetic conditions.

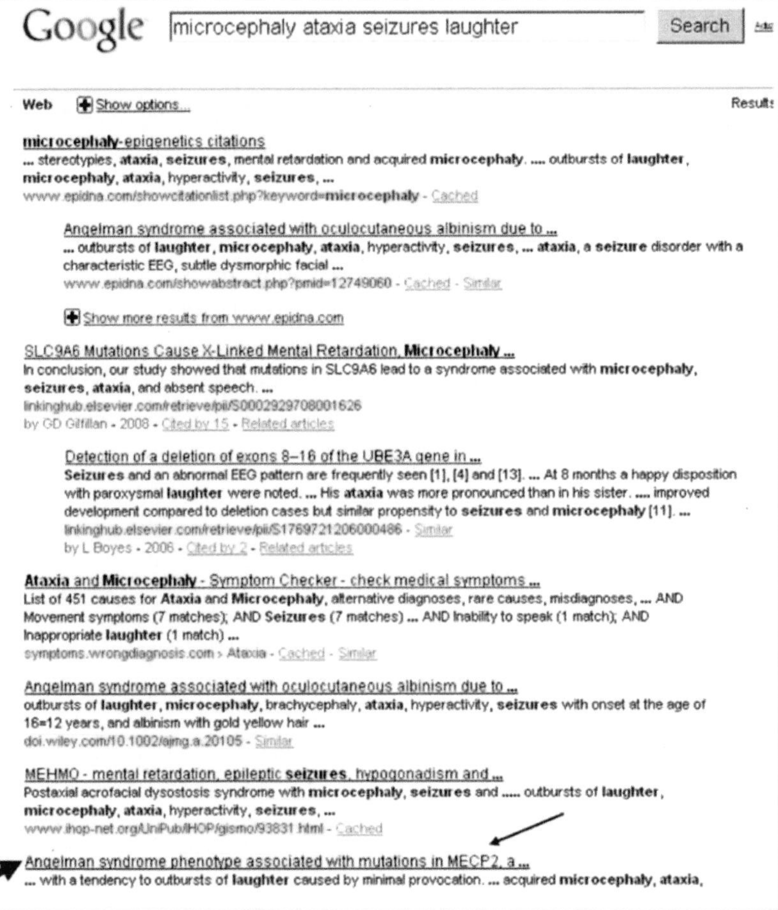

Figure 21-10. Google screen shot showing the "handles" used as search terms. Note mention of Angelman syndrome (thick arrow) and *MECP2,* the gene responsible for Rett syndrome (thin arrow).

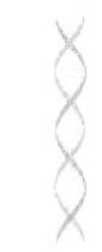

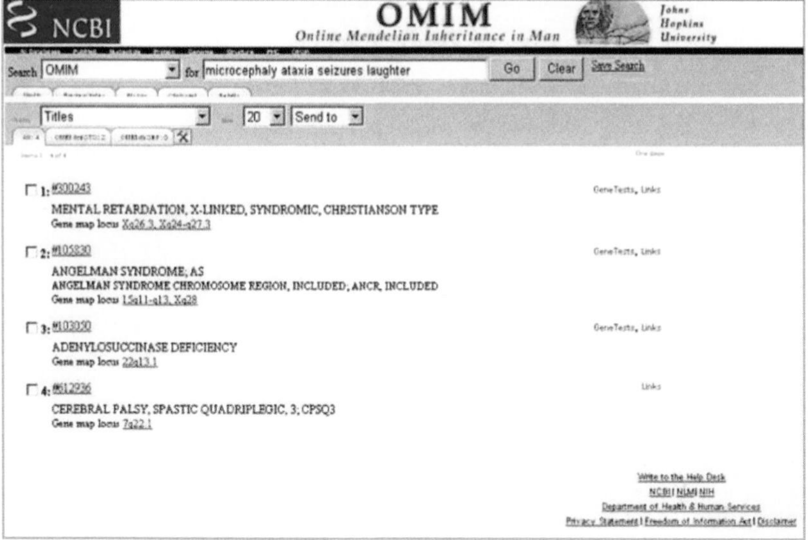

Figure 21-11. A screen shot from Online Mendelian Inheritance in Man using the same terms as in Figure 21-10. Angelman syndrome is identified, but *MECP2* or Rett syndrome is not. Removing the term "laughter" results in Angelman syndrome appearing as choice 8 and Rett syndrome as choice 6.

Key Points

- Medical information needed to care for patients is increasing in volume and complexity.
- Traditional methods of information acquisition will not allow clinicians to practice effectively.
- Point-of-care, just-in-time educational resources can rapidly provide information to clinicians without disrupting workflow.
- Passive and active CDS systems embedded in fully functional EHRs have the potential to improve the quality and efficiency of care.
- These systems do not replace physician thought processes, but should enhance them.

References

1. Schuster MA, McGlynn EA, Brook RH. How good is the quality of healthcare in the United States? *Milbank Quarterly*. 1998;76:517–563
2. Schuster MA, Duan N, Regalado M, et al. Anticipatory guidance: what information do parents receive? What information do they want? *Arch Pediatr Adolesc Med*. 2000;154(12):1191–1198
3. Mangione-Smith R, DeCristofaro AH, Setodji CM, et al. The quality of ambulatory care delivered to children in the United States. *N Engl J Med*. 2007;357:1515–1523
4. Ely JW, Osheroff JA, Gorman PN, et al. A taxonomy of generic clinical questions: classification study. *BMJ*. 2000;321(7258):429–432
5. Ely JW, Osheroff JA, Ebell MH, et al. Obstacles to answering doctors' questions about patient care with evidence: qualitative study. *BMJ*. 2002;324(7339):710
6. Ely JW, Osheroff JA, Chambliss ML, et al. Answering physicians' clinical questions: obstacles and potential solutions. *J Am Med Inform Assoc*. 2005;12(2):217–224
7. Cassidy SB, Allanson J, eds. *Management of Genetic Syndromes*. 2nd ed. Hoboken, NJ: John Wiley and Sons; 2005
8. Levy HP, LoPresti L, Siebert DC. Twenty questions in genetic medicine—an assessment of World Wide Web databases for genetics information at the point of care. *Genet Med*. 2008;10(9):659–667
9. InfoSourses.org. Clinical Decision Support System. http://www.infosources.org/what_is/Clinical_decision_support_system.html. Accessed November 23, 2010
10. Osheroff JA, Teich JM, Middleton BF, et al. A roadmap for national action on clinical decision support. *J Am Med Inform Assoc*. 2007;14(2):141–145
11. Online Mendelian Inheritance in Man. National Center for Biotechnology Information Web site. http://www.ncbi.nlm.nih.gov/omim. Accessed December 3, 2010

Glossary

-A-

acrocentric
When the centromere of a chromosome is positioned so that one chromosomal arm is much shorter than the other.

allele
One version of a gene at a given location (locus) along a chromosome.

aneuploidy
The occurrence of one or more extra or missing chromosomes leading to an unbalanced chromosome complement, or any chromosome number that is not an exact multiple of the haploid number.

anticipation
The tendency in certain genetic disorders for individuals in successive generations to present at an earlier age or with more severe manifestations; often observed in disorders resulting from the expression of a trinucleotide repeat mutation that tends to increase in size and have a more significant effect when passed from one generation to the next.

array comparative genomic hybridization (aCGH)
A method of examining multiple genes or loci simultaneously to identify genetic imbalance caused by the gain or loss of chromosomal material; may be designed as a multi-disorder (multigene) screening array to detect deletions or duplications across the genome; or it may be designed as a targeted array GH to interrogate a specific gene or chromosome segment.

autosome
Any chromosome that is not a sex-determining chromosome (ie, the X and Y chromosomes).

autosomal dominant

Describes a trait or disorder in which the phenotype is expressed in those who have inherited only one copy of a particular gene mutation (heterozygotes); specifically refers to a gene on 1 of the 22 pairs of autosomes (non–sex determining chromosomes).

autosomal recessive

Describes a trait or disorder requiring the presence of 2 copies of a gene mutation at a particular locus in order to express observable phenotype; specifically refers to genes on 1 of the 22 pairs of autosomes (non–sex determining chromosomes).

-B-

balanced chromosome translocations *See* translocation

band

A specific pattern of light and dark stripes that appear when chromosomes are stained at a particular stage in cell division using one of several types of preparations; bands help to identify the chromosome and evaluate its structure.

band level

The total number of bands estimated to be present in a haplotype set (23) of chromosomes. When cell division is arrested and cells are stained at prometaphase (early in mitosis), chromosomes appear longer, with approximately 700–1,200 bands. In metaphase (later in mitosis), chromosomes are more condensed, with approximately 300–600 bands. At higher band levels, the greater resolution increases the ability to identify more subtle chromosomal abnormalities and their breakpoints.

-C-

carrier

An individual who has a recessive, disease-causing gene mutation at a particular locus on one chromosome of a pair and a normal allele at that locus on the other chromosome; may also refer to an individual with a balanced chromosome rearrangement.

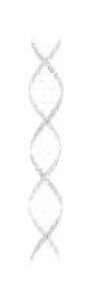

centromere
A constricted portion of the chromosome at which the chromatids (halves of the replicated chromosome) are joined and by which the chromosome is attached to the spindle during cell division. When aligning the chromosomes for analysis, each chromosome is placed with the short arms of chromosome oriented above the centromere and the long arms below.

chain terminator method
A common method of determining the sequence of DNA using a single-stranded DNA template; DNA primer; DNA polymerase, normal deoxynucleotide triphosphates (dNTPs); and radiolabeled, modified nucleotides (dideoxyNTPs or ddNTPs) that terminate DNA strand elongation.

chaperone therapy
Small pharmacological molecules that bind to and stabilize mutated enzymes, such as those found in some metabolic diseases (eg, cystic fibrosis).

chip *See* **gene chip**

chromatid
One of 2 identical halves of a replicated chromosome. Each half is called a sister chromatid. Chromatids are joined at the centromere.

chromatin
The combination of DNA and its packaging proteins that serve to condense DNA into a structure that prevents damage and controls DNA expression and replication. Three levels of chromatin organization are euchromatin (beads on a string, in which DNA wraps around histones), heterochromatin (the DNA and histones are tightly coiled into a 30 nm fiber), and the spatial organization of chromatin within the nucleus.

chromosome
Physical structure of genetic material consisting of a large DNA molecule organized into genes and supported by proteins, or chromatin.

classical genetics
The study of heredity based on the work of Gregor Mendel, who cross-pollinated pea plants. Also known as Mendelian genetics; it predates the advent of molecular biology.

clone

An identical copy of a DNA sequence or entire gene; one or more cells derived from and identical to a single ancestor cell; to isolate a gene or specific sequence of DNA.

coding region

All exons of a gene that contribute to the protein product(s) of the gene.

co-dominance

When both alleles (version of a gene at a given location) for a given gene are expressed.

codon

In DNA or RNA, a sequence of 3 nucleotides that codes for a specific amino acid or signals the termination of translation (ie, stop or termination codon).

cofactor

A non-protein component of an enzyme; organic cofactors are called coenzymes.

comparative genome hybridization

A technique that analyzes a sample of DNA for abnormal copy numbers (duplications and/or deletions) across the entire genome.

compound heterozygote

An individual who has 2 different abnormal alleles at a particular locus, one on each chromosome of a pair; usually refers to individuals affected with an autosomal recessive disorder.

congenital

Present from birth; not necessarily genetic.

consanguinity

Genetic relatedness between individuals descended from at least one common ancestor.

constitutional

A genetic abnormality present in each cell of the organism.

contiguous gene deletion syndrome

A syndrome caused by a microdeletion spanning 2 or more contiguous genes along a chromosome. Microdeletions may require FISH to be visualized, because they can be too small to be seen with conventional cytogenetic techniques.

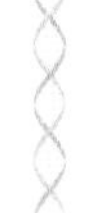

CpG islands
Short stretches of DNA that are rich in CG (cytosine-guanine), are found in approximately 70% of promoter regions of human genes, and are prone to methylation changes.

critical region
The specific portion of a chromosome or a gene that, when altered in some way (deleted, duplicated, or otherwise mutated), produces the characteristic set of phenotypic abnormalities associated with a particular syndrome or disorder.

cryptic deletion
A chromosome deletion too small to be observed with conventional cytogenetic techniques. These deletions are detectable with special techniques (eg, FISH or aCGH).

cytogenetics
The study of the structure, function, and abnormalities of human chromosomes.

cytokinesis
Division of the cytoplasm (extra-nuclear fluid containing organelles) within a cell following mitosis (somatic cell division).

-D-

daughter cell
The product of mitosis or somatic cell division.

de novo
A Latin term meaning new or from the beginning.

de novo mutation
An alteration in a gene that is present for the first time in one family member as a result of a mutation in a germ cell (egg or sperm) of one of the parents or in the fertilized egg itself. Synonyms: de novo gene mutation, new gene mutation, new mutation

deformation
An abnormal structure resulting from nondisruptive mechanical forces applied to a once normally formed structure.

deletion
A type of genetic mutation that results due to the loss of genetic material (eg, a single missing base pair or a segment of a chromosome) that may lead to abnormality or disease.

deletion/duplication analysis
Testing that identifies deletions/duplications of an entire exon, multiple exons, or a whole gene that are not readily detectable by sequence analysis of genomic DNA. A variety of methods may be used including quantitative PCR, long-range PCR, MLPA, and targeted array GH (gene or chromosome segment-specific). A full array GH analysis that detects deletions/duplications across the genome may also include a specific gene or chromosome segment of interest. Synonym: copy number analysis

diploid
The normal number of chromosomes in a somatic cell; in humans, 46 chromosomes (22 pairs of autosomes and 2 sex chromosomes).

disruption
Destruction of a once normally formed structure.

DNA
The molecules that encode the genes responsible for the structure and function of an organism and allow for transmission of genetic information from one generation to the next.

DNA banking
The process through which DNA is extracted from any of a number of possible cell sources and stored indefinitely by freezing or refrigerating for future testing.

DNA microchip *See* **gene chip**

DNA sequencing
A laboratory technique that determines the nucleotide progression of a strand of DNA.

dominant negative mutation
A mutation whose gene product adversely affects the normal, wild-type gene product within the same cell, usually by dimerizing (combining) with it. In cases of polymeric molecules, such as collagen, dominant negative mutations are often more deleterious than mutations causing the production of no gene product (null mutations or null alleles).

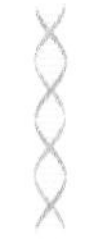

double heterozygote
An individual who is heterozygous for a mutation at each of 2 separate genetic loci.

duplication
The presence of an extra segment of DNA, resulting in redundant copies of a portion of a gene, an entire gene, or a series of genes, usually caused by unequal crossing over during gene replication, when gametes are formed in meiosis.

dysmorphology
The clinical study of abnormal structural (physical) features, including congenital malformations.

-E-

enhancer
Nucleic acid sequences within the DNA molecule that are necessary for proper gene expression, but do not code for genes.

epigenetics
The study of heritable, functionally relevant changes in gene expression or cellular phenotype by mechanisms other than changes in the nucleotide sequence.

epigenetic disorder
Disorders that arise from chemical modifications to a gene, primarily methylation and acetylation, that alter the transcription and expression of the gene.

epigenetic drift
Changes in gene expression (activation and deactivation) that occur over time due to a variety of reasons (eg, environmental factors or endogenous, random mechanisms).

exome sequencing
Sequencing of the entire protein-coding portion of the genome to identify the genetic cause of a single-gene disorder.

exon
Coding sequence of DNA that is translated to mature mRNA.

-F-

false paternity
The situation in which the alleged father of a particular individual is not the biological father. Synonyms: alternate paternity, nonpaternity, misattributed paternity

false-positive result
A test result that indicates that an individual is affected or has a certain gene mutation when he or she is actually unaffected or does not have the mutation (ie, a positive test result in an unaffected individual).

familial
Describes a phenotype that occurs in more than one family member; a familial phenotype may or may not be heritable in a classic Mendelian manner.

family history
The genetic relationships and medical history of a family; when represented in diagram form using standardized symbols and terminology, usually referred to as a pedigree.

first-degree relative
Any relative sharing 50% of genetic material with a particular individual in a family (ie, parent, sibling, offspring).

FISH *See* **fluorescent in situ hybridization**

fluorescent in situ hybridization (FISH)
A technique used to identify the presence of specific chromosomes or chromosomal regions through hybridization (attachment) of fluorescently labeled DNA probes to denatured chromosomal DNA. Examination under fluorescent lighting detects the presence of the hybridized fluorescent signal (and hence presence of the chromosome material) or absence of the hybridized fluorescent signal (and hence absence of the chromosome material).

founder effect
A gene mutation observed in high frequency in a specific population due to the presence of that gene mutation in a single ancestor or small number of ancestors.

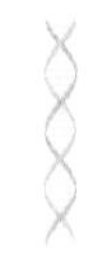

frameshift mutation
An insertion or deletion involving a number of base pairs that is not a multiple of 3 and consequently disrupts the triplet reading frame, usually leading to the creation of a premature termination (stop) codon and resulting in a truncated protein product. Synonyms: out-of-frame mutation, out-of-frame deletion

-G-

G-banded karyotype
A laboratory analysis used to analyze for chromosome abnormalities.

gamete
Mature reproductive cell, sperm or ovum, with haploid (1) set of genes (23 for humans).

gametogenesis
The meiotic process by which mature gametes (ova and sperm) are formed. Oogenesis is specifically the production of ova and spermatogenesis the production of sperm. Synonyms: spermatogenesis, oogenesis

gene
The basic unit of heredity, consisting of a segment of DNA arranged in a linear manner along a chromosome. A gene codes for a specific protein or segment of protein leading to a particular characteristic or function.

gene chip (also known as chip and DNA microchip)
Thousands of short, synthetic, single-stranded DNA sequences on the surface of a small glass plate. It is used in microarray technology for genomic analysis.

gene therapy
Experimental treatment of a genetic disorder by replacing, supplementing, or manipulating the expression of abnormal genes with normally functioning genes.

genetics
The study of heredity transmitted to offspring through the genes of their parents.

genetic counseling
A process, involving an individual or family, comprising evaluation to confirm, diagnose, or exclude a genetic condition, malformation syndrome, or isolated birth defect; discussion of natural history and the role of heredity; identification of medical management issues; calculation and communication of genetic risks; provision of or referral for psychosocial support.

genetic imprinting *See* **imprinting**

genome
The complete DNA sequence, supporting proteins, and associated metabolites (chemicals) comprising the entirety of the hereditary information.

genomics
The study of a person's genes including interaction of those genes with each other and the environment. The major tools and methods related to genomics studies are bioinformatics, genetic analysis, measurement of gene expression, and determination of gene function.

genomic imbalance
A condition where all or part of a chromosome has been deleted or duplicated.

genomic medicine
Using the interaction of genomic information and environmental factors (eg, diet, drugs) to predict, diagnose, and treat disease.

genomic microarray
A standard method of simultaneously assessing thousands of gene loci throughout the genome for deletions or duplications, using a computer to quantify fluorescent signals and hybridizing free DNA from the patient to individual probes. This method relies on both cytogenetic and molecular expertise.

genotype
The genetic constitution of an organism or cell; also refers to the specific set of alleles inherited at a locus.

genotype-phenotype correlation
The association between the presence of a certain mutation or mutations (genotype) and the resulting pattern of abnormalities or the expression of disease states (phenotype).

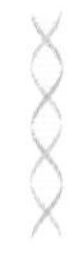

germline mosaicism
Two or more genetically different cell lines confined to the precursor (germline) cells of the egg or sperm; formerly called gonadal mosaicism.

-H-

haploid
Half the diploid or normal number of chromosomes in a somatic cell; the number of chromosomes in a gamete (egg or sperm) cell, which in humans is 23 chromosomes, one chromosome from each chromosome pairs (1–22) and one sex chromosome.

haploid insufficiency
The situation in which an individual who is heterozygous for a certain gene mutation or hemizygous at a particular locus, often due to a deletion of the corresponding allele, is clinically affected because a single copy of the normal gene is incapable of providing sufficient protein production to ensure normal function.

hemizygote
An individual who has only one member of a chromosome pair or chromosome segment rather than the usual 2; refers in particular to males who under normal circumstances have only one X chromosome and therefore are hemizygous for all their X-linked genes.

heteroplasmy
The situation in which, within a single cell, there is a mixture of mitochondria (energy-producing cytoplasmic organelles), some containing mutant DNA and some containing normal DNA.

heterozygote
An individual who has 2 different alleles at a particular locus, one on each chromosome of a pair; one allele is usually normal and the other abnormal.

histone
A structural protein associated with the DNA molecule.

homologous chromosomes
The 2 chromosomes from a particular pair, normally one inherited from the mother and one from the father, containing the same genetic loci in the same order. Synonym: homologs

homozygote
An individual who has 2 identical alleles at a particular locus, one on each chromosome of a pair.

horizontal transmission
A trait found in multiple individuals in the same generations; often due to autosomal recessive inheritance and compared to autosomal dominant transmission (vertical transmission).

-I-

imprinting
The process by which maternally and paternally derived chromosomes are uniquely chemically modified, leading to differential expression of a certain gene or genes on those chromosomes depending on their parental origin.

incomplete penetrance
A genetic mutation that produces no recognizable clinical manifestations, but can be transmitted and expressed in future generations.

informed consent
Permission given by an individual to proceed with a specific test or procedure, with an understanding of the risks, benefits, limitations, and potential implications of the procedure itself and its results.

institutional review board
A committee responsible for reviewing and approving biomedical research to ensure the safety of human subjects. It is typically composed of scientists, doctors, clergy, and consumers.

interphase
The resting phase between successive cell divisions.

intragenic
Being or occurring within a gene.

intron
Noncoding sequence of DNA.

inversion
A chromosomal rearrangement wherein a segment of genetic material breaks away from the chromosome, inverts end-to-end, and reinserts into the chromosome at the same breakage site.

isochromosome
A chromosome produced during cell division when the centromere splits transversely instead of longitudinally; the arms of the isochromosome are equal in length and genetically identical.

-K-

karyotype
A photographic representation of the chromosomes of a single cell, cut and arranged in pairs based on their size and banding pattern according to a standard classification.

-L-

linkage
The tendency for genes or segments of DNA closely positioned along a chromosome to segregate together at meiosis and therefore be inherited together.

linkage analysis
A method of locating a disease-causing mutation using several DNA sequence polymorphisms (normal variants) near or within the gene of interest. This technique is used in large, high-risk families to identify traits that are co-inherited with the disease.

linkage disequilibrium
In a population, co-occurrence of a specific DNA marker and a disease at a higher frequency than would be predicted by random chance.

loss of heterozygosity (LOH)
The result of a deletion or other mutational event at a particular locus heterozygous for a deleterious mutant allele and a normal allele; if the event occurs within the normal allele, it renders the cell hemizygous (one deleterious allele and one deleted allele).

lyonization
The phenomenon in females by which one X chromosome (either maternally derived or paternally derived) is randomly inactivated in early embryonic cells, with fixed inactivation in all descendant cells; first described by the geneticist Mary Lyon. Synonym: X-chromosome inactivation

-M-

malformation
A structural defect arising from an intrinsically abnormal development process during embryogenesis.

marker chromosome *See* **supernumerary chromosome**

matrilineal inheritance
Refers to mitochondrial DNA that is transmitted from the mother; fathers do not transmit mitochondrial DNA.

medical genomics *See* **genomic medicine**

meiosis
Cell division that results in the production of haploid (1 set of chromosomes; 23 in humans) gametes, sperm and ova.

Mendelian genetics
The study of inheritance based on the pea plant experiments of Gregor Mendel, published in 1866.

messenger RNA (mRNA)
A single-stranded RNA that is complementary to one of the DNA strands of a gene and serves as a template for protein synthesis.

methylation
The attachment of methyl groups to DNA at cytosine bases; correlated with reduced transcription of the gene and thought to be the principal mechanism in X-chromosome inactivation and imprinting.

methylation analysis
Testing that evaluates the methylation status of a gene (attachment of methyl groups to DNA cytosine bases); genes that are methylated are not expressed. Methylation plays a role in X-chromosome inactivation and imprinting.

microdeletion syndrome
A syndrome caused by a chromosomal deletion spanning several genes but is too small to be detected under the microscope using conventional cytogenetic methods. Depending on the size of the deletion, other methods of DNA analysis can sometimes identify the deletion. Synonym: contiguous gene deletion syndrome

microsatellite
Repetitive segments of DNA 2 to 5 nucleotides in length scattered throughout the genome in noncoding regions between genes or within genes (introns), often used as markers for linkage analysis because of the naturally occurring high variability in repeat number between individuals. These regions are inherently unstable and susceptible to mutations. Synonyms: satellite DNA, short tandem repeats

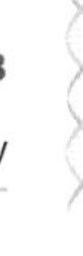

microsatellite instability (MSI)
The presence of a discrepancy between the size of microsatellites in DNA, resulting from mutations in a gene(s) in the DNA mismatch repair pathway that would normally correct these errors; often analyzed in tumor tissue. Synonyms: replication error phenotype or RER

missense mutation
A change of a single base pair that causes the substitution of a different amino acid in the resulting protein. This amino acid substitution may have no effect, or it may render the protein nonfunctional.

mitochondrial inheritance
Mitochondria, cytoplasmic organelles that produce the energy source ATP, contain their own distinct genome. Mutations in mitochondrial genes are responsible for several recognized syndromes and are always maternally inherited since ova contain mitochondria, whereas sperm do not.

mitosis
Division of a somatic cell (a body cell, ie, not sperm or ovum) resulting in genetically identical daughter cells.

molecular genetics
The study of the molecular processes underlying gene structure and function.

molecular reflex testing
A molecular test carried out in response to an analytical test result. This type of test is typically used to confirm results or to aid interpretation of the analytical test result.

monosomy
The presence of only one chromosome from a pair; partial monosomy refers to the presence of only one copy of a segment of a chromosome.

mosaicism
Within a single individual or tissue, the occurrence of 2 or more cell lines with different genetic or chromosomal constitutions.

mRNA *See* **messenger RNA**

multifactorial inheritance
The combined contribution of one or more often unspecified genes and environmental factors, often unknown, in the causation of a particular trait or disease. Synonym: polygenic inheritance

multiplex ligand-dependent probe assay (MLPA)
A PCR method that detects abnormal copies of DNA or RNA sequences that may differ in as little as only one nucleotide.

mutation
Any alteration in a gene from its natural state; may be disease-causing or a benign, normal variant.

-N-

nonsense mutation
A single nucleotide substitution that produces a stop codon in the gene, leading to a truncated protein product or to haploinsufficiency.

nuchal translucency
An increased thickness with translucency indicating subcutaneous fluid in the nuchal region of a fetus, noted on a fetal sonogram. It is associated with some genetic disorders (eg, Turner syndrome or Down syndrome).

nullisomic gamete
A sperm or ovum (egg) that lacks one or more pairs of homologous (identical) chromosomes.

-O-

obligate carrier
An individual who may be clinically unaffected but who must carry a gene mutation based on analysis of the family history; usually applies to disorders inherited in an autosomal recessive or X-linked recessive manner. Synonym: obligate heterozygote

oligonucleotide
A polymer of 2–20 nucleotides. It can be used as a probe in genetic testing when synthesized to match a region where a mutation is known to occur.

oocyte
An immature female reproductive cell that undergoes meiosis to become an ovum (egg).

-P-

patient-centered medical home (PC-MH)
A medical home model developed by the American Academy of Pediatrics that ensures care is accessible; continuous; comprehensive; family-centered; coordinated; compassionate; culturally effective; and meets preventive, primary, and tertiary needs.

pedigree
A diagram of the genetic relationships and medical history of a family using standard symbols and terminology.

penetrance
The proportion of individuals with a mutation causing a particular disorder who exhibit clinical symptoms of that disorder; most often refers to autosomal dominant conditions.

pericentric inversion
An inversion in which the breakpoints occur on both arms of a chromosome. The inverted segment spans the centromere.

pharmacogenomics
The study of inherited differences in drug metabolism and response using pharmacogenomic information. Pharmacogenomic information (eg, lack of an enzyme or metabolic variants) can be used to determine how an individual genetic variation will respond to some drugs.

phenotype
The observable physical and biochemical characteristics of the expression of a gene; the clinical presentation of an individual with a particular genotype.

pleiotropy
Multiple, often seemingly unrelated, physical effects caused by a single altered gene or pair of altered genes.

polymerase chain reaction (PCR)
A common procedure in molecular genetic testing and may be used to (1) generate a sufficient quantity of DNA to perform a test (eg, sequence analysis, mutation scanning) or (2) may be a test in and of itself (eg, allele-specific amplification, trinucleotide repeat quantification).

polymorphism
Natural variations in a gene, DNA sequence, protein, or chromosome that have no adverse effect on the individual and occur with fairly high frequency in the general population.

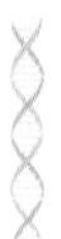

polyploidy

An increase in the number of haploid sets (23) of chromosomes in a cell. Triploidy refers to 3 whole sets of chromosomes in a single cell (in humans, a total of 69 chromosomes per cell); tetraploidy refers to 4 whole sets of chromosomes in a single cell (in humans, a total of 92 chromosomes per cell).

poor metabolizer (PM)

An individual with a predictably low rate of drug metabolism due to genetically determined drug-metabolizing enzymes.

population risk

The proportion of individuals in the general population who are affected with a particular disorder or who carry a certain gene; often discussed in the genetic counseling process as a comparison to the patient's personal risk given his or her family history or other circumstances. Synonym: background risk

post-translational modification

The final stage of protein production.

post-zygotic event

A mutational event or abnormality in chromosome replication or segregation that occurs after fertilization of the ovum by the sperm, often leading to mosaicism (2 or more genetically distinct cell lines within the same organism).

predictive testing

Testing offered to asymptomatic individuals with a family history of a genetic disorder and a potential risk of eventually developing the disorder.

preimplantation diagnosis

A procedure used to test for a particular genetic condition for which a fetus is specifically at risk by testing one cell removed from early embryos conceived by in vitro fertilization. Synonym: preimplantation testing

premutation

Found in disorders caused by trinucleotide repeat expansions (eg, fragile X syndrome), it is an abnormally large allele that is not associated with clinical symptoms, but can expand into a full mutation when transmitted to offspring. (Full mutations are associated with clinical symptoms of the disorder.)

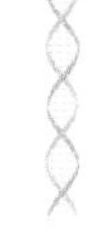

prenatal testing
Testing performed during pregnancy to determine if a fetus is affected with a particular disorder. Peripheral maternal blood testing, chorionic villus sampling (CVS), amniocentesis, and ultrasound are examples of procedures used either to obtain a sample for testing or to evaluate fetal anatomy.

presymptomatic testing
Testing of an asymptomatic individual in whom the discovery of a gene mutation might indicate certain development of findings related to a specific diagnosis at some future point.

primer
A short, single-stranded DNA sequence used in the PCR technique. The PCR method uses a pair of primers to hybridize with the sample DNA and define the region of the DNA that will be amplified. Primers are also referred to as oligonucleotides.

proband
The affected individual through whom a family with a genetic disorder is ascertained; may or may not be the individual presenting for genetic counseling. Synonyms: propositus, index case

promoter
A sequence of DNA that serves as the binding site for RNA polymerase, the enzyme to which mRNA binds to initiate transcription. It is usually found near the beginning of a gene.

pseudodominant inheritance
An autosomal recessive condition present in individuals in 2 or more generations of a family, thereby appearing to follow a dominant inheritance pattern. Common explanations include (1) a high carrier frequency and (2) birth of an affected child to an affected individual and a genetically related (consanguineous) reproductive partner.

-Q-

quantitative PCR
The use of PCR to determine the amount of DNA or RNA in a sample; commonly used to detect heterozygous deletion mutations and duplication mutations. Synonyms: real time quantitative PCR, kinetic quantitative PCR

-R-

real-time quantitative PCR
A molecular technique used to detect intragenic deletions and duplications.

rearrangement
A structural alternation in a chromosome, resulting in abnormal configuration (eg, breakage and reattachment of a segment of chromosomal material).

reciprocal translocation
A segment of one chromosome is exchanged with a segment of another chromosome of a different pair.

recombination
The exchange of a segment of DNA between 2 homologous chromosomes during meiosis leading to a novel combination of genetic material in the gamete. Synonym: crossing over

recurrence risk
The likelihood that a trait or disorder present in one family member will occur again in other family members in the same or subsequent generations.

restriction fragment length polymorphism analysis (RFLP analysis)
Fragment of DNA of predictable size resulting from digestion (cutting) of a strand of DNA by a given restriction enzyme. DNA sequence alterations (mutations) that destroy or create the sites at which a restriction enzyme cuts DNA change the size (and number) of DNA fragments resulting from digestion by a given restriction enzyme. Synonym: RFLP testing

ring chromosome
A structural rearrangement of a chromosome that occurs when a chromosome breaks in 2 places and the resulting pieces fuse to form a circular structure. Genetic material is often lost in this type of rearrangement.

risk assessment
Calculation of an individual's risk, using appropriate mathematical equations, of having inherited a certain gene mutation, of developing a particular disorder, or of having a child with a certain disorder based on analysis of multiple factors including family medical history and ethnic background.

RNA
The molecule synthesized from the DNA template; contains the sugar ribose instead of deoxyribose, which is present in DNA; 3 types of RNA exist: mRNA, transfer RNA (tRNA), and ribosomal RNA (rRNA).

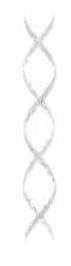

Robertsonian translocation
The joining of 2 acrocentric chromosomes at the centromeres with loss of their short arms to form a single abnormal chromosome; in acrocentric chromosomes the centromere is located near the end of the chromosome. Acrocentric chromosomes are chromosomes numbered 13, 14, 15, 21, and 22.

-S-

screening
Testing designed to identify individuals in a given population who are at higher risk of having or developing a particular disorder, or having a gene mutation for a particular disorder.

second-degree relative
Any relative sharing 25% of genetic material with a particular individual in a pedigree (ie, grandparent, grandchild, uncle, aunt, nephew, niece, half-sibling).

segregation
The separation of the homologous chromosomes and their random distribution to the gametes at meiosis.

sensitivity
The frequency with which a test yields a positive result when the individual being tested is actually affected or has the gene mutation in question.

sequence analysis
Process by which the nucleotide sequence is determined for a segment of DNA. Synonyms: gene sequencing, sequencing

sibship
A group of siblings; people related by a common ancestor.

simplex case
A single occurrence of a disorder in a family.

single-nucleotide polymorphism (SNP)
A natural variation in a single nucleotide at one loci in the genome. SNPs are used to correlate the genome with disease, drug response, and other phenotypes.

single-stranded conformational polymorphism (SSCP)
A type of mutation scanning; the identification of abnormally migrating single-stranded DNA segments on gel electrophoresis.

sister chromatid *See* **chromatid**

SNP *See* **single-nucleotide polymorphism**

somatic cell
A body cell, does not include reproductive cells sperm and ovum (egg).

somatic mosaicism
Two or more genetic or cytogenetic cell lines within the cells of the body (may or may not include the germline cells).

Southern blot
Molecular genetic testing technique used to detect differences in the lengths of DNA fragments following restriction enzyme digestion (commonly known as RFLPs). The lengths of restriction fragments can vary when mutations occur between 2 restriction sites (eg, large insertions, large deletions, and highly expanded trinucleotide repeats) or within a restriction site (eg, single base pair changes). Synonyms: Southern analysis, Southern blot analysis, Southern blotting, Southern blotting analysis

specificity
The probability that an individual who does not have the particular disease being tested for will be correctly identified as negative, expressed as the proportion of true-negative results to the total of true-negative and false-positive results.

spermatid
A haploid germ (reproductive) cell that is the product of meiosis II; the precursor cell to sperm during spermiogenesis.

spermatocyte
A diploid germ (reproductive) cell that is the product of meiosis I; the precursor cell to spermatid during spermatocytogenesis.

splice-site mutation
A mutation that alters or abolishes the specific sequence denoting the site at which the splicing of an intron takes place. Such mutations result in one or more introns remaining in the mature mRNA and can disrupt the generation of the protein product.

splicing
The process by which introns, noncoding regions, are excised out of the primary mRNA transcript and exons are joined together to generate mature mRNA. Synonym: splicing mutation

sporadic
The chance occurrence of a disorder or abnormality that is not likely to recur in a family.

stem cell
Unspecialized cells capable of mitosis (somatic cell division), sometimes after long periods of inactivity. Under certain physiological or experimental conditions, stem cells can be induced to become tissue- or organ-specific cells. There are 2 types of stem cells: embryonic and somatic adult stem cells.

subtelomeric region
The chromosomal region just proximal to the telomere (end of the chromosome) composed of highly polymorphic repetitive DNA sequences that are typically situated adjacent to gene-rich areas. Microdeletions and subtle rearrangements that disrupt genes in the subtelomeric regions can cause intellectual disability. Use of FISH to evaluate subtelomeric regions is usually required for detection of these abnormalities.

supernumerary chromosome
A small, extra chromosome containing a centromere occasionally seen in tissue culture, often in a mosaic state (present in some cells but not in others). This marker chromosome may be of little clinical significance or, if it contains material from one or both arms of another chromosome, may create an imbalance for whatever genes are present; establishing clinical significance, particularly if found in a fetal karyotype, is often difficult.

-T-

targeted mutation analysis
Testing for (1) a nucleotide repeat expansion (eg, the trinucleotide repeat expansion associated with Huntington disease) or (2) one or more specific mutations (eg, Glu6Val for sickle cell anemia, a panel of mutations for cystic fibrosis). Deletion or duplication analysis and family-specific mutation analysis are excluded from this definition. Synonym: allele-specific mutation analysis

telomere
The segment at the end of each chromosome arm, which consists of a series of repeated DNA sequences that regulate chromosomal replication at each cell division. Some of the telomere is lost each time a cell divides and, eventually, when the telomere is gone, the cell dies.

teratogen
Any agent that interferes with fetal development.

transcription
The process of synthesizing mRNA from DNA.

translation
The process of synthesizing an amino acid sequence (protein product) from mRNA.

translocation
A chromosome alteration in which a whole chromosome or segment of a chromosome becomes attached to or interchanged with another whole chromosome or chromosomal segment. The resulting hybrid segregates together at meiosis. Balanced translocations (in which there is no net loss or gain of chromosome material) are usually not associated with phenotypic abnormalities, although gene disruptions at the breakpoints of the translocation can, in some cases, cause adverse effects, including some known genetic disorders. Unbalanced translocations (in which there is loss or gain of chromosome material) nearly always yield an abnormal phenotype. Synonym: chromosome rearrangement

trinucleotide repeat
Sequences of 3 nucleotides repeated a number of times in tandem within a gene. Normal polymorphic variation in repeat number with no clinical significance commonly occurs between individuals. Abnormally large alleles are classified in increasing order of size as mutable normal alleles, reduced penetrance alleles, and full penetrance alleles.

trisomy
The presence of a single extra chromosome, yielding a total of 3 chromosomes of that particular type instead of a pair. Partial trisomy refers to the presence of an extra copy of a segment of a chromosome.

trisomy rescue
The phenomenon in which a fertilized ovum initially contains 47 chromosomes (ie, is trisomic), but loses one of the trisomic chromosomes in the process of cell division such that the resulting daughter cells and their descendants contain 46 chromosomes, the typical number.

-U-

ultra-rapid metabolizer (UM)
An individual with a rapid rate of drug metabolism due to genetically determined drug-metabolizing enzymes.

unbalanced chromosome translocation *See* **translocation**

unequal crossing over
Mispairing and exchange of DNA between genetically similar, nonhomologous chromosome regions that results in duplication or deletion of DNA in each daughter cell.

uniparental disomy (UPD)
The situation in which both members of a chromosome pair or segments of a chromosome pair are inherited from one parent and neither is inherited from the other parent. Uniparental disomy can result in an abnormal phenotype in some cases. Uniparental heterodisomy refers to 2 different homologous chromosomes inherited from one parent, instead of one from each parent, and uniparental isodisomy refers to 2 identical homologs from one parent.

-V-

variable expression
Variation in clinical features (type and severity) of a genetic disorder between affected individuals, even within the same family.

variable number tandem repeats (VNTR)
Linear arrangement of multiple copies of short repeated DNA sequences that vary in length and are highly polymorphic, making them useful as markers in linkage analysis.

vertical transmission
A trait found in multiple generations in a family.

-W-

wild-type allele
The normal, as opposed to a mutant, gene or allele.

-X-

X-chromosome inactivation
In females, the phenomenon by which one X chromosome (either maternally or paternally derived) is randomly inactivated in early embryonic cells, with fixed inactivation in all descendant cells; first described by the geneticist Mary Lyon. Synonym: lyonization

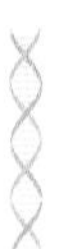

X-chromosome inactivation study (XCI study)
Molecular genetic testing to assess the relative proportion of methylated (inactive) X chromosomes to unmethylated (active) X chromosomes; used to determine if X-chromosome inactivation is random or skewed.

X-linked dominant
Describes a dominant trait or disorder caused by a mutation in a gene on the X chromosome. The phenotype is expressed in heterozygous females as well as in hemizygous males (who have one X chromosome); affected males tend to have a more severe phenotype than affected females.

X-linked lethal
A disorder caused by a dominant mutation in a gene on the X chromosome that is observed almost exclusively in females because it is almost always lethal in males who inherit the gene mutation.

X-linked recessive
A mode of inheritance in which a mutation in a gene on the X chromosome causes the phenotype to be expressed in males who are hemizygous for the gene mutation (ie, they have only one X chromosome) and in females who are homozygous for the gene mutation (ie, they have a copy of the gene mutation on each of their 2 X chromosomes). Carrier females who have only one copy of the mutation do not usually express the phenotype, although differences in X-chromosome inactivation can lead to varying degrees of clinical expression in carrier females.

-Z-

zygote
A fertilized ovum; the cell resulting from the union of gametes (ie, ovum and sperm).

zygosity testing
The process through which DNA sequences are compared to assess whether individuals born from a multiple gestation (twins, triplets, etc) are monozygotic (identical) or dizygotic (fraternal); often used to identify a suitable donor for organ transplantation or to estimate disease susceptibility risk if one sibling is affected.

Appendix A

Resources for the Pediatrician

Kim M. Keppler-Noreuil, MD

Introduction

To appropriately evaluate and manage a patient who may have a genetic diagnosis, the pediatrician must have knowledge of available resources and understand when a referral to a clinical geneticist is advisable.

The number and type of resources are vast. Resources are divided into 2 categories.

1. Resources available to the pediatrician when genetic factors are considered relevant in developing a differential diagnosis based on presenting clinical signs and/or symptoms
2. Resources for the pediatrician and patient/family once the specific genetics disorder or diagnosis is known

The resources suggested below are selected because they are accurate, dependable, and user-friendly. The genetic resources are provided in several formats, including textbooks, Internet resources, and software databases. Each resource has unique strengths and weaknesses, and an attempt has been made to help focus the pediatrician on those most relevant to the given topic.

Selected Resources Based on Clinical Symptoms and/or Signs

The genetic contribution to disease risk has been described as a continuum from diseases caused mostly by genetic factors, to diseases caused by a combination of genetic and environmental factors, to diseases caused mostly by environment influences.[1] Ascertainment or recognition of genetic factors relies on key characteristics in the medical history, including the prenatal, neonatal, and postnatal history, as well as a 3-generation family history. Clinical dysmorphology examination, in addition to medical and family history, can lead to a genetic diagnosis.

Family History

Family history can indicate a genetic diagnosis or genetic contribution to common diseases. The collection and evaluation of a detailed 3-generation family history or pedigree is essential for this purpose. Therefore, the family history can be used by the pediatrician as a triage tool in many clinical scenarios, such as in evaluation of the individual with developmental delay or intellectual disability.[1] As another example, suspicion of an underlying cancer genetic syndrome is raised with (1) earlier age of onset than typical for the cancer, (2) multiple individuals in at least 2 to 3 generations, (3) types of cancers/clusters, (4) histopathologic type of a particular cancer, and (5) bilateral versus unilateral disease.

Resources to obtaining a family history (Chapter 5) and providing basic risk calculations include

- March of Dimes: Genetics & Your Practice: "Family Health and Social History": www.marchofdimes.com/gyponline/index.bm2
- The American Society of Human Genetics—Health Provider Genetics Resources: www.ashg.org/press/healthprofessional.shtml

Prenatal History

In the prenatal history, the following key points raise concern about teratogenic effects: maternal illnesses (such as diabetes mellitus, hypertension, and infection) and maternal exposure to certain therapeutic medications, alcohol, drugs, and cigarettes. Other parts of the prenatal history that are helpful for determining an underlying genetic etiology include abnormal ultrasound findings (growth abnormalities or malformations), decreased movement, or abnormal prenatal screening results. Resources helpful for evaluating the implications of these historical findings include teratogen databases such as

- TERIS: http://depts.washington.edu/terisweb/teris/ (subscription database)
- Reprotox: reprotox.org (subscription database)
- *Smith's Recognizable Patterns of Human Malformation*, 6th ed. 2006
- *Human Malformations and Related Anomalies*, 2nd ed. 2006

Neonatal History

Neonatal historical clues to possible genetic contribution include growth retardation, overgrowth, abnormal Apgar scores, prematurity, poly- or anhydramnios, respiratory distress, and malformations. Resources to use when these findings are identified may include

- *Smith's Recognizable Patterns of Human Malformation,* 6th ed. 2006 (organized by sign-specific syndromes and by index in the back of book for symptoms/signs with listing of syndromes)
- Online Mendelian Inheritance of Man (OMIM): www.ncbi.nlm.nih.gov/OMIM

Postnatal History

Postnatal history and findings may include, but not be limited to, poor feeding, developmental delay, hypotonia, hypertonia, abnormal newborn hearing screen, abnormal newborn screening test, and the presence of single or multiple malformations. Several studies highlight the usefulness of the physical examination findings, in particular the presence of minor malformations in signaling the presence of a likely genetic diagnosis. Valuable resources to search for potential diagnoses with a presence of a particular malformation or neurologic finding may include

- OMIM: www.ncbi.nlm.nih.gov/OMIM
- *Inherited Metabolic Diseases (Core Handbooks in Pediatrics)* (for abnormal newborn screening test or signs like hypotonia)
- *Human Malformations and Related Anomalies* (for structural malformations)

Some pediatricians may order appropriate initial studies then seek consultation with a clinical geneticist, while others may choose to proceed directly to consult the clinical geneticist to start the diagnostic evaluation. Either way, knowing what is likely to be involved in the clinical genetics diagnostic evaluation allows the pediatrician to prepare the family for what to expect during the evaluation and to integrate a diagnosis into the care provided to the child and the family.[1] A partnership between genetics and the pediatrician ensures a smooth transition between care provided by the 2 specialties.[2]

Selection of Resources and Available Formats Based on Known Diagnoses

When a specific diagnosis is identified, there are a multitude of available resources for the pediatrician. The initial source will depend on whether there is a specific question regarding the disease characteristics, natural history, complications, and etiology of the disorder, and/or for diagnostic testing, which includes a growing number of biochemical, cytogenetic, and DNA-based tests. Choice of one or more of these resources may also be based on the format or presentation of the information, as well as the intended audience and the application of the information (eg, whether for the physician or for the patient and family). For instance, the pediatrician may choose a textbook, Internet resource(s), or software program, or all of these.

Each of the different formats has somewhat unique qualities and emphases, but naturally there is some overlap of information within these resources. Most physicians should use each of these resources in Table 1 and Table 2, recognizing their potential strengths and weaknesses.

Textbooks will have the advantage of presenting a comprehensive review of information, often written by experts in the field and in a particular area. Possible disadvantages of using a textbook include (1) not easily accessible or portable, (2) costly (eg, may be limited to whether a physician has chosen to purchase this resource), (3) outdated information depending on date of publication, (4) it may not specifically address the question asked or be difficult to find the information in the presenting format, and (5) it may not be appropriate for sharing with the patient or family.

There are hundreds of Internet resources, with the advantages of being (1) easily accessible for those with computer access, (2) free for the user for many of these, (3) able to find answers to specific questions, (4) updated regularly for some. Disadvantages of Internet resources may include (1) reliability and accuracy of the information (the user must know the source of the information provided) and (2) some require a subscription or membership fee.

Finally, software programs have the advantage of providing search protocols to generate differential diagnoses and can be accessed on the computer without having an unwieldy textbook; however, they can also be costly and may not be updated as frequently as some of the Internet resources. In addition, many are written by and for geneticists, and non-geneticists may find them difficult to understand and use.

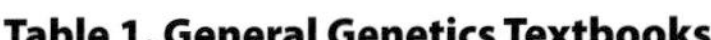

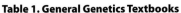

Table 1. General Genetics Textbooks

Textbook	Description
Cassidy SB, Allanson JE. *Management of Genetic Syndromes*. 3rd ed. New York, NY: Wiley-Blackwell; 2010	Description of the more commonly encountered syndromes, including an overview of the characteristic findings, etiology, and natural history, followed by a discussion of the evaluation and management/treatments organized by organ system involvement for each syndrome. Useful information for the clinician that can be shared with the patient/family as well.
Hennekam RCM, Allanson J, Krantz I. *Gorlin's Syndromes of the Head & Neck*. 5th ed. New York, NY: Oxford University Press; 2010	This textbook presents a comprehensive delineation of multiple syndromes with unusual facies grouped into useful categories. Besides excellent narrative descriptions and photographs, molecular aspects of the syndromes are also addressed.
Jones KL. *Smith's Recognizable Patterns of Human Malformation*. 6th ed. Philadelphia, PA: Saunders-Elsevier; 2006	A primary source for thorough yet concise descriptions of syndromes, sequences, and associations organized by the most commonly recognized chromosomal, single gene, teratogenic, and unknown etiologic disorders. Descriptions include associated findings organized by frequency in different organ systems, known etiology(ies), natural history, pertinent references, and useful photographs and diagrams.
Nussbaum R, Innes R, Willard H. *Thompson and Thompson Genetics in Medicine*. 7th ed. Philadelphia, PA: Saunders-Elsevier; 2007	Application of basic genetic concepts and principles to clinical genetics. It provides illustrative 2-page case summaries with overview of etiology and inheritance, with reference to the text for more in-depth discussion of basic concepts.
Rimoin DL, Connor JM, Pyeritz RE, Korf BR. *Emery and Rimoin's Principles and Practice of Medical Genetics*. 5th ed. New York, NY: Churchill Livingstone; 2007	A comprehensive and up-to-date textbook of clinical genetics, presenting basic and general principles of genetics, approaches to clinical problems, and specific disorders, organized by organ systems. Disease-gene discovery as it clarifies the pathways, network, and systems in which these genes normally interact to result in emergent phenotypes in clinical genetics is discussed in this text.
Seashore MR, Wappner RS. *Genetics in Primary Care & Clinical Medicine*. Stanford, CA: Appleton & Lange; 1996	A well-written, concise book that covers a wide range of genetic disorders, including a large number of inborn errors of metabolism. Excellent introduction to clinical genetics.

Table 1. General Genetics Textbooks *(continued)*

Textbook	Description
Stevenson RE, Hall JG, Goodman RM. *Human Malformations and Related Anomalies*. 2nd ed. New York, NY: Oxford University Press; 2006	Structural malformations within each organ system are reviewed by experts in the field of genetics, with descriptions including epidemiology of the defect, embryologic pathogenesis, etiology, natural history, prognosis, and listings of associated syndromes/disorders. Helpful figures, photographs, and tables are used.
Stevenson RE, Schwartz CE, Rogers RC. *X-linked Intellectual Disability Syndromes*. 2nd ed. New York, NY: Oxford University Press; 2012	A clinical presentation of known syndromic forms of intellectual disability having X-linked patterns of inheritance.
Chromosomal Abnormalities	
Schinzel A. *Catalogue of Unbalanced Chromosome Aberrations in Man.* New York, NY: Walter de Gruyter; 2001	Source book on chromosome abnormalities.
Connective Tissue and Skeletal Dysplasias	
Beighton P. *McKusick's Heritable Disorders of Connective Tissue.* 5th ed. St Louis, MO: Mosby; 1993	A comprehensive reference text on both generalized and heritable inherited disorders of connective tissue. The book is intended for geneticists, genetic counselors, and medical specialists (orthopedists, ophthalmologists, dermatologists, cardiologists, and others) who are involved in the care or study of patients with inherited disorders of connective tissue. The author and contributors are all acknowledged experts in this field.
Spranger JW, Brill PW, Superti-Furga A, Unger S, Nishimura G. *Bone Dysplasias: An Atlas of Genetic Disorders of Skeletal Development.* 3rd ed. New York, NY: Oxford University Press; 2012	Definitive resource containing 160 chapters on individual disorders, common and rare, that are grouped by families of conditions according to the *International Nomenclature and Classification of the Osteochondrodysplasias*. Each chapter puts its condition into the current context of genetic diseases. The chapters review clinical, laboratory, radiographic, demographic, pathologic, and genetic findings; discuss prognosis, treatment, and differential diagnosis; and supply pertinent references. The radiologic and clinical images in each chapter are characteristic and instructive.

Table 1. General Genetics Textbooks *(continued)*

Textbook	Description
Teratology	
Briggs GG, Freeman RK, Yaffe SJ. *Drugs in Pregnancy and Lactation.* 6th ed. Baltimore, MD: Lippincott, Williams & Wilkins; 2002	Reference guide to fetal and neonatal risk. Discusses risk potential to the fetus of maternal drugs ingested during pregnancy and risk potential to the infant of maternal drugs with breastfeeding. It evaluates the research literature, animal and human, applied and clinical. It provides recommendations for the use of drugs based on review of the risks to benefits.
Shepard TH. *Catalog of Teratogenic Agents.* 13th ed. Baltimore, MD: Johns Hopkins University Press; 2010	A valuable reference on the known fetal outcomes of human and animal maternal exposure to drugs, chemicals, and infectious agents and outcomes secondary to maternal disease. It features about 3,000 agents, including 1,200 additions of drugs and other agents to which pregnant women may be exposed; there are 250 newly listed agents.
Cancer Syndromes	
Lindor NM, McMaster ML, Lindor CJ, Greene MH; National Cancer Institute, Division of Cancer Prevention, Community Oncology and Prevention Trials Research Group. Concise handbook of familial cancer susceptibility syndromes—second edition. *J Natl Cancer Inst Monogr*. 2008;(38):1–93	Clinically accessible catalog of recognizable family cancer syndromes designed for busy clinicians who only occasionally need this information. This handbook presents summaries of cancer genetic syndromes in alphabetical order organized into subtopics: OMIM number, inheritance pattern, gene and chromosomal location, mutations, incidence, diagnosis, laboratory features, associated malignant neoplasms, associated benign neoplasms, cancer risk management, comments, and references.
Inherited Metabolic Diseases	
Hoffman GF, Nyhan WL, Zschocke J, et al. *Inherited Metabolic Diseases (Core Handbooks in Pediatrics).* Philadelphia, PA: Lippincott Williams & Wilkins; 2002	Presents rational approaches for investigations of patients based on their history, symptoms, and signs and puts emphasis on acutely presenting disorders and emergency situations. It provides a system-based and symptom-based approach to inherited metabolic diseases designed to help colleagues come to the appropriate diagnoses and to arrange an optimal therapy program.

Table 2. Online Genetics Resources

Organization/Resource	URL	Description
American Academy of Pediatrics (AAP) Committee on Genetics	www.aap.org/visit/cmte18.htm	This site contains links to various topics and resources on clinical genetics. It includes links to current AAP policy statements authored by the Committee on Genetics (eg, health supervision guidelines for various disorders including Down syndrome, Williams syndrome, fragile X syndrome, and many others). It also contains links to a selected list of other genetics-related AAP policy documents, patient education brochures and other materials related to genetics issues, and selected links (AAP links, external links).
American Medical Association (AMA)	www.ama-assn.org/ama/pub/physician-resources/medical-science/genetics-molecular-medicine/news.shtml	The AMA Web site provides a wealth of genetics information, materials, and continuing medical education program resources that inform health providers about the basic science of genetics and describe how knowledge gained from research advances and discoveries in the field can be applied to general medical practice. Some genetics resources of interest featured on the AMA Web site include • Basic genetics FAQs for health care professionals • Family history information for health care professionals • "Genetics and Molecular Medicine" (2007)—information for health providers on the latest research in medical • Genetics and molecular medicine • "Genetics: Education and Research" (2007)—information for health providers regarding genetics education initiatives and recent research developments • "Genetics and Common Disorders: Implications for Primary Care and Public Health Providers" (2006)

Organization/Resource	URL	Description
American Society of Human Genetics (ASHG)—Genetics Resources for Health Professionals	www.ashg.org/press/healthprofessional.shtml	This Web site contains multiple links to a number of genetic topics for the health professional, including • Genetics education resources for practitioners • Quick reference resources for practitioners • Incorporating genetics in clinical practice • Personalized medicine and pharmacogenetics • Genetic testing • Family history • Glossaries and definitions of genetics terms • Audio clips and podcasts • Presentation resources
Dartmouth Medical School: "Genetics in Clinical Practice: A Team Approach"	http://iml.dartmouth.edu/education/cme/Genetics/	The CME program resources featured on this Web site are intended for health care providers who see patients that may have genetic disorders and/or risk factors for developing such disorders. The resources from this CME program provide information about genetic testing and other basic clinical genetics concepts. They also explain how knowledge of clinical genetics can positively affect patient health outcomes and improve disease prevention and treatment methods on a larger scale.
eMedicine	http://emedicine.medscape.com/pediatrics_genetics	Medscape's continually updated clinical reference with 6,500 articles and 10,000 physician contributors providing pediatrics-focused genetics and metabolic disease articles.
GeneReviews and GeneTests	www.geneclinics.org	This expert-written, peer-reviewed medical database contains descriptions of genetic disorders, including information on diagnosis, treatment, and genetic testing for these conditions. The information is very useful, particularly for clinicians. It also provides links to other genetic resources for the clinician and for families. It has educational modules on clinical genetics.

Table 2. Online Genetics Resources *(continued)*

Organization/Resource	URL	Description
Genetics Alliance and ASHG: "Guide to Understanding Genetics"	www.geneticalliance.org/understanding.genetics	A group of experts from Genetic Alliance and ASHG worked in partnership to create a straightforward guide for the general public, health care providers, and their patients. The guide covers basic information about genetics concepts and provides in-depth information about genetic conditions, newborn screening, family history gathering, genetic counseling, and an overview of different types of genetic tests and their applications.
Genetics Resources on the Web (GROW)	http://bioethics.od.nih.gov/grow.html	The mission of the GROW site and search engine is to optimize the use of the Web to provide health professionals and the public with high-quality information related to human genetics, with a particular focus on genetic medicine and health.
InfoGenetics	www.infogenetics.org	This site is designed to assist providers in the daily care of their patients and on how to use constantly changing genetics information and testing in clinical care. It was developed with support from Genetic Services Branch, Maternal and Child Health, Department of Health and Human Services and Children's Hospital of The King's Daughters Health System, Norfolk, VA. It has links to many different genetic Web sites. The listing of Web sites includes • University of California, San Diego Biochemical testing • Clinical guidelines • Clinical trial (National Institutes of Health) • Prenatal genetics—www.reprotox.org (current information about teratogens) • Cancer genetics—www.cancer.gov/cancerinfo/prevention-genetics-causes (information about genetic cancer syndromes) • Support groups (support group information for patients and families) • Parent to parent (family contacts through the National Parent to Parent Support and Information System) • Newborn screening (information about newborn screening programs in all 50 states) • Ethical issues (ethical and legal issues that are important in taking care of individuals with genetic problems)

Organization/Resource	URL	Description
March of Dimes—Genetics and Your Practice	www.marchofdimes.com/gyponline/index.bm2	Founded by Franklin D. Roosevelt to fight polio, the March of Dimes' expanded mission is to prevent premature births and birth defects through research and advocacy. This is a global organization with local chapters and extensive networks. Local programs include Centering Pregnancy (providing access to group prenatal care) and NICU Family Support (providing education and support to parents of infants in the NICU).
National Coalition for Health Professional Education in Genetics (NCHPEG)	www.nchpeg.org	Established by the AMA, the American Nurses Association, and the National Human Genome Research Institute, the NCHPEG is committed to a national effort to promote health professional education and access to information about advances in human genetics. NCHPEG members are an interdisciplinary group of leaders from more than 140 diverse health professional organizations, consumer and volunteer groups, government agencies, private industry, managed care organizations, and genetics professional societies.
National Human Genome Research Institute	www.genome.gov	This site presents educational materials about genetics and genomics for educators and the general public.
National Library of Medicine (NLM)—Genetics Home Reference	http://ghr.nlm.nih.gov	Guide to understanding genetic conditions, genes, chromosomes, and newborn screening and testing. It also provides links to other resources.
National Organization of Rare Disorders (NORD)—The Rare Disease Database	http://www.rarediseases.org	This is one of the largest clinical databases, containing information on more than 1,000 rare disorders. It is maintained by NORD, a federation of voluntary health organizations.
Newborn Screening ACT Sheets and Confirmatory Algorithms	www.acmg.net/resources/policies/ACT/condition-analyte-links.htm	The contents describe the interrelationships between the conditions screened in newborn screening laboratories and the markers (analytes) used for screening. For each marker(s), there is (1) an action (ACT) sheet that describes the short-term actions a health professional should follow in communicating with the family and determining the appropriate steps in the follow-up of the infant that has screened positive and (2) an algorithm that presents an overview of the basic steps involved in determining the final diagnosis in the infant.

Table 2. Online Genetics Resources *(continued)*

Organization/Resource	URL	Description
Online Mendelian Inheritance in Man (OMIM)	www.ncbi.nlm.nih.gov/omim	This is the online version of *Mendelian Inheritance in Man*. OMIM is a comprehensive, authoritative, and timely compendium of human genes and genetic phenotypes. The full-text, referenced overviews in OMIM contain information on all known Mendelian disorders and more than 12,000 genes. OMIM focuses on the relationship between phenotype and genotype. It is updated daily, and the entries contain copious links to other genetics resources. It is freely available from the National Center for Biotechnology Information. It has clinical data that are useful in daily practice. It also contains links to various resources, including PubMed, which is useful to access scientific publications.
Rare Genetic Diseases in Children	http://mcrcr2.med.nyo.edu/murphp01	This site contains links to various sources of information on rare genetic disease that affect children.
Reprotox	www.reprotox.org	Database of teratogens.
Society for the Study of Inborn Errors of Metabolism (SSIEM)	www.ssiem.org.uk/	The home page of the SSIEM provides excellent links to various Internet resources that deal with inborn errors of metabolism, including laboratory directories.
TERIS database (teratogen information system database)	http://depts.washington.edu/terisweb/teris/	Developed by the University of Washington and updated with information from Shepard. As part of TERIS, 6 nationally recognized clinical teratologists rate the magnitude of teratogenic risk to a child born after gestational exposure and the quality and quantity of data used for risk estimates and offer qualifying comments. Requires 1 yearly subscription fee.

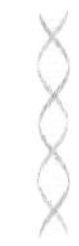

Dysmorphology Databases

The Web sites below link to information about these databases. The databases are available by subscription only.

- POSSUM (www.possum.net.au)
  Database that assists clinicians in diagnosing dysmorphic syndromes in patients. It contains multiple malformations and metabolic, teratogenic, chromosomal, and skeletal syndromes and their images—for learning and diagnosis.
- London Medical Databases (www.lmdatabases.com/about_lmd.html)
  Currently consists of a dysmorphology, a neurogenetics, and an ophthalmic genetics database for clinicians.

Web Sites for Ethical Issues in Medical Genetics

www.faseb.org/genetics/ashg/ashgmenu.htm
www.acmg.net
www.nsgc.org/
www.nhgri.nih.gov/ELSI

Resources for Patients and Families

See Table 3 for a list of resources that can be shared with patients and families.

Using the Tools of the Trade

The clinical geneticist often uses dysmorphology databases, particularly when there are structural malformations in addition to neurobehavioral findings. However, genetics resources can be used by both the clinical geneticist and pediatrician. In order to illustrate how these tools are put into practice, an example that a pediatrician might encounter is in Box 1.

Table 3. Resources for Patients and Families

Resource	URL	Description
Ask the Geneticist	http://askthegen.org	This Web site posts answers to questions from the public about genetic concepts and the etiology, treatment, research, and testing of and predisposition to genetic disorders. Developed by Emory University Department of Human Genetics and University of Alabama at Birmingham Department of Genetics.
Chromosome Deletion Outreach	www.chromodisorder.org	Information and support for families and professionals affected by chromosome deletions, trisomies, inversions, translocations, and rings.
Family Village	www.familyvillage.wisc.edu/index.htmlx	Information, resources, and communication opportunities for individuals/families with cognitive and other disabilities for consumers and health professionals.
Genetic Alliance	http://geneticalliance.org	Directory of genetic support groups and assistance for consumers and professionals in identifying support groups, self-help groups, community organizations, information resources, clinical research studies, and genetics centers.
Genetic and Rare Disease Information Center	www.rarediseases.nih.gov/html/resources/info_cntr.html	Experienced specialists available to answer questions (in English or Spanish) from consumers, health professionals, and biomedical researchers; established by the National Human Genome Research Institute and the Office of Rare Diseases, National Institutes of Health.
Genetics and Rare Conditions	www.kumc.edu/gec/support	Links to lay advocacy groups, support groups, and information on genetic conditions and birth defects for professionals, educators, and consumers. Developed by the University of Kansas.

Table 3. Resources for Patients and Families

Resource	URL	Description
National Organization for Rare Disorders	www.rarediseases.org	Three searchable databases (Index of Rare Diseases, Organizational Database, and Orphan Drug Database).
New York Online Access to Health	www.noah-health.org	Provides access to current, full-text consumer health information in English and Spanish.
Unique: Rare Chromosome Disorder Support Group	www.rarechromo.org	Source of information, mutual support, and self-help to families of children with any rare chromosome disorders, including deletions, trisomy, balanced translocations, unbalanced translocations, rings, inversions, duplications, tetrasomy, monosomy, triploidy, isodicentric, marker, mosaic, and sex chromosome aneuploidy.
Chromosomal Disorders		
• American Association for Klinefelter Syndrome and Support • Klinefelter Syndrome Support Group	• www.aaksis.org • klinefeltersyndrome.org	Klinefelter syndrome (47,XXY) is the result of an extra "X" chromosome. Klinefelter syndrome is the most common sex chromosome variation, occurring in 1 out of 500 males.
• National Down Syndrome Society • National Down Syndrome Congress	• www.ndss.org • www.ndsccenter.org	Down syndrome, also known as trisomy 21, results from an extra 21 chromosome in all, or a portion, of cells. The extra set of the genes present on the 21 chromosome produces the physical and developmental characteristics present in individuals with Down syndrome.
Turner Syndrome Society of the United States	www.turner-syndrome-us.org	Condition occurring in girls and women (1/2,000 live female births) resulting from a partial or complete missing "X" chromosome. Affected females are generally of short stature, need hormone therapy to enter puberty, and usually are infertile.

Box 1. Case Report: 3-Year-Old Boy, TJ, Presenting With Delayed Speech

His mother reports that he says only 10 single words and no sentences. He also has autistic-like behaviors with hand flapping, poor adaptability to changes in his environment, and poor social interactions. You, as the pediatrician, obtain a family history using a 3-generation pedigree. A pedigree taken using resources like the Web site www.ashg.org/press/healthprofessional.shtml (Family History Resources for Practitioners) or www.ama-assn.org/ama/pub/physician-resources/(Family History Information) elicits further information that TJ has one sister, who has normal development. His mother had "reading problems" but graduated from high school. She has 2 brothers, and 1 sister, age 30 years, who has a son with attention-deficit/hyperactivity disorder and learning problems. One of her brothers has mild intellectual disability.

Physical examination reveals normal growth parameters, macrocephaly, prominent ears, long chin, but is otherwise normal.

Based on the patient history of developmental delay, autistic-like features, physical examination findings of macrocephaly and large ears, and the family history of affected males related through unaffected or mildly affected females, you consider a diagnosis of a possible X-linked inherited genetic syndrome.

What is the next step? Resources like "Guide to Understanding Genetics" from the Genetics Alliance and American Society of Human Genetics (ASHG) provide information about basic genetic concepts and genetic evaluations.

What other resources should you consult? OMIM, using search terms of "macrocephaly, intellectual disability" provides a list of possible diagnoses. Because of the possible X-linked pattern of inheritance for learning problems in the family, you may choose the text *X-linked Mental Retardation*, or the American Academy of Pediatrics (AAP) publication on evaluation of the child with developmental disability or intellectual disability. With your patient's symptoms of autistic-like behaviors, you might choose *GeneReviews,* searching under the entry of "Autism Overview."

What initial testing or evaluations should be performed? From the listed resources above, you elect to obtain the following testing: chromosome analysis, chromosome microarray analysis, and DNA testing for fragile X syndrome. GeneTests provides information about these studies and laboratories that offer these tests. In addition, it would be warranted to consult the clinical geneticist.

Testing for fragile X syndrome is positive. Your patient, TJ, has 200 CAG trinucleotide repeats, indicating a full mutation causative of fragile X syndrome.

What resources are useful for understanding etiology, associated complications, and management for the physician? What about counseling regarding risk of recurrence and need to test other family members? Again *GeneReviews* is an excellent choice to address these questions. There are also useful texts, including *Management of Genetic Syndromes*, and other Web sites, like eMedicine or AAP guidelines on fragile X syndrome. Referral to the clinical geneticist in your area is indicated.

What resources are there for the family? Genetic Alliance (http://geneticalliance.org) and Genetic and Rare Disease Information Center (http://rarediseases.info.nih.gov/Resources/Rare_Diseases_Information.aspx) are 2 choices. On the Web site genetests.org, under the *GeneReviews* section on "Resources" there are useful referral resources for the family as well.

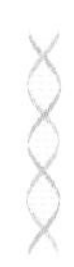

How to Stay Current

As reviewed in the preceding discussion, pediatricians need to constantly update their clinical knowledge, and the previously listed Web sites are recommended and designed particularly for the purpose of allowing the pediatrician to stay current with genetics information pertinent for patient care. The American College of Medical Genetics and Genomics, American Society of Human Genetics, National Human Genome Research Institute/National Institutes of Health, Centers for Disease Control and Prevention, March of Dimes, and National Coalition for Health Professional Education in Genetics provide excellent educational modules and continuing medical education (CME) programs.

In addition, there are a number of resources developed by general pediatricians that have sections on genetics for CME, including GeneralPediatrics.com, AAP PediaLink, and *Pediatrics in Review.* PubMed can be used to search for recent publications regarding a specific question on genetic disorders as well. The impact of genetics in pediatrics will certainly continue to grow, and access to reliable resources will be essential for optimal evaluation and management of patients.

References

1. Burke W. Genetic testing in primary care. *Annu Rev Genom Human Genet.* 2004;5:1–14
2. Moeschler JB, Shevell M; American Academy of Pediatrics Committee on Genetics. Clinical genetic evaluation of the child with mental retardation or developmental delays. *Pediatrics.* 2006;117(6):2304–2316

Appendix B

Newborn Screening ACT Sheets

The American College of Medical Genetics ACT sheets are 1- or 2-page sheets that provide a brief differential diagnosis for genetic conditions, a short description of each condition, a bulleted list of actions for the primary care physician to take immediately after the positive newborn screen, the process to confirm the diagnosis, and a short paragraph about the expected course of the condition. In addition, the ACT sheets provide links to more information about testing, treatment, and outcomes. Individual newborn screening programs may add additional information about local resources for diagnosis and treatment.

The American Academy of Pediatrics has developed guidance that defines the steps required for short-term follow-up, including a description of how to incorporate newborn screening ACT sheets into practice. (See American Academy of Pediatrics Newborn Screening Authoring Committee. Newborn screening expands: recommendations for pediatricians and medical homes—implications for the system. *Pediatrics.* 2008;121:197–217.)

A sample of ACT sheets and algorithms for 5 conditions are included in this appendix.

- Primary congenital hypothyroidism
- Thyroxine-binding globulin deficiency
- Sickle cell anemia
- Cystic fibrosis
- Galactokinase deficiency

The full range of ACT sheets is available at www.acmg.net/AM/Template.cfm?Section=ACT_Sheets_and_Confirmatory_Algorithms&Template=/CM/HTMLDisplay.cfm&ContentID=5661.

Abbreviations

2M3HBA, 2-Methyl-3-hydroxybutyric aciduria

3MCC, 3-Methylcrotonyl-CoA carboxylase

3MGA, 3-methylglutaconic aciduria

CACT, carnitine-acylcarnitine translocase

CAH, congenital adrenal hyperplasia

CoA, coenzyme A

CPT, carnitine palmitoyltransferase

GALT, galactose-1-phosphate uridyl transferase

GNMT, guanidinoacetate methyltransferase

HMG, 3-hydroxy-3-methylglutaryl

IRT, immunoreactive trypsinogen

LCHAD, long-chain 3-hydroxyacyl-CoA dehydrogenase

MCAD, medium-chain acyl-CoA dehydrogenase

M/SCHAD, medium- and short-chain 3-hydroxyacyl-CoA dehydrogenase

MSUD, maple syrup urine disease

PKU, phenylketonuria

SCAD, short-chain acyl-CoA dehydrogenase

SCID, severe combined immunodeficiency

SUAC, succinylacetone

TBG, thyroxine-binding globulin

TFP, trifunctional protein

TSH, thyroid-stimulating hormone

VLCAD, very long-chain acyl-CoA dehydrogenase

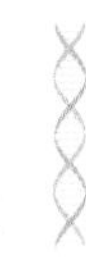

American College of Medical Genetics *ACT SHEET*

Newborn Screening ACT Sheet
[Elevated TSH (Primary TSH test)]
Congenital Hypothyroidism

Differential Diagnosis: Primary congenital hypothyroidism (CH); transient CH.

Condition Description: Lack of adequate thyroid hormone production..

YOU SHOULD TAKE THE FOLLOWING ACTIONS:

- Contact family to inform them of the newborn screening test result.
- Consult pediatric endocrinologist; refer to endocrinologist, if considered appropriate.
- Evaluate infant (see clinical considerations below).
- Initiate timely confirmatory/diagnostic testing as recommended by the specialist.
- Initiate treatment as recommended by consultant as soon as possible.
- Educate parents/caregivers that hormone replacement prevents mental retardation.
- Report findings to state newborn screening program.

Diagnostic Evaluation: Diagnostic tests should include serum free T4 and thyroid stimulating hormone (TSH); consultant may also recommend total T4 and T3 resin uptake. Test results include reduced free T4 and elevated TSH in primary hypothyroidism; if done, reduced total T4 and low or normal T3 resin uptake

Clinical Considerations: Most neonates are asymptomatic, though a few can manifest some clinical features, such as prolonged jaundice, puffy facies, large fontanels, macroglossia and umbilical hernia. Untreated congenital hypothyroidism results in developmental delay or mental retardation and poor growth.

Additional Information:
American Academy of Pediatrics
Genetics Home Reference

Referral (local, state, regional and national):
Testing
Clinical Services
Lawson Wilkins Pediatric Endocrine Society "Find A Doc"
Find Genetic Services

Disclaimer: This guideline is designed primarily as an educational resource for clinicians to help them provide quality medical care It should not be considered inclusive of all proper procedures and tests or exclusive of other procedures and tests that are reasonably directed to obtaining the same results. Adherence to this guideline does not necessarily ensure a successful medical outcome. In determining the propriety of any specific procedure or test, the clinician should apply his or her own professional judgment to the specific clinical circumstances presented by the individual patient or specimen. Clinicians are encouraged to document the reasons for the use of a particular procedure or test, whether or not it is in conformance with this guideline. Clinicians also are advised to take notice of the date this guideline was adopted, and to consider other medical and scientific information that become available after that date.

 (Funded in part through MCHB/HRSA/HHS grant #U22MC03957)

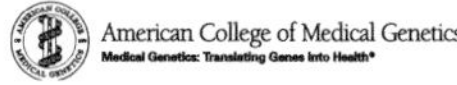

American College of Medical Genetics *ACT SHEET*

LOCAL RESOURCES: Insert State newborn screening program web site links

State Resource site *(insert state newborn screening program website information)*

Name

URL

Comments

Local Resource Site *(insert local and regional newborn screening website information)*

Name

URL

Comments

APPENDIX: Resources with Full URL Addresses

Additional Information:

American Academy of Pediatrics
http://pediatrics.aappublications.org/cgi/content/full/117/6/2290?maxtoshow=&HITS=10&hits=10&RESULTFORMAT=&fulltext=congenital+hypothyroidism&searchid=1&FIRSTINDEX=0&sortspec=relevance&resourcetype=HWCIT

Genetics Home Reference
http://ghr.nlm.nih.gov/condition=congenitalhypothyroidism

Referral (local, state, regional and national):

Testing
http://www.ncbi.nlm.nih.gov/sites/GeneTests/lab/clinical_disease_id/20744?db=genetests&country=United%20Statezs

Clinical Services
Lawson Wilkins Pediatric Endocrine Society "Find a Doc"
http://lwpes.org

Find Genetic Services
http://www.acmg.net/GIS/Disclaimer.aspx

Disclaimer: This guideline is designed primarily as an educational resource for clinicians to help them provide quality medical care It should not be considered inclusive of all proper procedures and tests or exclusive of other procedures and tests that are reasonably directed to obtaining the same results. Adherence to this guideline does not necessarily ensure a successful medical outcome. In determining the propriety of any specific procedure or test, the clinician should apply his or her own professional judgment to the specific clinical circumstances presented by the individual patient or specimen. Clinicians are encouraged to document the reasons for the use of a particular procedure or test, whether or not it is in conformance with this guideline. Clinicians also are advised to take notice of the date this guideline was adopted, and to consider other medical and scientific information that become available after that date.

 (Funded in part through MCHB/HRSA/HHS grant #U22MC03957)

American College of Medical Genetics
Medical Genetics: Translating Genes Into Health®

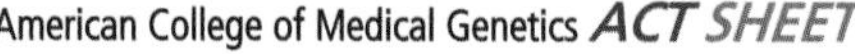

Newborn Screening ACT Sheet
[Low T4 and/or elevated TSH (Primary T4 follow-up TSH test)]
Congenital Hypothyroidism

Differential Diagnosis: Primary and secondary congenital hypothyroidism (CH), transient CH, thyroxine binding globulin (TBG) deficiency.

Condition Description: Lack of adequate thyroid hormone production..

YOU SHOULD TAKE THE FOLLOWING ACTIONS:

- Contact family to inform them of the newborn screening test result.
- Consult pediatric endocrinologist; refer to endocrinologist if considered appropriate.
- Evaluate infant (see clinical considerations below).
- Initiate timely confirmatory/diagnostic testing as recommended by the specialist.
- Initiate treatment as recommended by consultant as soon as possible.
- Educate parents/caregivers that hormone replacement prevents mental retardation.
- Report findings to newborn screening program.

Diagnostic Evaluation: Diagnostic tests should include serum free T4 and thyroid stimulating hormone (TSH); consultant may also recommend total T4 and T3 resin uptake. Test results include reduced free T4 and elevated TSH in primary hypothyroidism. TSH is reduced or inappropriately normal in secondary (hypopituitary) hypothyroidism. Low total T4 and elevated T3 resin uptake are consistent with TBG deficiency.

Clinical Considerations: Most neonates are asymptomatic, though a few can manifest some clinical features, such as prolonged jaundice, puffy facies, large fontanels, macroglossia and umbilical hernia. Untreated congenital hypothyroidism results in developmental delay or mental retardation and poor growth.

Additional Information:
American Academy of Pediatrics
Genetics Home Reference

Referral (local, state, regional and national):
Testing
Clinical Services
Lawson Wilkins Pediatric Endocrine Society "Find A Doc"
Find Genetic Services

Disclaimer: This guideline is designed primarily as an educational resource for clinicians to help them provide quality medical care It should not be considered inclusive of all proper procedures and tests or exclusive of other procedures and tests that are reasonably directed to obtaining the same results. Adherence to this guideline does not necessarily ensure a successful medical outcome. In determining the propriety of any specific procedure or test, the clinician should apply his or her own professional judgment to the specific clinical circumstances presented by the individual patient or specimen. Clinicians are encouraged to document the reasons for the use of a particular procedure or test, whether or not it is in conformance with this guideline. Clinicians also are advised to take notice of the date this guideline was adopted, and to consider other medical and scientific information that become available after that date.

 (Funded in part through MCHB/HRSA/HHS grant #U22MC03957)

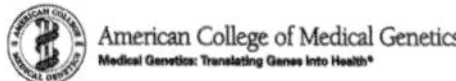

American College of Medical Genetics *ACT SHEET*

LOCAL RESOURCES: Insert State newborn screening program web site links

State Resource site *(insert state newborn screening program website information)*

Name	
URL	
Comments	

Local Resource Site *(insert local and regional newborn screening website information)*

Name	
URL	
Comments	

APPENDIX: Resources with Full URL Addresses

Additional Information:

American Academy of Pediatrics
http://pediatrics.aappublications.org/cgi/content/abstract/91/6/1203

Genetics Home Reference
http://ghr.nlm.nih.gov/condition=congenitalhypothyroidism

Referral (local, state, regional and national):

Testing
http://www.ncbi.nlm.nih.gov/sites/GeneTests/lab/clinical_disease_id/20744?db=genetests&country=United%20States

Clinical Services
Lawson Wilkins Pediatric Endocrine Society "Find A Doc"
http://lwpes.org/

Find Genetic Services
http://www.acmg.net/GIS/Disclaimer.aspx

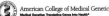

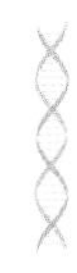

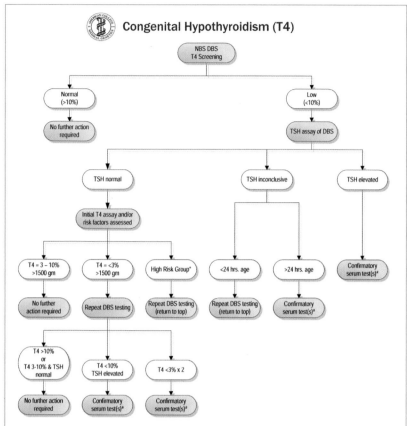

Congenital Hypothyroidism (T4)

- NBS DBS T4 Screening
  - Normal (>10%)
    - No further action required
  - Low (<10%)
    - TSH assay of DBS
      - TSH normal
        - Initial T4 assay and/or risk factors assessed
          - T4 = 3 – 10% >1500 gm
            - No further action required
          - T4 = <3% >1500 gm
            - Repeat DBS testing
              - T4 >10% or T4 3-10% & TSH normal
                - No further action required
              - T4 <10% TSH elevated
                - Confirmatory serum test(s)[a]
              - T4 <3% x 2
                - Confirmatory serum test(s)[a]
          - High Risk Group*
            - Repeat DBS testing (return to top)
      - TSH inconclusive
        - <24 hrs. age
          - Repeat DBS testing (return to top)
        - >24 hrs. age
          - Confirmatory serum test(s)[a]
      - TSH elevated
        - Confirmatory serum test(s)[a]

Actions are shown in shaded boxes, while results are in the unshaded boxes.

Abbreviations/Key
NBS = Newborn screening
DBS = Dried Blood Spot
T4 = Thyroxine or total thyroxine
TSH = Thyroid Stimulating Hormone
CHD = Congenital Heart Disease

*** High risk group**
<1500 gm
NICU admission
Same-sex twin
Transfusion
CHD/other severe congenital anomaly
Drugs: dopamine, steroids, iodine

[a]Confirmatory Serum Tests
Free T4 [or] T4 and T3 resin uptake (T3RU)
TSH

Disclaimer: *This guideline is designed primarily as an educational resource for clinicians to help them provide quality medical care It should not be considered inclusive of all proper procedures and tests or exclusive of other procedures and tests that are reasonably directed* to obtaining the same results. *Adherence to this guideline does not necessarily ensure a successful medical outcome. In determining the propriety of any specific procedure or test, the clinician should apply his or her own professional judgment to the specific clinical circumstances presented by the individual patient or specimen. Clinicians are encouraged to document the reasons for the use of a particular procedure or test, whether or not it is in conformance with this guideline. Clinicians also are advised to take notice of the date this guideline was adopted, and to consider other medical and scientific information that become available after that date.*

(Funded in part through MCHB/HRSA/HHS grant #U22MC03957)

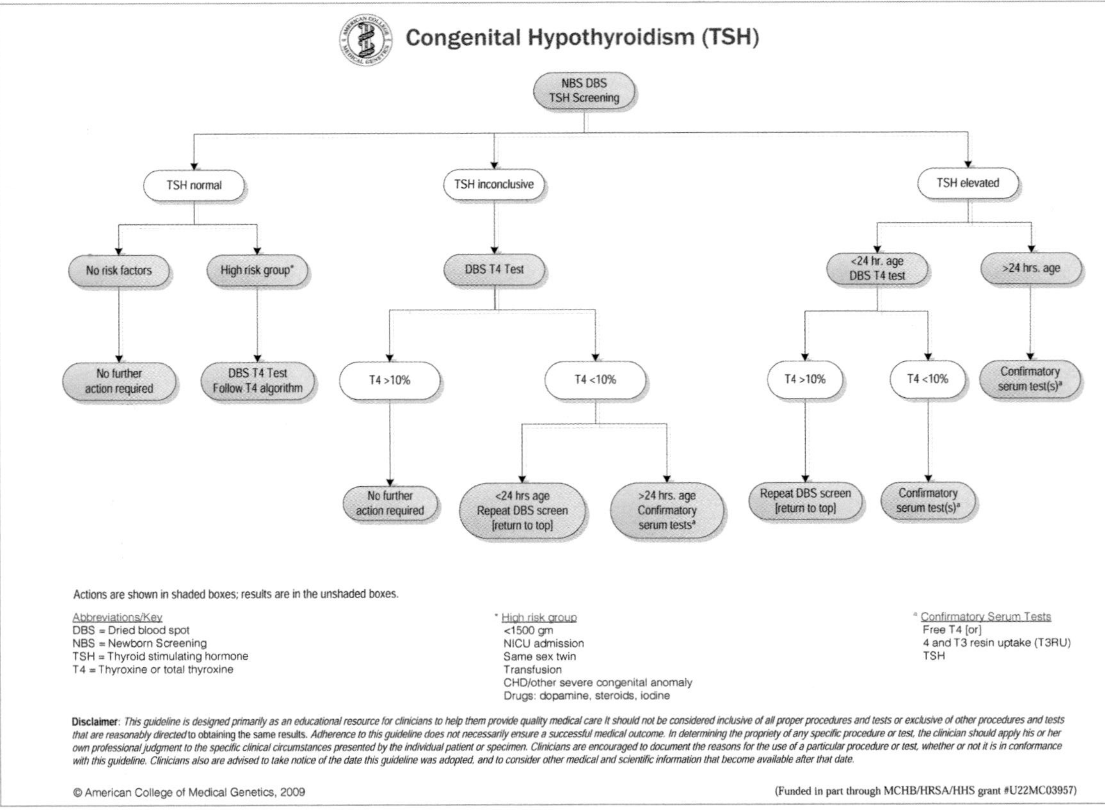
Congenital Hypothyroidism (TSH)
NBS DBS TSH Screening
TSH normal
TSH inconclusive
TSH elevated
No risk factors
High risk group*
DBS T4 Test
<24 hr. age DBS T4 test
>24 hrs. age
No further action required
DBS T4 Test Follow T4 algorithm
T4 >10%
T4 <10%
T4 >10%
T4 <10%
Confirmatory serum test(s)a
No further action required
<24 hrs age Repeat DBS screen [return to top]
>24 hrs. age Confirmatory serum testsa
Repeat DBS screen [return to top]
Confirmatory serum test(s)a
Actions are shown in shaded boxes; results are in the unshaded boxes.
Abbreviations/Key
DBS = Dried blood spot
NBS = Newborn Screening
TSH = Thyroid stimulating hormone
T4 = Thyroxine or total thyroxine
* High risk group
<1500 gm
NICU admission
Same sex twin
Transfusion
CHD/other severe congenital anomaly
Drugs: dopamine, steroids, iodine
a Confirmatory Serum Tests
Free T4 [or]
4 and T3 resin uptake (T3RU)
TSH
Disclaimer: This guideline is designed primarily as an educational resource for clinicians to help them provide quality medical care It should not be considered inclusive of all proper procedures and tests or exclusive of other procedures and tests that are reasonably directed to obtaining the same results. Adherence to this guideline does not necessarily ensure a successful medical outcome. In determining the propriety of any specific procedure or test, the clinician should apply his or her own professional judgment to the specific clinical circumstances presented by the individual patient or specimen. Clinicians are encouraged to document the reasons for the use of a particular procedure or test, whether or not it is in conformance with this guideline. Clinicians also are advised to take notice of the date this guideline was adopted, and to consider other medical and scientific information that become available after that date.
© American College of Medical Genetics, 2009
(Funded in part through MCHB/HRSA/HHS grant #U22MC03957)

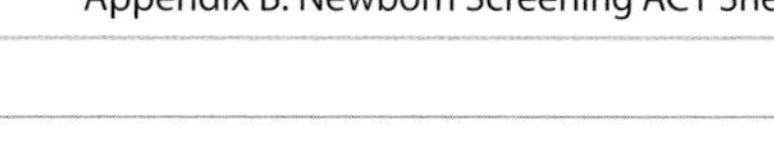

Newborn Screening ACT Sheet
[Elevated IRT +/- DNA]
Cystic Fibrosis

Differential Diagnosis: Cystic fibrosis (CF); gastrointestinal abnormalities are also causes of increased IRT.

Condition Description: The cystic fibrosis transmembrane conductance regulator (CFTR) protein regulates chloride transport that is important for function of lungs, upper respiratory tract, pancreas, liver, sweat glands, and genitourinary tract. CF affects multiple body systems and is associated with progressive damage to respiratory and digestive systems.

YOU SHOULD TAKE THE FOLLOWING ACTIONS:

- Contact family to inform them of the newborn screening result and to ascertain clinical status (meconium ileus, failure to thrive, recurrent cough, wheezing and chronic abdominal pain).
- Contact CF Center for consultation with CF specialist.
- Determine sweat chloride (sweat test) through experienced sweat test laboratory.
- If cystic fibrosis is confirmed, clinical evaluation and genetic counseling are indicated.
- Report findings to newborn screening program.

Diagnostic Evaluation: Varies with screening test. Infants with highly elevated immunoreactive trypsinogen (IRT) may be considered screen positive. Elevated IRT results are followed with second tier tests for either additional IRT measurement or CFTR mutation panels. If screen positive, follow up with sweat chloride test to confirm diagnosis.

Clinical Considerations: Deficient chloride transport in lungs causes production of abnormally thick mucous leading to airway obstruction, neutrophil dominated inflammation and recurrent and progressive pulmonary infections. Pancreatic insufficiency found in 80 – 90% of cases. Some males may be infertile in adulthood.

Additional Information:

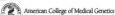

Gene Reviews
Cystic Fibrosis Foundation
OMIM
Genetics Home Reference
American College of Medical Genetics

Referral (local, state, regional and national):

Testing
Clinical Services
Find Genetic Services

Disclaimer: This guideline is designed primarily as an educational resource for clinicians to help them provide quality medical care It should not be considered inclusive of all proper procedures and tests or exclusive of other procedures and tests that are reasonably directed to obtaining the same results. Adherence to this guideline does not necessarily ensure a successful medical outcome. In determining the propriety of any specific procedure or test, the clinician should apply his or her own professional judgment to the specific clinical circumstances presented by the individual patient or specimen. Clinicians are encouraged to document the reasons for the use of a particular procedure or test, whether or not it is in conformance with this guideline. Clinicians also are advised to take notice of the date this guideline was adopted, and to consider other medical and scientific information that become available after that date.

 (Funded in part through MCHB/HRSA/HHS grant #U22MC03957)

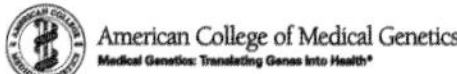

American College of Medical Genetics *ACT SHEET*

LOCAL RESOURCES: Insert State newborn screening program web site links

State Resource site *(insert state newborn screening program website information)*

Name	
URL	
Comments	

Local Resource Site *(insert local and regional newborn screening website information)*

Name	
URL	
Comments	

APPENDIX: Resources with Full URL Addresses

Additional Information:

Gene Reviews
http://www.ncbi.nlm.nih.gov/bookshelf/br.fcgi?book=gene&part=cf

Cystic Fibrosis Foundation
http://www.cff.org/AboutCF/

OMIM
http://www.ncbi.nlm.nih.gov/entrez/dispomim.cgi?id=219700

Genetics Home Reference
http://ghr.nlm.nih.gov/condition=cysticfibrosis

American College of Medical Genetics
http://www.acmg.net/StaticContent/StaticPages/CF_Mutation.pdf

Referral (local, state, regional and national):

Testing
http://www.ncbi.nlm.nih.gov/sites/genetests/clinic?db=genetests

Clinical Services
http://www.cff.org/LivingWithCF/CareCenterNetwork/CFFoundation-accreditedCareCenters/

Find Genetic Services
http://www.acmg.net/GIS/Disclaimer.aspx

Disclaimer: This guideline is designed primarily as an educational resource for clinicians to help them provide quality medical care It should not be considered inclusive of all proper procedures and tests or exclusive of other procedures and tests that are reasonably directed to obtaining the same results. Adherence to this guideline does not necessarily ensure a successful medical outcome. In determining the propriety of any specific procedure or test, the clinician should apply his or her own professional judgment to the specific clinical circumstances presented by the individual patient or specimen. Clinicians are encouraged to document the reasons for the use of a particular procedure or test, whether or not it is in conformance with this guideline. Clinicians also are advised to take notice of the date this guideline was adopted, and to consider other medical and scientific information that become available after that date.

 (Funded in part through MCHB/HRSA/HHS grant #U22MC03957)

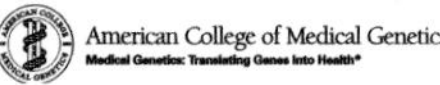

Immunoreactive Trypsinogen (IRT Elevated)

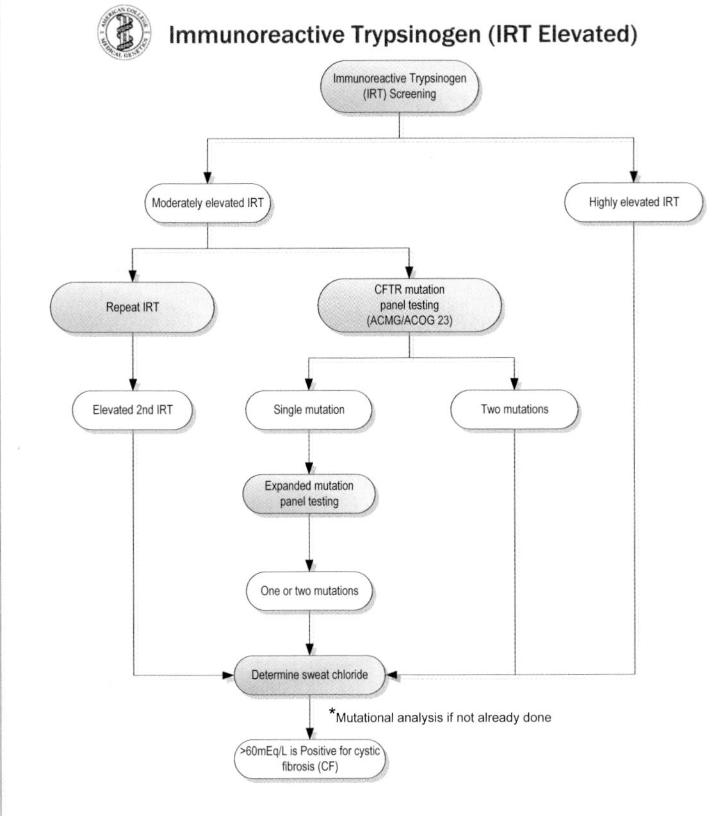

Actions are shown in shaded boxes; results are in the unshaded boxes.

Disclaimer: These standards and guidelines are designed primarily as an educational resource for physicians to help them provide quality clinical services. Adherence to these standards and guidelines does not necessarily ensure a successful medical outcome. These standards and guidelines should not be considered inclusive of all proper procedures and tests or exclusive of other procedures and tests that are reasonably directed to obtaining the same results. In determining the propriety of any specific procedure or test, the healthcare provider should apply his or her own professional judgment to the specific clinical circumstances presented by the individual patient or specimen. It may be prudent, however, to document in the patient record the rationale for any significant deviation from these standards and guidelines.

(Funded in part through MCHB/HRSA/HHS grant #U22MC03957)

American College of Medical Genetics *ACT SHEET*

Newborn Screening ACT Sheet

[Increased Total Galactose with normal GALT]

Primary or Secondary Hypergalactosemia

Differential Diagnosis: Galactokinase (GALK) deficiency; UDP-galactose-4 epimerase deficiency; undefined increase.

Condition Description: Galactose comes from the lactose of breast milk or formula. Galactokinase deficiency is caused by a defect in conversion of galactose to galactose-1-phosphate. Epimerase deficiency limits the production of UDP-galactose, a co-substrate of GALT.

YOU SHOULD TAKE THE FOLLOWING ACTIONS:

- Contact family to inform them of the newborn screening result.
- See and evaluate the infant. Check for reducing substance in urine.
- Consult/refer to a metabolic specialist to determine appropriate follow-up.
- If clinical evaluation is normal and urinary reducing substance is negative, collect and send repeat dried blood specimen to the newborn screening program.
- Report the findings to the newborn screening program.

Diagnostic Evaluation: The diagnosis of galactokinase and epimerase deficiencies is established by quantitation of the respective enzyme activity in erythrocytes.

Clinical Considerations: The neonate is usually normal. If GALK deficiency is untreated, cataracts develop. Treatment is withdrawal of milk. Epimerase deficiency is usually benign.

Additional Information:

Gene Reviews
Genetics Home Reference

Referral (local, state, regional and national):

Testing
Clinical Services
Find Genetic Services

Disclaimer: This guideline is designed primarily as an educational resource for clinicians to help them provide quality medical care It should not be considered inclusive of all proper procedures and tests or exclusive of other procedures and tests that are reasonably directed to obtaining the same results. Adherence to this guideline does not necessarily ensure a successful medical outcome. In determining the propriety of any specific procedure or test, the clinician should apply his or her own professional judgment to the specific clinical circumstances presented by the individual patient or specimen. Clinicians are encouraged to document the reasons for the use of a particular procedure or test, whether or not it is in conformance with this guideline. Clinicians also are advised to take notice of the date this guideline was adopted, and to consider other medical and scientific information that become available after that date.

 (Funded in part through MCHB/HRSA/HHS grant #U22MC03957)

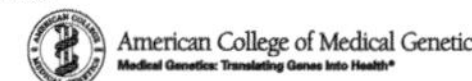

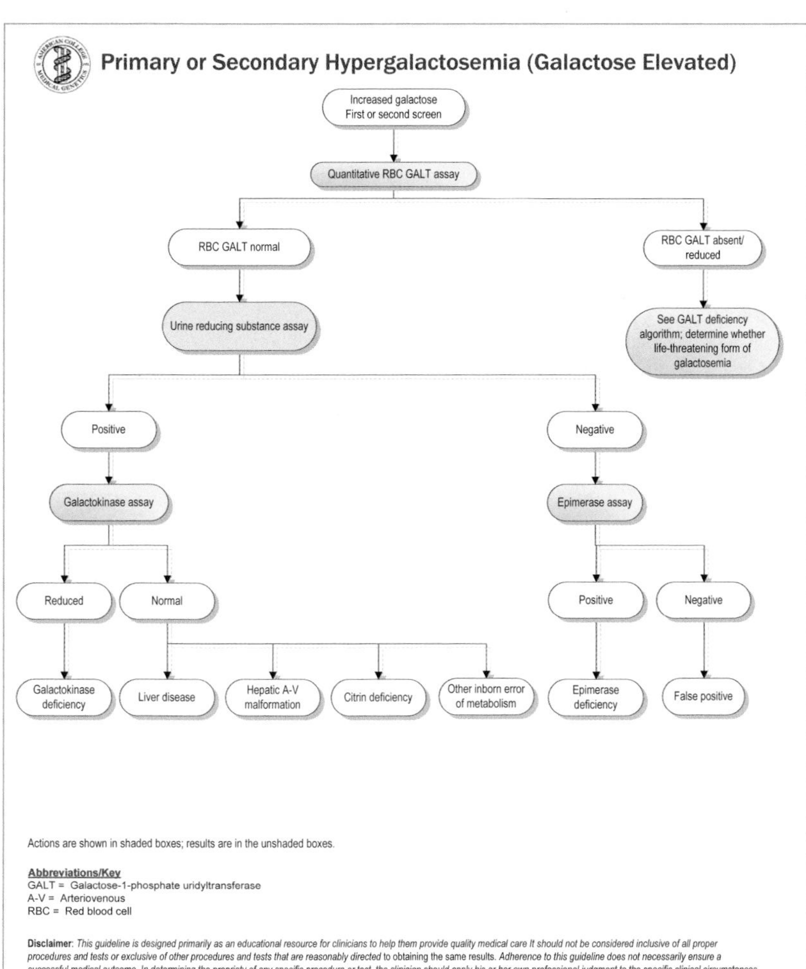

Actions are shown in shaded boxes; results are in the unshaded boxes.

Abbreviations/Key
GALT = Galactose-1-phosphate uridyltransferase
A-V = Arteriovenous
RBC = Red blood cell

Disclaimer: *This guideline is designed primarily as an educational resource for clinicians to help them provide quality medical care It should not be considered inclusive of all proper procedures and tests or exclusive of other procedures and tests that are reasonably directed to obtaining the same results. Adherence to this guideline does not necessarily ensure a successful medical outcome. In determining the propriety of any specific procedure or test, the clinician should apply his or her own professional judgment to the specific clinical circumstances presented by the individual patient or specimen. Clinicians are encouraged to document the reasons for the use of a particular procedure or test, whether or not it is in conformance with this guideline. Clinicians also are advised to take notice of the date this guideline was adopted, and to consider other medical and scientific information that become available after that date.*

(Funded in part through MCHB/HRSA/HHS grant #U22MC03957)

American College of Medical Genetics *ACT SHEET*

LOCAL RESOURCES: Insert State newborn screening program web site links

State Resource site *(insert state newborn screening program website information)*

Name	
URL	
Comments	

Local Resource Site *(insert local and regional newborn screening website information)*

Name	
URL	
Comments	

APPENDIX: Resources with Full URL Addresses

Additional Information:

Gene Reviews
http://www.ncbi.nlm.nih.gov/bookshelf/br.fcgi?book=gene&part=galactosemia

Genetics Home Reference
http://ghr.nlm.nih.gov/condition=galactosemia

Referral (local, state, regional and national):

Testing
http://www.ncbi.nlm.nih.gov/sites/GeneTests/lab/clinical_disease_id/2229?db=genetests&country=United%20States

Clinical Services
http://www.ncbi.nlm.nih.gov/sites/genetests/clinic?db=genetests

Find Genetic Services
http://www.acmg.net/GIS/Disclaimer.aspx

Disclaimer: This guideline is designed primarily as an educational resource for clinicians to help them provide quality medical care It should not be considered inclusive of all proper procedures and tests or exclusive of other procedures and tests that are reasonably directed to obtaining the same results. Adherence to this guideline does not necessarily ensure a successful medical outcome. In determining the propriety of any specific procedure or test, the clinician should apply his or her own professional judgment to the specific clinical circumstances presented by the individual patient or specimen. Clinicians are encouraged to document the reasons for the use of a particular procedure or test, whether or not it is in conformance with this guideline. Clinicians also are advised to take notice of the date this guideline was adopted, and to consider other medical and scientific information that become available after that date.

 (Funded in part through MCHB/HRSA/HHS grant #U22MC03957)

American College of Medical Genetics
Medical Genetics: Translating Genes Into Health®

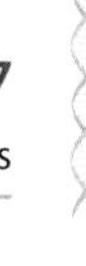

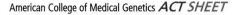

American College of Medical Genetics *ACT SHEET*

Newborn Screening ACT Sheet
[FS]
Sickle Cell Anemia (HbSS Disease or HbS/Beta Zero Thalassemia)

Differential Diagnosis: Homozygous sickle cell disease (Hb SS), sickle beta-zero thalassemia, or sickle hereditary persistence of fetal hemoglobin (S-HPFH).

Condition Description: A red blood cell disorder characterized by presence of fetal hemoglobin (F) and hemoglobin S in the absence of hemoglobin A. The hemoglobins are listed in order of the amount of hemoglobin present (F>S). This result is different from FAS which is consistent with sickle carrier.

YOU SHOULD TAKE THE FOLLOWING ACTIONS:

- Contact the family to inform them of the screening result.
- Consult a specialist in hemoglobin disorders; refer if needed.
- Evaluate infant and assess for splenomegaly; do complete blood count (CBC) with mean corpuscular volume (MCV), and reticulocyte count.
- Order hemoglobin profile analysis (usually performed by electrophoresis).
- Initiate timely confirmatory/diagnostic testing as recommended by consultant.
- Initiate daily penicillin VK (125mg po bid) prophylaxis and other treatment as recommended by the consultant.
- Educate parents/caregivers regarding the risk of sepsis, the need for urgent evaluation if fever of $\geq 38.5°$ C ($101°$ F) or signs and symptoms of splenic sequestration.

Diagnostic Evaluation: CBC, MCV, and reticulocyte count. Hemoglobin separation by electrophoresis, isoelectric focusing or high performance liquid chromatography (HPLC) shows FS pattern. DNA studies may be used to confirm genotype. Sickledex is not appropriate for confirmation of diagnosis in infants.

Clinical Considerations: Newborn infants are usually well. Hemolytic anemia and vaso-occlusive complications develop during infancy or early childhood. Complications include life-threatening infection, splenic sequestration, pneumonia, acute chest syndrome, pain episodes, aplastic crisis, dactylitis, priapism, and stroke. Comprehensive care including family education, immunizations, prophylactic penicillin, and prompt treatment of acute illness reduces morbidity and mortality. S-HPFH is typically benign.

Additional Information:

Grady Comprehensive Sickle Cell Center
Management and Therapy of Sickle Cell Disease
Sickle Cell Disease in Children and Adolescents: Diagnosis, Guidelines for Comprehensive Care, and Protocols for Management of Acute and Chronic Complications
American Academy of Pediatrics
Sickle Cell Disease Association of America

Referral (local, state, regional and national):

Testing
Clinical Services
Comprehensive Sickle Cell Center Directory
Sickle Cell Information Center
Find Genetic Services

Disclaimer: This guideline is designed primarily as an educational resource for clinicians to help them provide quality medical care. It should not be considered inclusive of all proper procedures and tests or exclusive of other procedures and tests that are reasonably directed to obtaining the same results. Adherence to this guideline does not necessarily ensure a successful medical outcome. In determining the propriety of any specific procedure or test, the clinician should apply his or her own professional judgment to the specific clinical circumstances presented by the individual patient or specimen. Clinicians are encouraged to document the reasons for the use of a particular procedure or test, whether or not it is in conformance with this guideline. Clinicians also are advised to take notice of the date this guideline was adopted, and to consider other medical and scientific information that become available after that date.

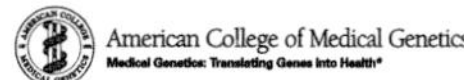

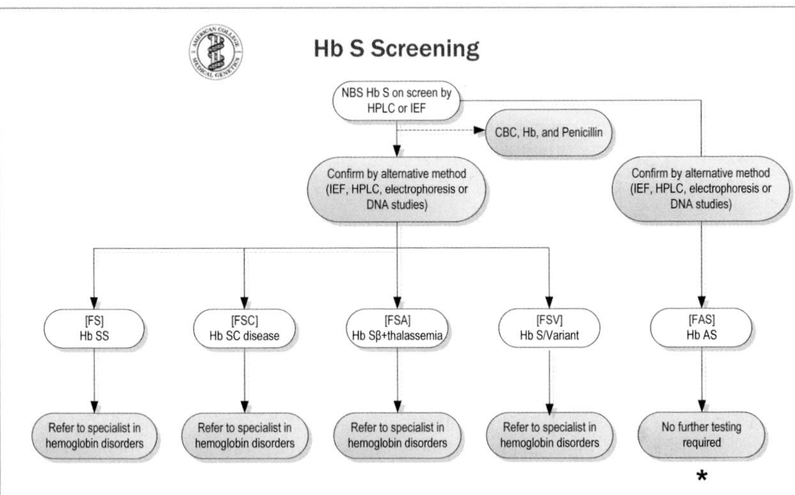

* Offer family members referral for hemoglobin disorders testing and genetic counseling.

Action steps are shown in shaded boxes; results are in the unshaded boxes.

Abbreviations/ Key
F, S, A, C, and V = The hemoglobins seen in neonatal screening.
HPLC: High performance liquid chromatography
IEF: Isoelectric focusing
‡ = Repeat testing at 6 months age is required if genotyping to confirm the newborn screening result is not done.

Disclaimer: *This guideline is designed primarily as an educational resource for clinicians to help them provide quality medical care It should not be considered inclusive of all proper procedures and tests or exclusive of other procedures and tests that are reasonably directed to obtaining the same results. Adherence to this guideline does not necessarily ensure a successful medical outcome. In determining the propriety of any specific procedure or test, the clinician should apply his or her own professional judgment to the specific clinical circumstances presented by the individual patient or specimen. Clinicians are encouraged to document the reasons for the use of a particular procedure or test, whether or not it is in conformance with this guideline. Clinicians also are advised to take notice of the date this guideline was adopted, and to consider other medical and scientific information that become available after that date.*

(Funded in part through MCHB/HRSA/HHS grant #U22MC03957)

American College of Medical Genetics *ACT SHEET*

LOCAL RESOURCES: Insert State newborn screening program web site links

State Resource site *(insert state newborn screening program website information)*

Name

URL

Comments

Local Resource Site *(insert local and regional newborn screening website information)*

Name

URL

Comments

APPENDIX: Resources with Full URL Addresses

Additional Information:

Grady Comprehensive Sickle Cell Center
http://www.scinfo.org/index.php?option=com_content&view=article&id=218:hemoglobins-what-the-results-mean&catid=11&Itemid=21

Management and Therapy of Sickle Cell Disease
http://www.nhlbi.nih.gov/health/prof/blood/sickle/index.htm

Sickle Cell Disease in Children and Adolescents: Diagnosis, Guidelines for Comprehensive Care, and Protocols for Management of Acute and Chronic Complications
http://www.dshs.state.tx.us/newborn/pdf/sedona02.pdf

American Academy of Pediatrics
http://pediatrics.aappublications.org/cgi/content/full/109/3/526

Sickle Cell Disease Association of America
http://www.sicklecelldisease.org/

Referral (local, state, regional and national):

Testing
http://www.ncbi.nlm.nih.gov/sites/GeneTests/lab/clinical_disease_id/2028?db=genetests&country=United%20States

Clinical Services

Comprehensive Sickle Cell Center Directory
http://www.scinfo.org/index.php?option=com_content&view=article&id=197&Itemid=34

Sickle Cell Information Center
http://www.scinfo.org/

Find Genetic Services
http://www.acmg.net/GIS/Disclaimer.aspx

Disclaimer: This guideline is designed primarily as an educational resource for clinicians to help them provide quality medical care. It should not be considered inclusive of all proper procedures and tests or exclusive of other procedures and tests that are reasonably directed to obtaining the same results. Adherence to this guideline does not necessarily ensure a successful medical outcome. In determining the propriety of any specific procedure or test, the clinician should apply his or her own professional judgment to the specific clinical circumstances presented by the individual patient or specimen. Clinicians are encouraged to document the reasons for the use of a particular procedure or test, whether or not it is in conformance with this guideline. Clinicians also are advised to take notice of the date this guideline was adopted, and to consider other medical and scientific information that become available after that date.

 (Funded in part through MCHB/HRSA/HHS grant #U22MC03957)

American College of Medical Genetics
Medical Genetics: Translating Genes Into Health®

Appendix C

Initial Genetics Screening Evaluation

Section 1

The family history information is be entered by the patient's parent/guardian on arrival at the primary care physician's office or collected by a key office person (nurse, assistant, other) at the time of check-in. Of note is the suggested weighting of family history information. Section 1 is more heavily weighted—a "yes" response to any of the questions deserves consideration for obtaining additional information and/or a genetic referral. The second series of question is less heavily weighted, and a "yes" response to 2 or more of the questions deserves consideration for obtaining additional information and/or a genetic referral. Both lists that follow are not comprehensive and hence not applicable for the evaluation of a complete family history that would be pertinent for more thorough evaluations.

Section 2

Key system involvement highlights issues that are worthy of consideration for further evaluation by the primary care physician, possibly including subspecialty referral. The disorders are subdivided into 4 categories (growth, development, morphology, and neuromuscular function).

Note—The primary care physician should use a combination of the family history tool (#1) and the key system involvement tool (#2) at the end of the evaluation (#3) to assess whether additional information, further evaluation, and/or genetic referral should be considered.

1. Family History

Family history questions—The following questions provide an initial basis for the evaluation of potentially genetic or genetically related disorders and are designed as a screening tool only. Clinical judgment regarding the interpretation of family history questions is critical to the use of that information. The list below is not comprehensive and hence not applicable for the evaluation of a complete family history that would be pertinent for more thorough evaluations.

More Heavily Weighted

Birth defects?	Y	N
Unusual physical features?	Y	N
Global developmental delay?	Y	N
Intellectual disability?	Y	N
Vision impairment?	Y	N
Hearing impairment?	Y	N
Early sudden deaths?	Y	N
Multiple miscarriages?	Y	N
Premature menopause?	Y	N

Summary—One or more "yes" answers deserves consideration for obtaining additional information and/or a genetic referral.

Number of "Yes" Answers ______________________

Less Heavily Weighted

Organ abnormalities?	Y	N
Heart disease?	Y	N
Respiratory disease?	Y	N
Stroke?	Y	N
Hypertension?	Y	N
Cancers?	Y	N
Obesity?	Y	N
Infertility?	Y	N

Summary—Two or more "yes" answers deserves consideration for obtaining additional information and/or a genetic referral.

Number of "Yes" Answers ______________________

2. Key System Involvement

a. Disorder of growth	Y	N
i. Short stature	Y	N
1. Isolated	Y	N
2. Associated with other findings	Y	N
3. Disproportionate (limb segments [proximal, middle distal] are disproportionate or left/right limb asymmetry)	Y	N
ii. Tall stature	Y	N
b. Disorder of development	Y	N
i. Global developmental delay	Y	N
ii. Intellectual disability	Y	N
iii. Autism spectrum disorders	Y	N
c. Disorder of morphology (dysmorphology)	Y	N
i. Craniofacial	Y	N
ii. Truncal	Y	N
iii. Genitalia	Y	N
iv. Extremities	Y	N
d. Disorder of neuromuscular function	Y	N
i. Altered consciousness	Y	N
ii. Seizures—early onset	Y	N
iii. Ataxia	Y	N
iv. Regression	Y	N

Summary—The information above is noted by medical history and/or by physical examination to aid in the consideration of the necessity of additional evaluation and/or genetic referral—clinical and/or metabolic.

Number of "Yes" Answers ____________________

3. Final Summary

Additional information, further evaluation, and/or genetic evaluation recommended	Y	N
Based on family history information	Y	N
Based on clinical assessment	Y	N
Based on family history <u>and</u> clinical assessment	Y	N

Index

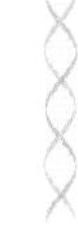

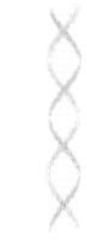

H

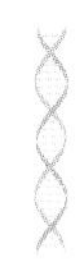

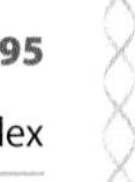

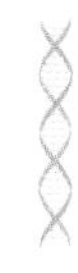

P

T

U